Edward D. Churchill's
Surgeon to Soldiers

Diary and Records of the Surgical Consultant, Allied Force Headquarters, World War II

2024 EDITION WITH MODERN COMMENTARY

Edward D. Churchill's
Surgeon to Soldiers

Diary and Records of the Surgical Consultant, Allied Force Headquarters, World War II

2024 EDITION WITH MODERN COMMENTARY

Edward D. Churchill, MD

John Homans Professor Emeritus of Surgery
Harvard University
Former Chief, General Surgical Services
Massachusetts General Hospital
Boston, Massachusetts

COMMENTARY EDITORS

Jeremy W. Cannon, MD, SM, FACS, Col (Ret.), USAF Reserve, MC

Professor of Surgery
Division of Traumatology, Surgical Critical
Care & Emergency Surgery
Department of Surgery
Perelman School of Medicine at the University
of Pennsylvania
Philadelphia, Pennsylvania

Eric A. Elster, MD, FACS, FRCSEng (Hon.), CAPT, MC, USN (Ret.)

Dean, School of Medicine
Professor of Surgery
Professor in Molecular and Cell Biology
Uniformed Services University of the Health
Sciences
Bethesda, Maryland

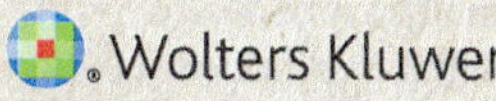

Philadelphia · Baltimore · New York · London
Buenos Aires · Hong Kong · Sydney · Tokyo

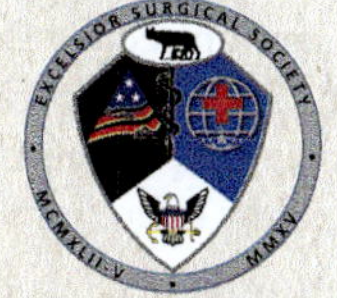

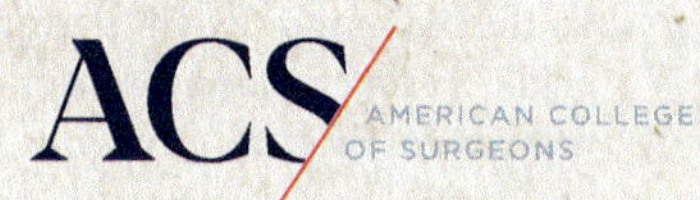

Senior Acquisitions Editor: Keith Donnellan
Senior Development Editor: Ashley Fischer
Editorial Coordinator: Priyanka Alagar
Marketing Manager: Kirsten Watrud
Senior Production Project Manager: Catherine Ott
Managers, Graphic Arts & Design: Stephen Druding, Leslie Caruso
Manufacturing Coordinator: Lisa Bowling
Prepress Vendor: S4Carlisle Publishing Services

9 8 7 6 5 4 3 2 1

Printed in the United States of America

Library of Congress Cataloging-in-Publication Data

ISBN-13: 978-1-9752-4114-8

Cataloging in Publication data available on request from publisher.

---

shop.lww.com

MPP0724

FOREWORD

Dr. Edward D. Churchill's "Surgeon to Soldiers" is a must read for historians and military medical and line leadership. Originally published nearly 30 years after the United States entered World War II, it provides a timeless and relevant context for how to prepare for the next large-scale conflict and advance medical and surgical care.

Written from the extensive diary and personal notes Churchill kept throughout his military service from 1943 to 1945, it provides detailed and intimate insights into the medical and surgical challenges during the war, the need for organizational reforms, and the importance of research on the battlefield. As Churchill states, "What was not generally understood was that experience in the field could point the way toward immediate and radical changes of methods and equipment and that quick footwork in making these changes spell survival." The U.S. Joint Trauma System, which helped produce the highest rates of survival during the Iraq and Afghanistan wars, was built on this very concept.

Churchill's chapters on "Wound and Shock," "Thermal Burns," and "Management of Surgical Wounds" should be of great historical interest to any surgeon, and his discussion of communication up the chain of command and connection with allies is relevant today for novice and senior military officers.

The book presents many personal profiles of icons in American surgery who contributed to the war effort and in doing so should inspire current and future generations of academic surgeons to be involved in supporting military medicine.

Churchill, through his description of the alignment of leading academic medical centers and schools with reserve military units, allows us to learn from the past as we organize military medical support for the future. We are also given an appreciation for how to integrate and adapt civilian surgical expertise to military organizations.

The Excelsior Society, originally born out of research efforts of the surgical consultants at the end of World War II and now reborn as an integral part of the American College of Surgeons-Military Health System Partnership, has done a valuable service to a new generation of civilian and military surgeons by republishing Churchill's book. I have read and reread "Surgeon to Soldiers" over the years and as a senior surgeon, academic and military medical leader charged with the responsibility to prepare military medical officers to "Care for those in Harm's Way" I continue to gain valuable insights.

Jonathan Woodson, MD, MSS, FACS
President, Uniformed Services University of the Health Sciences
Major General (Ret.)

Two inescapable risks characterize each new generation of military surgeons: (1) failing to learn from experiences of the past and (2) fighting the last war by mindlessly following practices from the most recent conflict. We believe this republished monograph that documents and reflects upon surgical best practice in World War II will help minimize these risks.

This project originated from a few different threads. First, the inspiration of the primary author, Colonel Edward Delos Churchill, MD. A small handful of surgeons have carried the torch of optimal combat casualty care from generation to generation. The role played by Dr. Churchill in this capacity became apparent to the first author (JWC) while preparing a talk for the 2008 meeting of the Halsted Society titled "Combat Consultants from Edward D. Churchill to the Senior Visiting Surgeons." Background research for this talk included reviewing a microfiche copy of the August 1943 *New York Times* article on the inadequacy of plasma alone for combat casualty resuscitation. Churchill's refreshing candor and willingness to risk his professional reputation for the benefit of his patients leapt from the scratchy facsimile of this now infamous article. These same qualities fill the pages of *Surgeon to Soldiers*.

The second thread is the unwavering commitment to surgical excellence and the importance of mentorship modeled by Dr. Norman Rich, Dr. Josef E. Fischer, and Dr. C. William Schwab in the mold of Churchill. As the founding chair of the Uniformed Services University Department of Surgery, honorary member of the Excelsior Surgical Society, and mastermind behind the Vietnam Vascular Registry, few have done more to improve the care of the combat wounded in modern history than Dr. Rich. We all owe him an enormous debt of gratitude for faithfully curating the lessons of history and for training many generations of expert combat surgeons.

Dr. Fischer contributed in a different way. He was one of Churchill's last chief residents and then joined the MGH faculty concurrent with the publication of *Surgeon to Soldiers* and Churchill's death. Years later, as chair of Surgery at Beth Israel Deaconess Medical Center, he ensured his own chief residents (including JWC) knew of Churchill's numerous surgical contributions. Dr. Fischer also edited *Mastery of Surgery* in which he amplified the message of each chapter with expert commentary. The format of this republication of *Surgeon to Soldiers* emulates *Mastery* by placing these indispensable precepts into a modern context.

One of the current standard-bearers in military surgical mentorship is Dr. C. William Schwab. Throughout the arc of his career, Dr. Schwab has personally groomed over 20 military trauma fellows, and he has shaped both of our careers in countless ways. As a servant-leader, he was the first senior visiting surgeon to travel to Landstuhl in support of Operation Iraqi Freedom and Operation Enduring Freedom, and his fingerprints are all over many of the *Essential Readings*. May we all aspire to this high level of commitment and personal investment in future generations of military surgeons.

The final thread is the theme of taking a journey through a refining crucible. In reading *Surgeon to Soldiers*, one can sense Churchill's transformation from ivory tower academic to seasoned expeditionary consultant as he endures battlefield hardships along with his surgeons. Churchill labored on this path for 2½ years broken up with very occasional Châteauneuf-du-Pape and filet mignon at various Excelsior Hotels and officer messes (perhaps an earlier version of "surf and turf" Fridays at the DFAC). Few today can imagine such an intense deployment experience. For those interested in the nonmedical history of the North African-Mediterranean campaign, we commend to you the exceptionally well-written and imminently readable *Liberation Trilogy* by Rick Atkinson. To augment Churchill's original work, we have provided a map (**Figure P.1**) of the most significant locations in this epic journey and a timeline (**Figure P.2**) of his deployment. Also note that to avoid duplication in the references at the end of each commentary, we have assembled an *essential reading* list in a special section in this frontmatter. Thank you for taking the time to carefully read Churchill's reflections and the accompanying commentaries as part of your own surgical journey. We truly believe this endeavor will pay dividends in lives saved on battlefields of the future.

Jeremy W. Cannon, MD, SM, FACS, Col (Ret.), USAF Reserve, MC
Professor of Surgery
Division of Traumatology, Surgical Critical Care & Emergency Surgery
Department of Surgery
Perelman School of Medicine at the University of Pennsylvania
Philadelphia, Pennsylvania

Eric A. Elster, MD, FACS, FRCSEng (Hon.), CAPT, MC, USN (Ret.)
Dean, School of Medicine
Professor of Surgery
Professor in Molecular and Cell Biology
Uniformed Services University of the Health Sciences
Bethesda, Maryland

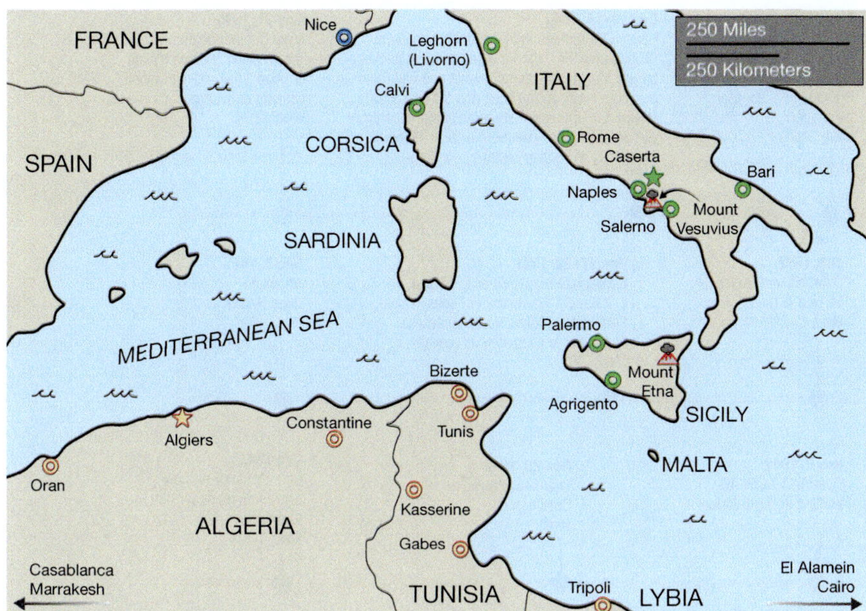

Figure P.1 Map: As chief surgical consultant to the Mediterranean and North African theaters, Colonel Edward "Pete" Churchill's area of responsibility extended across the entirety of North Africa and included the various Mediterranean islands as well as the mainland of Italy and southern France. These theaters were marked by some of the most lethal fighting in World War II.

By all accounts, Colonel Churchill was a "surgeon's surgeon," preferring time spent in the field observing and analyzing conditions on the ground to sitting back in his office. This style of leadership generated a grueling travel schedule: within 2 months of his arrival in theater in March 1943, he had visited more than 15 different American and British medical facilities in some of the locations marked on this map. Living conditions on these tours were austere for the most part. Algiers, Algeria, served as Colonel Churchill's operational headquarters from his arrival through July 4, 1944, when he moved to the relatively cozier billeting of the Royal Palace at Caserta, Italy. This spectacular structure, built by Charles of Bourbon in the early 1700s, served as the administrative and cultural center of Naples. From this location, Colonel Churchill continued his travels to the various field hospitals of the Mediterranean theater while also preparing for the invasion of Southern France. Following the defeat of the Axis powers, Churchill remained actively engaged as a surgical consultant up to his departure for New York on a hospital ship in October 1945.

Circles denote key cities mentioned throughout *Surgeon to Soldiers* while stars indicate Colonel Churchill's two headquarter sites.

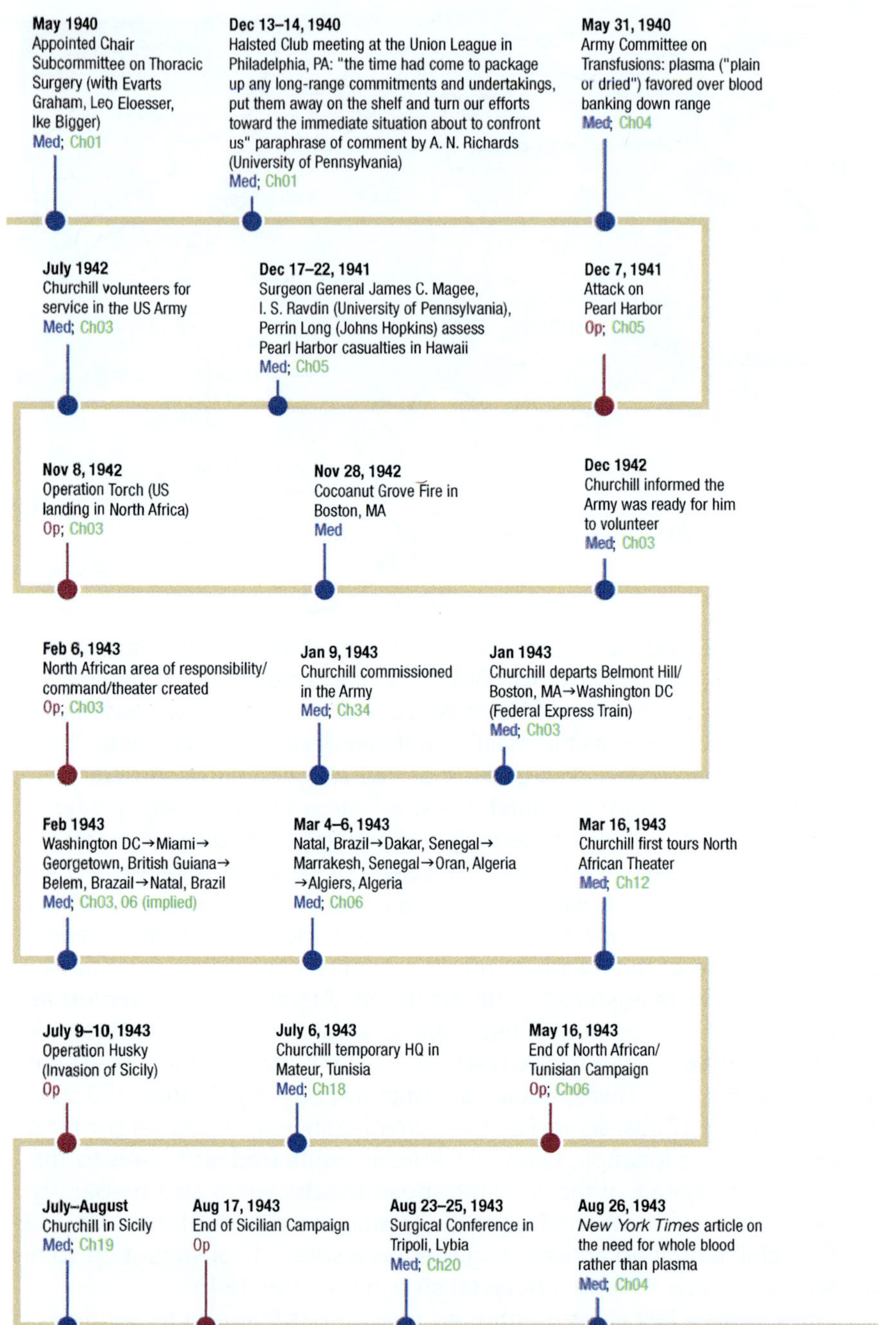

Figure P.2 Timeline: This timeline indicates both the key medical and operational events described in *Surgeon to Soldiers*. Med, Medical Event; Op, Operational Event.

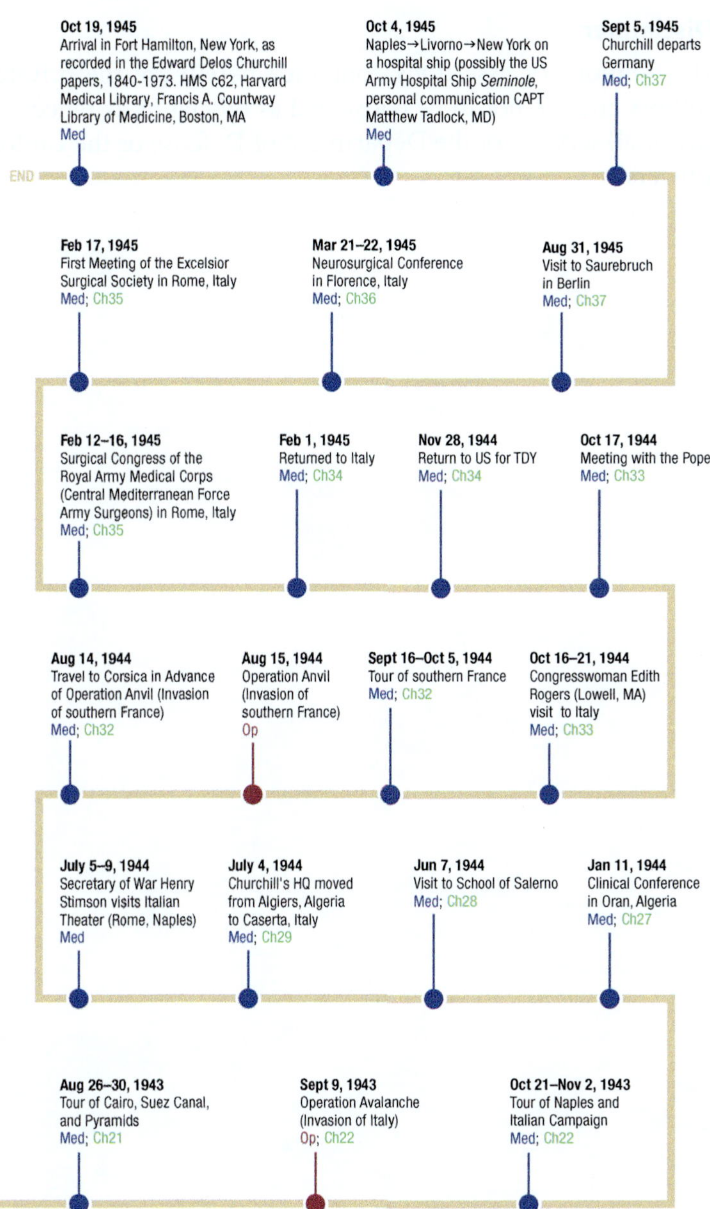

Figure P.2 (continued)

Disclaimer

The opinions or assertions contained herein are the private views of the authors and are not to be construed as official or as reflecting the views of any or all services of the Department of Defense or the Uniformed Services University.

Book Reviews on *Surgeon to Soldiers*

King LS. Surgeon to soldiers: diary and records of the Surgical Consultant, Allied Force Headquarters, World War II. *JAMA*. 1972;220(4):595.

Stewart JD. Surgeon to soldiers: diary and records of the Surgical Consultant, Allied Force Headquarters, World War II. *Ann Surg*. 1973;177(1):132.

Zero Preventable Death Report and Editorials

Berwick DM, Downey AS, Cornett EA. A national trauma care system to achieve zero preventable deaths after injury: recommendations from a National Academies of Sciences, Engineering, and Medicine Report. *JAMA*. 2016;316(9):927-928.

National Academies of Sciences, Engineering, and Medicine. *A National Trauma Care System: Integrating Military and Civilian Trauma Systems to Achieve Zero Preventable Deaths after Injury*. The National Academies Press; 2016.

Rasmussen TE, Kellermann AL. Wartime lessons—shaping a national trauma action plan. *N Engl J Med*. 2016;375(17):1612-1615.

The Walker Dip and Military Readiness

Cannon JW, Gross KR, Rasmussen TE. Combating the peacetime effect in military medicine. *JAMA Surg*. 2021;156(1):5-6.

DeBakey ME. History, the torch that illuminates: lessons from military medicine. *Mil Med*. 1996;161(12):711-716.

Elster EA, Bowyer MW, Knudson MM. Assessing clinical readiness: a paradigm shift in medical education. *JAMA Surg*. 2021;156(11):999-1000.

Kellermann AL, Kotwal RS, Rasmussen TE. Military medicine's value to us health care and public health: bringing battlefield lessons home. *JAMA Netw Open*. 2023;6(9):e2335125.

Knudson MM, Elster EA, Woodson J, Kirk G, Turner P, Hoyt DB. A shared ethos: the Military Health System Strategic Partnership with the American College of Surgeons. *J Am Coll Surg*. 2016;222(6):1251-1255.

Schwab CW. Winds of war: enhancing civilian and military partnerships to assure readiness: white paper presented at the American College of Surgeons 100th Annual Clinical Congress, San Francisco, CA, October 2014. *J Am Coll Surg*. 2015;221(2):235-254.

Walker AJ. The 'Walker dip.' *J R Nav Med Serv*. 2018;104:173-176.

Edward D. Churchill and the Senior Visiting Surgeon Program 2005-2012

Cannon JW, Fischer JE. Edward D. Churchill as a combat consultant: lessons for the senior visiting surgeons and today's military medical corps. *Ann Surg*. 2010;251(3):566-572.

Knudson MM, Evans TW, Fang R, et al. A concluding after-action report of the Senior Visiting Surgeon program with the United States Military at Landstuhl Regional Medical Center, Germany. *J Trauma Acute Care Surg*. 2014;76(3):878-883.

Moore EE, Knudson MM, Schwab CW, Trunkey DD, Johannigman JA, Holcomb JB. Military-civilian collaboration in trauma care and the senior visiting surgeon program. *N Engl J Med*. 2007;357(26):2723-2727.

Moore FD. Edward Delos Churchill: 1895-1972. *Ann Surg*. 1973;177(4):507-508.

Combat Casualty Care Texts and Joint Trauma System Practice Management Guidelines

Emergency War Surgery. 5th ed. Office of the Surgeon General, Borden Institute; 2018.

Out of the Crucible: How the US Military Transformed Combat Casualty Care in Iraq and Afghanistan. Kellermann AL, Elster E, eds. Office of the Surgeon General, Borden Institute; 2017.

Joint Trauma Systems. Clinical Practice Guidelines (CPGs). https://jts.health.mil/index.cfm/PI_CPGs/cpgs

Clinical Care Monographs

Barr J, Cherry KJ, Rich NM. Vascular surgery in World War II: the shift to repairing arteries. *Ann Surg*. 2016;263(3):615-620.

Cancio LC, Lundy JB, Sheridan RL. Evolving changes in the management of burns and environmental injuries. *Surg Clin North Am*. 2012;92(4):959-986.

Cannon JW, Hofmann LJ, Glasgow SC, et al. Dismounted complex blast injuries: a comprehensive review of the modern combat experience. *J Am Coll Surg*. 2016;223(4):652-664.

Churchill ED. The surgical management of the wounded in the Mediterranean theater at the time of the fall of Rome. *Ann Surg*. 1944;120(3):268-283.

Holcomb JB, Jenkins D, Rhee P, et al. Damage control resuscitation: directly addressing the early coagulopathy of trauma. *J Trauma*. 2007;62(2):307-310.

Hoyt DB. Blood and war–lest we forget. *J Am Coll Surg*. 2009;209(6):681-686.

Rotondo MF, Schwab CW, McGonigal MD, et al. 'Damage control': an approach for improved survival in exsanguinating penetrating abdominal injury. *J Trauma*. 1993;35(3):375-82.

CONTRIBUTORS

Hasan B. Alam, MD, FACS
Loyal and Edith Davis Professor of Surgery
Professor of Cell & Developmental Biology
Chair, Department of Surgery
Northwestern University Feinberg School of Medicine
Surgeon-in-Chief, Northwestern Memorial Hospital
Chicago, Illinois

Zarina S. Ali, MD, FACS, FAANS
Chief, Penn Presbyterian Medical Center
Co-Director, Penn Nerve Center
Vice Chair, Inclusion, Diversity and Equity
Department of Neurosurgery
Perelman School of Medicine at the University of Pennsylvania
Philadelphia, Pennsylvania

Douglas H. Anderson, DO
Cardiac Surgeon
Department of Surgery
United States Air Force/University of Maryland
Baltimore, Maryland

Scott B. Armen, MD, FACS, COL, MC, USAR
Chief, Division of Trauma, Acute Care and Critical Care Surgery
Department of Surgery and Neurosurgery
Penn State University College of Medicine
Hershey, Pennsylvania

Rocco A. Armonda, MD, FAANS
Director of Neuroendovascular Surgery
Department of Neurosurgery
Georgetown University Hospital
Washington, District of Columbia

Juan A. Asensio, MD, PhD (Hon), DABS, FACS, FCCM, FRCS (England), FSVS, FAIM, FISS, KM
Professor and Vice-Chairman of Surgery
Chief, Division of Trauma Surgery and Surgical Critical Care
Director of Trauma Center and Trauma Program
Department of Surgery, Creighton University School of Medicine
Professor of Clinical and Translational Science
Department of Translational Science, Creighton University School
    of Medicine
Creighton University Medical Center
Adjunct Professor of Surgery, Uniformed Services University of the
    Health Sciences
F. Edward Hébert School of Medicine
Walter Reed National Military Medical Center
Bethesda, Maryland
Adjunct Professor of Surgery
Department of Surgery
Rush Medical College
Chicago, Illinois

Jeffrey A. Bailey, MD, FACS
Professor
Department of Surgery
Washington University School of Medicine
St Louis, Missouri

Christopher D. Barrett, MD
Assistant Professor of Surgery
Department of Surgery
Assistant Professor of Cellular and Integrative Physiology
Department of Cellular and Integrative Physiology
University of Nebraska Medical Center
Omaha, Nebrask

Gary Alan Bass, MD, MSc, MBA, PhD, FEBS (Em Surg)
Assistant Professor of Surgery
Division of Traumatology, Surgical Critical Care and Emergency Surgery
Perelman School of Medicine at the University of Pennsylvania
Philadelphia, Pennsylvania

Andrew Neil Beckett, MD, MSc, FRCSC, FACS
Associate Professor
Department of Surgery
University of Toronto
Toronto, Ontario, Canada

Linda C. Benavides, MD, FACS
General Surgeon
Department of General Surgery
Madigan Army Medical Center
Tacoma, Washington

Carl A. Beyer, MD
Assistant Professor of Surgery
Department of Surgery
University of South Florida Morsani College of Medicine
Tampa, Florida

Matthew J. Bradley, MD, MS, FACS
Program Director, General Surgery Residency
Department of Surgery
Uniformed Services University of the Health Sciences
Walter Reed National Military Medical Center
Bethesda, Maryland

Karen J. Brasel, MD, MPH, FACS
Professor
Program Director in Surgery
Department of Surgery
Oregon Health & Science University
Portland, Oregon

Christopher J. Burns, MD, FACS
Trauma Medical Director
Department of Surgery
South Shore Hospital
South Weymouth, Massachusetts

Dale F. Butler, MD, MBA, FACS
Assistant Professor
Department of Surgery
UT Southwestern Medical School
Dallas, Texas

Leopoldo C. Cancio, MD, FACS
Director
US Army Burn Center
US Army Institute of Surgical Research
Fort Sam Houston, Texas

Jeremy W. Cannon, MD, SM, FACS, Col (Ret.), USAF Reserve, MC
Professor of Surgery
Division of Traumatology, Surgical Critical Care &
  Emergency Surgery
Department of Surgery
Perelman School of Medicine at the University of Pennsylvania
Philadelphia, Pennsylvania

Paul K. Carlton, Jr, MD, FACS
Retired Air Force Surgeon General
Department of Medical Service
United States Air Force
College Station, Texas

Renford Cindass, Jr, MD, FACS
Trauma Medical Director
Department of General Surgery
A. T. Augusta Military Medical Center
Fort Belvoir, Virginia

William G. Cioffi, MD, FACS
Professor, Chair, Chief of Surgery
Department of Surgery
Alpert Medical School of Brown University
Rhode Island Hospital
Providence, Rhode Island

Dawn M. Coleman, MD, FACS, LTC, MC, USAR
Professor, Surgery
Chief, Division of Vascular and Endovascular Surgery
Duke University School of Medicine
Durham, North Carolina

Miguel A. Cubano, MD, MBA, FACS
Clinical Professor of Surgery
Uniformed Services University of the Health Sciences
Staff General Surgeon
Department of Surgery
Naval Hospital Jacksonville
Jacksonville, Florida

Mary A. Decoteau, MD, FACS

General Surgeon
Department of Trauma
Perelman School of Medicine at the University of Pennsylvania
Philadelphia, Pennsylvania

Bradley A. Dengler, MD, FACS

Director, Military Traumatic Brain Injury Initiative
Department of Surgery
Uniformed Services University of the Health Sciences
Bethesda, Maryland

Warren C. Dorlac, MD, FACS

Associate Clinical Professor of Surgery
Trauma Surgeon
Department of Surgery
School of Medicine at Colorado State University
Fort Collins, Colorado

Joseph J. DuBose, MD, FACS, Col (Ret.), USAF, MC

Professor of Surgery
Department of Surgery and Perioperative Care
Dell Medical School of the University of Texas
Austin, Texas

Juan C. Duchesne, MD, FACS, FCCP, FCCM

The William Henderson Chair of Surgery Endowed Professor of
    Trauma
Chief, Division of Trauma, Acute Care, and Critical Care Surgery
Department of Surgery
Tulane School of Medicine
New Orleans, Louisiana

Alexander L. Eastman, MD, MPH, FACS, FAEMS

Senior Medical Officer—Operations
Office of Health Security
U.S. Department of Homeland Security
Associate Professor of Surgery
Department of Surgery
Uniformed Services University of the Health Sciences
Washington, District of Columbia

Brian J. Eastridge, MD, FACS
Chief, Division of Trauma and Emergency General Surgery
Department of Surgery
UT Health San Antonio
San Antonio, Texas

Matthew J. Eckert, MD, FACS, COL (Ret.), US Army
Program Director, Surgical Critical Care Fellowship
Chief, Trauma and Acute Care Surgery
University of North Carolina School of Medicine
Chapel Hill, North Carolina

Mary J. Edwards, MD, MBA, FACS, COL (Ret.), MC, USA
Professor, Pediatric Surgery
Department of Surgery
Albany Medical College
Albany, New York

Joel B. Elterman, MD, FACS, COL, USAFR, MC, FS
IMA to Command Surgeon, US Space Command
Medical Director, Department of Trauma
Medical Center of the Rockies
Loveland, Colorado

Joseph M. Galante, MD, MBA, FACS
Interim Chief Medical Officer
Department of Surgery
UC Davis Health
Sacramento, California

Margaret E. Gallagher, MD, FACS
Pediatric and General Surgeon
Department of Surgery
Blanchfield Army Community Hospital
Fort Campbell, Kentucky

Brian J. Gavitt, MD, MPH, FACS
Commander 88th Surgical Operations Squadron
Department of United States Air Force
Wright-Patterson Medical Center
Dayton, Ohio

Daniel J. Grabo, MD
Professor, Trauma, Acute Care Surgery and Surgical Critical Care
Department of Surgery
West Virginia University School of Medicine
Morgantown, West Virginia

Kirby R. Gross, MD, FACS
Attending Surgeon
Division of Trauma, Department of Surgery
Cooper Medical School of Rowan University
Camden, New Jersey

Ronald I. Gross, MD, FACS
Professor of Surgery
Frank H. Netter School of Medicine at Quinnipiac University
East Haddam, Connecticut

Rathnayaka M. K. D. Gunasingha, MD
General Surgeon
Department of Surgery
Womack Army Medical Center
Fort Liberty, North Carolina

Jennifer M. Gurney, MD, FACS
Chief, Joint Trauma System
Department of Surgery
Brook Army Medical Center
San Antonio, Texas

Daniel A. Hammer, DDS, FACS
Vice Chair
Department of Oral and Maxillofacial Surgery
Naval Medical Center San Diego
San Diego, California

Reynold Henry, MD, MPH, Lt Col, USAF, MC
Assistant Professor
Division of Acute Care Surgery
University of Nebraska Medical Center
Omaha, Nebraska

Luke J. Hofmann, DO, FACS
Director, Surgical Trauma ICU
Department of Surgery
Brooke Army Medical Center
San Antonio, Texas

John B. Holcomb, MD, FACS
Professor of Surgery
Department of Surgery
University of Alabama at Birmingham Marnix E. Heersink
  School of Medicine
Birmingham, Alabama

Danielle B. Holt, MD, MSS, FACS
Associate Dean for Admissions
Associate Professor of Surgery
Department of Surgery
Uniformed Services University of the Health Sciences
Bethesda, Maryland

John D. Horton, MD, FACS
Chief, Pediatric Surgery
Deputy Consultant to the Surgeon General for General Surgery
Department of Surgery
Madigan Army Medical Center
Tacoma, Washington

Susanna D. Howard, MD
Resident
Department of Neurosurgery
Perelman School of Medicine at the University of Pennsylvania
Philadelphia, Pennsylvania

Kenji Inaba, MD, FRCSC, FACS
Professor and Vice Chair of Surgery
Chief of Trauma and Surgical Critical Care
Department of Surgery
Keck School of Medicine of the University of Southern California
Los Angeles, California

Donald H. Jenkins, MD, FACS
Professor of Surgery
Uniformed Services University of the Health Sciences
Professor/Clinical, Division of Trauma and Emergency Surgery
Vice Chair for Quality, Department of Surgery
Betty and Bob Kelso Distinguished Chair in Burn and Trauma Surgery
Associate Deputy Director, Military Health Institute
Division of Trauma and Emergency Surgery
Department of Surgery
UT Health San Antonio
San Antonio, Texas

Elliot M. Jessie, MD, MBA, FACS
Chief, Section of Acute Care Surgery & Surgical Critical Care
Department of Surgery
Ochsner Medical Center New Orleans
New Orleans, Louisiana

Jay A. Johannigman, MD, FACS
Professor
Department of Surgery
Uniformed Services University of the Health Sciences
Bethesda, Maryland

Lewis J. Kaplan, MD, FACS, FCCP, FCCM
Section Chief, Surgical Critical Care
Director, Surgical ICU
Corporal Michael J. Crescenz VA Medical Center
Philadelphia, Pennsylvania

Jane J. Keating, MD, FACS
Assistant Professor of Surgery
Department of Surgery
UConn School of Medicine
Hartford Hospital
Hartford, Connecticut

Jeffrey D. Kerby, MD, PhD, FACS
Director, Division of Trauma and Acute Care Surgery
Department of Surgery
University of Alabama at Birmingham Marnix E. Heersink
    School of Medicine
Birmingham, Alabama

M. Margaret "Peggy" Knudson, MD, FACS
Professor of Surgery
Department of Surgery
UCSF School of Medicine
San Francisco, California

Stephen J. Kovach III, MD, FACS
Herndon B. Lehr Endowed Associate Professor of Plastic Surgery
Associate Professor of Surgery, Division of Plastic Surgery
Associate Professor of Surgery, Department of Orthopaedic Surgery
Perelman School of Medicine at the University of Pennsylvania
Chief of Plastic Surgery, Penn Presbyterian Medical Center
Director, Microsurgery Fellowship
University of Pennsylvania Health System
Philadelphia, Pennsylvania

Rosemary A. Kozar, MD, PhD, FACS
Professor and Director of Translational Research Shock Trauma
Department of Surgery
R Adams Cowley Shock Trauma Center
University of Maryland School of Medicine
Baltimore, Maryland

Peter A. Learn, MD, FACS
System Division Chief for Surgical Oncology
Department of Surgery
Inova Health System
Fairfax, Virginia

L. Scott Levin, MD, FACS
Chairman
Department of Orthopaedic Surgery
Hospital of the University of Pennsylvania
Philadelphia, Pennsylvania

Keith D. Lillemoe, MD, FACS
W. Gerald Austen Professor of Surgery
Department of Surgery
Harvard Medical School
Chief, Department of Surgery
Massachusetts General Hospital
Boston, Massachusetts

Robert B. Lim, MD, FACS
Vice Chair of Education
Department of Surgery
Wake Forest University School of Medicine
Atrium Carolinas Medical Center
Charlotte, North Carolina

Jonathan B. Lundy, MD, FACS, LTC (Ret.), US Army
Trauma/General Surgeon
Department of General Surgery
Capital Surgeons Group
Austin, Texas

Matthew J. Martin, MD, FACS, FASMBS
Chief, Emergency General Surgery
Division of Acute Care Surgery
Los Angeles General Medical Center
Keck School of Medicine of the University of Southern California
Los Angeles, California

Kenneth L. Mattox, MD, FACS
Distinguished Service Professor
Michael E. DeBakey Department of Surgery
Baylor College of Medicine
Houston, Texas

John C. Mayberry, MD, FACS
Trauma Medical Director
Department of Surgery
West Valley Medical Center
Caldwell, Idaho

Emily Mayhew, MSc, PhD
Historian in Residence
Department of Bioengineering
Imperial College London
London, England

Jeffrey D. McNeil, MD, FACS
Cardiothoracic Surgeon
Cardiothoracic & Vascular Surgical Associates, P.A.
Austin, Texas

Ernest E. Moore, MD, FACS
Director of Research
Department of Surgery
Ernest E. Moore Shock Trauma Center at Denver Health
Denver, Colorado

Marc A. de Moya, MD, FACS
Professor
Department of Surgery
Medical College of Wisconsin
Chief of Trauma, Acute Care Surgery
Froedtert Trauma Center
Milwaukee, Wisconsin

Clinton K. Murray, MD
Commanding General
Department of US Army Medical Center of Excellence
Joint Base San Antonio
Fort Sam, Houston, Texas

Matthew D. Nealeigh, DO, MHPE, FACS
Director, Breast Care and Research Center
Assistant Professor of Surgery
Assistant Professor of Health Professions Education
Norman M. Rich Department of Surgery
Uniformed Services University of the Health Sciences
Bethesda, Maryland

Jamison S. Nielsen, DO, MBA, MCR, FACS, FAWM
Colonel, Medical Corps, United States Army Reserve
Commander, 7451 Medical Operational Readiness Unit, JBLM, WA
Associate Trauma Medical Director
St. Joseph Medical Center
Tacoma, Washington

Timothy P. Plackett, DO, MPH, FACS
Assistant Professor of Surgery
Department of Surgery
Pritzker School of Medicine at the University of Chicago
Chicago, Illinois

Travis M. Polk, MD, FACS, CAPT, MC, USN
Director
DoD Combat Casualty Care Research Program Institution
US Army Medical Research and Development Command
Fort Detrick, Maryland

Benjamin K. Potter, MD, FACS, COL, MC, USA (Ret.)
Norman M. Rich Professor and Chair
Department of Surgery
Uniformed Services University of Health Sciences
Bethesda, Maryland

Joseph F. Rappold, MD, FACS
Trauma/Critical Care Surgeon
Department of Surgery
Maine Medical Center
Portland, Maine

Todd E. Rasmussen, MD, FACS
Professor of Surgery
Department of Vascular Surgery
Mayo Clinic
Rochester, Minnesota

Peter M. Rhee, MD, MPH, FACS
Director of Surgical Critical Care
Department of Surgery
Saint Barnabas Hospital
Bronx, New York

Norman M. Rich, MD, FACS
Leonard Heaton and David Packard Professor of Surgery
Department of Surgery
Uniformed Services University of the Health Sciences
Walter Reed National Military Medical Center
Bethesda, Maryland

Julie A. Rizzo, MD, FACS
Trauma Research Overlord
Department of Trauma
Brooke Army Medical Center City
JBSA-Fort Sam Houston, Texas

Omar A. Rokayak, DO, FACS
Assistant Professor of Surgery
Department of Surgery
Virginia Commonwealth University School of Medicine
Richmond, Virginia

Rachel M. Russo, MD, MS, NHDP-BC, FACS, LT COL, USAF, MC
Voluntary Assistant Clinical Professor
Division of Trauma, Acute Care Surgery, and Surgical Critical Care
Department of Surgery
University of California Davis Medical Center
Sacramento, California

Valerie G. Sams, MD, FACS
Director, Center for Sustainment of Trauma and Readiness Skills
    (CSTARS) Cincinnati
Department of Surgery
University of Cincinnati Medical Center
Cincinnati, Ohio

Thomas M. Scalea, MD, FACS
The Honorable Francis X. Kelly Distinguished Professor of
    Trauma Surgery
Physician in Chief
R Adams Cowley Shock Trauma Center
University of Maryland School of Medicine
Baltimore, Maryland

Andrew T. Schlussel, DO, FACS, FASCRS
Colon and Rectal Surgeon
Department of Surgery
HCA Memorial Hospital
Jacksonville, Florida

Martin A. Schreiber, MD, FACS, FCCM
Professor of Surgery
Head, Division of Trauma, Critical Care and Acute Care Surgery
Department of Surgery, Donald D. Trunkey Center for Civilian and
    Combat Casualty Care
Oregon Health & Science University
Portland, Oregon

C. William Schwab, MD, FACS
Emeritus Professor
Department of Surgery
Hospital of the University of Pennsylvania
Philadelphia, Pennsylvania

Stacy A. Shackelford, FACS, COL, USAF, MC
Trauma Medical Director
Defense Health Agency Colorado Springs Market
San Antonio, Texas

Rob L. Sheridan, MD, FACS
Burn Unit Director and Chief of Staff
Department of Surgery
Shriners Children's Boston
Boston, Massachusetts

R. Stephen Smith, MD, FACS, CAPT, MC, USNR (Ret.)
Professor of Surgery and Anesthesiology
Department of Surgery
University of Florida College of Medicine
Gainesville, Florida

Mary F. Stuever, DO, FACS, Lt Col, USAF, MC
Trauma Medical Director
Department of Surgery
Landstuhl Regional Medical Center
Landstuhl, Germany

Michael J. Sutherland, MD, FACS
Director, Division of Member Services
American College of Surgeons
Chicago, Illinois

Matthew D. Tadlock, MD, FACS
Associate Professor of Surgery
Department of Surgery
Uniformed Services University of the Health Sciences
Trauma/Critical Care Surgeon
Naval Medical Center San Diego
San Diego, California

Nigel R. M. Tai, CBE, MB, BS, MS, FRCS, COL
Consultant in Vascular and Trauma Surgeon
Academic Department of Military Surgery and Trauma
Research and Clinical Innovation
HQ Surgeon General
UK Defence Medical Services
London, England

Eric H. Twerdahl, MD, FACS
Staff Vascular Surgeon
Division of Vascular and Cardiothoracic Surgery
Walter Reed National Military Medical Center
Bethesda, Maryland

Alex B. Valadka, MD, FACS
Professor
Department of Neurological Surgery
University of Texas Southwestern Medical Center
Dallas, Texas

Ian L. Valerio, MD, MS, MBA, FACS, CAPT, MC, USN
Plastic and Reconstructive Surgeon
Director of the Advanced Peripheral Nerve and Microsurgery
    Fellowship
Division of Plastic and Reconstructive Surgery
Department of Surgery
Harvard Medical School
Massachusetts General Hospital
Boston, Massachusetts

John Devin B. Watson, MD, FACS, FSVS
Vascular Surgeon
Department of Cardiac, Thoracic, and Vascular Surgery
LewisGale Medical Center
Salem, Virginia

Gordon G. Wisbach, MD, MBA, FACS, FASMBS
Professor of Surgery
Department of General Surgery
Navy Medicine Readiness and Training Command, San Diego
San Diego, California

James E. Wiseman, MD, MBA, FACS
Assistant Professor of Surgery
Department of Trauma and Surgical Critical Care
University of Maryland School of Medicine
Baltimore, Maryland

Jonathan Woodson, MD, MSS, FACS, Major General (Ret.), MC, USAR
President
Department of Defense
Uniformed Services University of the Health Sciences
Bethesda, Maryland

Tamara J. Worlton, MD, FACS
Associate Professor of Surgery
Department of Surgery
Uniformed Services University of the Health Sciences
Bethesda, Maryland

Jay A. Yelon, DO, FACS, FCCM
Trauma Surgeon
Bureau of Medicine and Surgery
United States Navy
Philadelphia, Pennsylvania

The reprinting of *Surgeon to Soldiers* represents the culmination of more than a decade of effort by numerous members of the Military Medical Corps and the American College of Surgeons (ACS) trauma community. This shared introduction affords the opportunity to detail the journey that began in the first decade of Operation Iraqi Freedom/Operation Enduring Freedom (OIF/OEF) and concludes with the re-presentation of the journal of a truly great American surgeon soldier, Colonel Edward D. Churchill, MD.

Jay A. Johannigman, MD, FACS

During my first deployment as a surgeon to Balad Air Base, Iraq, I enjoyed a visit from Colonel John Holcomb. This visit was early in the conflict during a very challenging time as the Joint Trauma System (JTS) existed as only a concept, not an official program. Colonel Holcomb held the informal title of "JTS Forward Surgeon," and like Churchill, he was making the rounds across his area of responsibility (AOR). During this visit, Colonel Holcomb shared early data from the nascent Joint Theater Trauma Registry to support our desire as medics to "Get It Right." I also recall he mentioned Churchill's memoir to me as a "must read" for all deployed surgeons.

Upon my return to CONUS, I secured an original copy that has remained close at hand ever since. To this day, this timeless book serves as a quiet reminder of the truism that the principles of military medicine that bring our injured home are rarely innovated, but rather have more likely just been forgotten by each successive generation. If ever I am so naïve to think that I have chanced upon an innovative improvement or insight into the care of the injured service member, I simply reach for my copy of *Surgeon to Soldiers* and realize that Dr. Churchill—and those that came before him—faced these same issues. As CAPT Frank Butler, MD, FACS (chair of the CoTCCC) so succinctly stated, "These lessons were written in blood, and it is our profound responsibility to learn them and integrate them into our practice."

M. Margaret "Peggy" Knudson, MD, FACS

Churchill's major contribution to both military and civilian surgery was defining the role of a consultant surgeon. In that role, he observed and described several important lessons learned that are still applicable both on and off the battlefield today: the importance of a far forward surgical facility within 60 minutes of the injury, the need for staged surgical procedures to ensure best outcomes, and the importance of red blood cell transfusions in addition to plasma during the immediate resuscitation period.

If these lessons sound familiar they are! You will recognize in this work the concepts of the Golden Hour, Damage Control Surgery, and Damage Control Resuscitation. Churchill warned that military surgery was a "discontinuous specialty" as lessons learned during wartime are frequently forgotten until the next war, resulting in limbs and lives lost. His message of changing military surgery into a continuous specialty begins by studying the many important lessons captured in *Surgeons to Soldiers*.

John B. Holcomb, MD, FACS

Colonel Churchill's *Surgeon to Soldiers*, as well as Major Harvey Cushing's *From a Surgeons Journal* should be mandatory reading for every deployed surgeon. I read them both before and during deployments and learned so much. As described in their books from the two world wars, very little has changed in war wounds, and while the instruments we use are fancier, the wounds, triage, and levels of care are similar. Their words eloquently describe the strong emotions, bonds, and passion that we experience when caring for the combat wounded. Thank you to the leaders that made this new edition of *Surgeon to Soldiers* available to the next generation of combat surgeons.

Juan A. Asensio, MD, PhD (Hon), DABS, FACS, FCCM, FRCS (England), FSVS, FAIM, FISS, KM

Man's inhumanity for man knows no limits and given the cyclical nature of war, it is no small wonder that lessons learned at a great cost in blood, pain, and lives are frequently forgotten. I am forever grateful to my mentor Dr. Norman M. Rich who introduced me to this book as a source of wisdom applicable to all surgeons. Dr. Churchill's pen clearly crystallized an account of the difficulties, polarizing opinions/factions, and controversies that at times posed a threat to the best possible care of the wounded. Churchill persevered and prevailed just like his political contemporary Winston Churchill who famously stated, "Never give in, never, never, never, never—in nothing great or small, large, or petty—never give in except to convictions of honor and good sense. Never yield to force, never yield to the apparently overwhelming might of the enemy."

Michael J. Sutherland, MD, FACS

This reproduction with commentary of Colonel Churchill's book provides contemporary military surgeons and leaders with the ability to see the lessons of our past framed in the challenges of 21st-century conflict. We have all heard the famous quote from George Santayana: "Those who cannot remember the past are condemned to repeat it." The greater challenge is to contextualize the lessons of the past in the current setting. This enables leaders to see the applicability of history and create policies and processes that avoid the folly of having to learn from our own mistakes. I hope that you find that this edition demonstrates the durability of lessons learned from our past.

The content that follows is an exact reproduction of the original text first published in 1972, with only a few annotated errata. Most chapters are followed by expert commentaries to place these invaluable insights into a modern context. We hope the reader will take full advantage of this seminal work.

CONTENTS

APPENDICES 417

To our mentors past and present who, like Churchill, inspired us through their example and pushed us to do more than we thought possible in caring for the combat wounded.

PART ONE

Medical Mobilization

1

National Research Committees

Medical Mobilization of World War II began for me at a dinner party held by the Halsted Club in Philadelphia in December 1940. A. N. Richards, of the University of Pennsylvania, was invited to speak. Richards was already involved in the scientific mobilization in Washington. He became a member of the Medical Research Committee, one of the high-level coordinating groups active throughout the war. At the dinner Richards, in his quiet way, said that so far as he could see, the time had come to package up any long-range commitments and undertakings, put them away on the shelf and turn our efforts toward the immediate situation about to confront us.

The moment selected as the beginning of the war is an arbitrary one. Quincy Howe, writing in 1946, chose September 19, 1931, when Japanese troops marched into Manchuria and seized key points on various railroad lines ceded by Russia to Japan after the Russo-Japanese War of 1905. China did not even break off relations with Japan.

In January 1932, Secretary of State Henry Stimson tried to invoke the Nine-Power Treaty, declaring that Japan had in fact encroached upon the territorial integrity of China. This agreement dated from the Washington Naval Conference of 1932 at which a 5:5:3 ratio among the American, British and Japanese navies was established. The purpose was to reduce the likelihood of offensive naval warfare being carried beyond the recognized sphere of influence of the signatory nations. Secretary Stimson's lead was not followed by Sir John Simon, the British Foreign Secretary, and this Anglo-American split played into Japanese hands. On February 2, 1932, at the Geneva Conference of the League of Nations, Japan proposed that the British and Americans cut their navies in two and promised to reduce hers to the same level, thus gaining equality. The American delegation proposed cutting all armies in half and outlawing bombers, tanks, chemical warfare and heavy artillery. Italy and Russia accepted the program; France and Britain rejected it.

A convenient date for the beginning of World War II in Europe is September 1, 1939, when at 4:40 in the morning the *Luftwaffe* bombed

Polish airfields and Nazi Germany followed the bombing with the blitzkrieg invasion.

In the spring of 1940, the Allied armies in Europe suffered reverses that were reflected in the United States by a sense of growing national danger. In May, a state of national emergency was proclaimed. With a rapid expansion of the armed services inevitable, the Surgeon General called upon the National Research Council (N.R.C.) for help in the many medical problems that lay ahead. Dr. Lewis H. Weed, Chairman of the Division of Medical Sciences, assembled a number of advisory committees to serve during the emergency.

I found myself on the Subcommittee on Thoracic Surgery, as chairman, with Evarts Graham, Leo Eloesser and Ike Bigger. We were given the responsibility of drawing up a guide for the surgical treatment of wounds of the chest. Evarts Graham had been overseas during World War I but, as I recall, never had any real experience in treating chest wounds, although he had been sent over with an evacuation hospital. Ike Bigger was our authority on wounds of the heart, for he had had some actual experience in Richmond, but this chiefly concerned stab wounds in which the ice pick was a favorite weapon in Saturday night fights.

PROBLEM OF MANUALS

One of the first activities of the N.R.C. was to prepare various medical and surgical manuals. This was an excellent idea on paper but not significant as it turned out. One great difficulty was defining the type of document we were to produce. Leo Eloesser, with experience in the Spanish Civil War, felt that we should prepare a field manual that a medical officer could have in his pocket and review when he was confronted with casualties; in other words, a "medical cookbook." Eloesser's thought was all toward didactic, concise "recipes." For a man with a wound in his chest that had mobilized the chest wall the recipe would instruct: "Take two towel clips, anchor them around the ribs and suspend the towel clips."

We had many arguments how we might best instruct medical officers. We found it almost impossible to plan a manual without being able to visualize the type of wound that would be encountered in battle. The manuals as a whole were far from satisfactory to those of us who prepared them, and had best be forgotten.

When I look back at the manual on thoracic surgery, I must admit that it was as good as could be expected. At least it did not contain many errors—except those of omission. The one prepared by our committee was short, so it was bound in a cover with a couple of others. This activity in the preparation of manuals at least made us do some thinking.

The manuals were not revised and, after medical officers had experience in combat, were discarded. The best manuals dealt only with broad principles and the sequence of procedures without specifying a precise time factor—an important factor I shall discuss shortly.

Our committee worked only a few months in preparing the text, and many items were omitted. One important omission was the treatment of the contaminated and infected hemothorax. This was because some of us were beginning to glimpse the possibility of removing blood and damaged tissues from an infected hemothorax followed by primary closure rather than the universal employment of drainage. The sulfonamides were already available, although penicillin had not yet appeared. Evarts Graham, being a classicist from World War I where he had experienced the hemolytic streptococcus infections of the pleura following influenza, could not tolerate the conception that an infected pleural space could be closed without drainage. He was influenced by the experience of the Empyema Commission. (See Appendix B, pp. 437 to 455.) Even after the vast experience of World War II, I had to defend primary closure of an infected hemothorax at one of the first meetings of the American Association for Thoracic Surgery. Evarts Graham still could not accept this because it was a departure from a principle he had stood for in the era when streptococcus empyema was rampant.

The manual on thoracic surgery was designed to teach medical officers how to treat chest injuries in the field. This introduced immediately a prime consideration in military surgery, namely, working in terms of *timing*. Military surgery differs from civilian surgery in that a paramount consideration is the introduction of the dimension of *time* as the all-important element in carrying out surgical procedures. Under the conditions of combat one has little idea whether a wounded man will reach a specified medical installation one, five, twelve or twenty-four hours after he has been struck by a missile. In wound management these are just as important variables as whether a missile hit him in the head, the chest, the abdomen or leg. They are equally unforeseeable until a particular combat situation exists. Even then it is only possible to plan in terms of the average. A plan may assume that a wounded man will arrive at a specified position four hours after being hit and will reach another place twelve hours later. Also, all planning has to be in terms of the greatest good for the greatest number. Planning, therefore, is theoretic until one assumes a position both in time and in place. This must be derived from actual experience in the specific situation.

The following note from Leo Eloesser on March 23, 1943, shows what we really thought of manuals: "Have you seen the manual? To my mind it is the amalgamated and condensed Fritz. Every time I think of yours and my name on the cover it gives me the chills. Any interne would be able to tell that the set-up figured on page 265 is a Rube Goldberg apparatus without any purpose. The piffle in the figure is only exceeded by that in the last half of page 263. If anybody knows what the authors of the last half of this page are talking about they are good. The trocar in figure 4 is wrong. Figure 11 looks like something Mary got up to sail on the pond at Belmont. The other figures are equally illuminating. In short, it makes me sick to my stomach."

These manuals ranged from the cookbook level to pure textbook presentations. Most far afield was a section on hematogenous osteomyelitis in the orthopedic manual. It was a section someone had written for a textbook and the author had probably thought, "You're going to see osteomyelitis, take this and put it in the manual." Some of the manuals were submitted to a committee. A committee will always iron out and eliminate controversial details. It is even impossible to have a committee of cooks write a good cookbook. Consequently the instructions in the manuals frequently came to a dead center.

Once in a while, I found in my consulting work in the field overseas that the manual on shock would be quoted—much to my annoyance because the ideas cited were usually fallacious.

ACTIVITY—AND SECRECY

Preceding our entry into World War II there was a long period of frantic but somewhat fruitless activity in Washington, D.C. It became a matter of personal prestige to know things of importance and yet not say that one knew. Merely to travel to Washington "on the Federal" made one's friends prick up their ears. It carried the implication that you were important and must know many things. Nearly everyone was jockeying for a position of importance "on the inside." Any experimental laboratory work that had a remote connection with the war effort was hush-hush.

But a gap existed between actual experience in the field and the activities of the N.R.C. Experience in the field was limited to that which the British were having in Ethiopia and, later, in the desert warfare. Any written document, any report regarding the care of the British wounded was a carefully guarded secret. The Office of the Surgeon General of the Army would not allow even the N.R.C. to see such records. All information was filed away under lock and key.

During this period there was an elderly British officer—Colonel Gillespie—who had access to these documents through the War Office in London and gave us anything he thought might further the war effort. Gillespie described the England of this period as a "drunk leaning against a lamppost—in need of both support and light."

This frantic effort of secrecy was not so noticeable at the higher levels of government but pervaded the lower levels of activity where it contributed to the prestige of those "in the know." Even information on the bombing of London was scarcely obtainable. John Fulton of Yale made a trip to London and brought back news of the so-called blast injury which was being encountered. He wrote rather a good article about it which was published in the *New England Journal of Medicine*. Much of our knowledge about blast injury was based on rumor and much of it was exaggerated and distorted. Facts, even if one is on the scene, are difficult to extract, so in part this situation was due to secrecy and, in part, merely lack of facts. This was to become apparent to me later when I arrived in North Africa. One of the most difficult tasks was to identify the facts in a situation because one saw the situation itself with an emotional coloration that was often intensified by other observers. This subjectivity interfered with any semblance of scientific exactitude.

It is impossible to plan for war with intuition the sole guide. It must be planned on the basis of experience. When no one comes forward with such experience, except that derived long ago in another war in another place, even the writing of a simple manual becomes difficult. World War II was quite a different kind of a war than World War I, and the participation of American surgeons in World War I was limited and spotty. No one was able to sift out which surgeons who wrote about World War I were correct and which ones were in error. In retrospect, there were some very sound writings but others that were pathetically inadequate.

Military surgery is a subspecialty of surgery, but a discontinuous one. It can be compared to a hypothetical situation in which all neurological surgeons today would close their operating rooms, pack up their instruments, destroy their books or bury them on a dusty shelf, and all neurological surgery would come to a halt. Twenty-five years later, someone has the idea suddenly to start neurological surgery again. Some young fellow who has never seen the living human brain might go to these vast storehouses of dusty volumes and face the task of sifting what was true from what was not true. That would be the first task in the revival of neurosurgery. Military surgery suffers from this type of discontinuity.

FILTERING IDEAS

Indeed, when the Division of Medical Sciences and the N.R.C. set up its top Committee of Surgery before the United States entered World War II, the committee was not only faced by the problem of extrapolation and projection of ideas, but also by the task of filtering out gross errors. In addition to the sincere and sound efforts that were being made, the committee had to deal with any number of misguided and crackpot ideas.

In setting up this committee, the Division of Medical Sciences and the N.R.C. had to do so on the basis of "window dressing." I do not use the words window dressing in a derogatory sense because it was essential to have well-known surgeons backing up the Surgeon General by the prestige of their names—elder statesmen in the hierarchy of surgery, many of whom were supposed to have had extensive experience in World War I.

OBSERVERS ON THE BATTLEFIELD

Not only was it hard for the N.R.C. to get useful surgical information based on experience in World War I, there was a time after our entry into World War II when the N.R.C. didn't even get as useful information from the field as it might have.

Prevailing United States Army doctrines in 1942 held that a combat force could best be supported by activating methods and procedures generally known at the outbreak of war. Exception was made for new developments expected to emerge from the intense scientific effort in this country, specifically that fostered by the Office of Scientific Research and Development, with the advice of the N.R.C. Otherwise, combat-support was pictured as calling for the replacement of personnel and supplies when needed, and a reasonable modicum of skill in adapting standardized procedures to specialized situations as they were encountered. What was not generally understood was that experience in the field could point the way toward immediate and radical changes of methods and equipment, and that quick footwork in making these changes spelled survival. To be sound, changes of this type required as much factual evidence as could be assembled.

As a consequence, no provision was made for the collection and analysis of surgical evidence so that corrective measures might be devised by those on the spot when confronted with the unexpected. The idea of sending out skilled observers to identify new problems and solve them then and there was not entertained. In fact, such an idea smacked of the academic and was dismissed with the stern reminder that medicine was on the march to help fight a war, not to indulge in research.

Interestingly enough, it was the combat units that pointed the way by using the services of experts to observe and report on the performance of machines of war. Many were the "bugs" that remained in new tanks, planes and missiles, and these defects were constantly being ironed out. Precise and scientific measurement of novel developments by the enemy required alert and expert intelligence. One recalls, for instance, the encounter with magnetic mines that threatened shipping in the North Atlantic. Combat commanders and their conventional military staffs cannot be expected to solve such problems unaided and, in fact, may not be able to define them in terms that can lead to a solution elsewhere. The same may be said of a wound surgeon confronted by a case of anuria in a forward hospital.

Beginning in the North African campaign and continuing through Sicily, Italy, and southern France, the surgeons of the theater were hard pressed by the need for surgical evidence to guide their daily work. Some of the first compilations of the records of patients who had disappeared into the evacuation stream were made as follow-up studies by members of the 2nd Auxiliary Surgical Group. This was partly because the surgical teams had periods of relative inactivity that could be devoted to such pursuits and partly because of the wise insistence of their Commanding Officer, Colonel James H. Forsee, M.C., on maintaining duplicated clinical records. It could have been so easy to let down standards and be too busy to keep records adequate for analysis.

The theater was also fortunate in the assignment of affiliated hospital units from leading teaching hospitals with chiefs of surgery who insisted on the maintenance of high standards. A professor of surgery from Oslo, after three weeks in the forward area in Italy, said: "You are holding to the standards of university clinic surgery under fire and in tents with mud floors."

Finally, the small group of peripatetic officers who were identified as consultants were not deployed with the mission of commissars or Gauleiters. They were searching for surgical evidence by direct observation and inquiry. The achievement of a consultant was aptly described by Sir Patrick Berkeley Moynihan following World War I: "I have gathered a posie of other men's flowers and nothing but the thread that binds them is mine own."

The North African-Mediterranean Theater of Operations provided a favorable environment for such undertakings. It was an experimental laboratory not only for surgery but also for medicine as a whole, for ordnance, for equipment and, as many are reluctant to recall, even for rations. It was vital that wound surgery be carried on within a framework of inquiry, for this theater was the proving ground for the greater task that was to come.

National Research Committees
COMMENTARY

Rachel M. Russo, Todd E. Rasmussen, and C. William Schwab

Upon volunteering to serve as a surgical consultant during World War II, Churchill committed to preserving the most valuable military asset—warfighters. Military medicine optimizes warfighter health and ensures these men and women will fight without hesitation, knowing they will receive the best medical care possible if injured. In a combat setting, delivering the best possible care requires focused empiricism, evolving practice as new insights are gained from *data-driven analysis* of outcomes. Churchill most assuredly believed in this approach, beginning his memoir with this first chapter on National Research Committees.

The National Research Council (NRC) was founded in 1916 against the backdrop of World War I in response to growing sentiment that the United States was unprepared for a large-scale combat engagement. The nascent NRC quickly marshalled "all scientific forces of the country for national defense." Despite the relatively short period of direct US engagement in the war, the prolific scientific advancements of the NRC led President Woodrow Wilson to issue an executive order establishing an enduring role for the NRC to harness American expertise across the sciences to maintain our competitive advantage.

By the time of Churchill's involvement with the NRC, the nation had undergone the tribulations of the Great Depression, leading to severe curtailment of the NRC's activities due to inadequate funding. After being tasked to produce a guide for the surgical treatment of chest wounds, Churchill laments the misdirected activities of the NRC. He proclaims that the real problem with combat surgical care was the lack of military surgeons with relevant experience in a deployed environment, even among authors of the manual. Such challenges are typical during an interwar period, as combat-weary personnel complete their service and are replaced by eager but inexperienced junior officers. His frustration with the discontinuous nature of military surgery, which inevitably erodes combat surgical skills during peacetime, has come to be known as the Walker Dip or "peacetime effect."

More recently, addressing the Walker Dip has been a major focus of the National Academies of Sciences, Engineering, and Medicine (NASEM), for which the NRC serves as the operational arm. The 2016 NASEM report, *A National Trauma Care System: Integrating Military and Civilian Trauma Systems to Achieve Zero Preventable Deaths After Injury*, provides a blueprint for national health policy changes to preserve the medical advances of war and to improve care in civilian settings. Almost prophetically, in this opening chapter of *Surgeon to Soldiers* Churchill makes many observations and recommendations consistent with the NASEM report. Common themes include reducing obstacles that preclude information sharing, standardizing data collection, and collating medical records for outcomes research and performance improvement. He praises the documentation practices of civilian hospitals that enable the determination of the most common injuries and the most effective treatments. Churchill also proposed the solution of placing expert observers along the continuum of care to gather information, identify problems, and generate an improvement plan. These solutions would ultimately be implemented in the American military some 60 years later in the form of the Joint Trauma Systems' Department of Defense Trauma Registry. For medicine to remain the victor of war, these vital advancements must be preserved.

SUGGESTED READINGS

Agarwal D, Barker CF, Naji A, Schwab CW. Reciprocal learning between military and civilian surgeons: past and future paths for medical innovation. *Ann Surg.* 2021;274(5): e460-e464.

Cannon JW, Gross KR, Rasmussen TE. Combating the peacetime effect in military medicine. *JAMA Surg.* 2021;156(1):5-6.

Lockwood JS. War-time activities of the National Research Council and the Committee on Medical Research: with particular reference to team-work on studies of wounds and burns. *Ann Surg.* 1946;124(2):314-327.

National Academies of Sciences, Engineering, and Medicine. *A National Trauma Care System: Integrating Military and Civilian Trauma Systems to Achieve Zero Preventable Deaths After Injury.* The National Academies Press; 2016.

Rasmussen TE, Coleman DM. Leave no one behind: invited commentary on Association of Time from Injury to Initial Hospital Arrival, Emergency Trauma Surgery, and Survival in U.S. Military Casualties. *Ann Surg.* 2023;279(1):11-12.

Walker AJ. The 'Walker dip'. *J Roy Nav Med Serv.* 2018;104:173-176.

2

Thermal Burns

Before Entering the Army, I also served on the N.R.C. Subcommittee for Thermal Burns. Our goal was to find the most effective treatment possible for burns, a goal that researchers, over the years, have taken many paths—often, strange paths—to try to reach.

HISTORIC BACKGROUND

An example of the empiric management of burns will be drawn from the history of surgery. Anyone might be amazed today to have spirits of turpentine applied to a fresh burn. One does not have to go very far back in history to find that this was a popular remedy advocated in surgical monographs. A surgeon, like most everyone else, likes to have a rational explanation for what he does. But a rational explanation does not mean, of course, that his treatment is a correct one. Why was turpentine put on a burned surface? At the time this was popular, the concept was that the injured tissues were thrown into a violent vibratory activity. This can be envisioned by comparing it to the vibration of a bell after it has been struck by its clapper. The thermal injury was supposed to initiate this action in the tissues and it continued after the source of heat had been removed.

Two schools of treatment arose. One held that this increased activity of the tissues should be suppressed by putting on a cold application—ice or cold water. The other held that tissue vibration or reverberation should be allowed to continue and only diminish slowly, the way the sound of the vibration of a bell fades slowly away. It was considered harmful to counteract the reverberation of the tissues with a sudden and violent reversal, so efforts were made to sustain it and let it subside slowly. The argument for putting on turpentine was based on this theory. It was obvious that turpentine was an irritant to the tissues. At least the physician could hear the patient scream when it was applied, and since the patient probably screamed when he was burned initially, this was evidence that turpentine was maintaining the activity induced by the boiling water or hot iron.

Again, there was the theory that a burned patient absorbed broken-down tissue elements. This merged with the traumatic toxemia concept of shock that Walter Cannon and others sponsored in World War I and was only superseded when Underhill pointed out the local loss of fluid and the hemoconcentration that were proportionate to the surface area of the burn. The inevitable implantation of pyogenic bacteria on tissues injured by a burn was not understood.

At that time our medical colleagues were still talking of the deleterious effects of a focus of infection such as a tiny apical abscess at the root of a tooth. It was widely accepted that such a focus was the cause of arthritis and other ailments. Physicians were busy trying to ferret out hidden foci of infection. The comparable doctrine in surgery centered on dead or injured tissue which gave forth products of its decomposition. These ideas were linked with some of the pre-Listerian and pre-Pasteurian concepts of miasmas that found origin in decomposing organic matter; miasmas that were transmitted by the air and could deleteriously affect the wounds of a patient in an adjacent bed. It was generally believed that dead tissue itself, produced by thermal or other trauma, gave rise to *toxins*. This concept was held by Davidson, who had the opportunity of seeing a great many burns during the industrial development of the Detroit area. Davidson, who worked at the Henry Ford Hospital, proposed putting tannic acid on the surface of a burn, the thought being that it would precipitate the poisonous broken-down proteins and fix them on the surface of the burn rather than allow them to be absorbed into the body. Tannic acid was supposedly noncorrosive and bound the proteins into a dense coagulum.

The application of tannic acid to the surface of burns was popular for a period, and when I worked in the emergency ward of the Massachusetts General Hospital (M.G.H.) in 1921, we were provided with a "burn kit" developed for this purpose.

When Cannon announced the toxic mechanism of wound shock during World War I, he postulated that a broken-down product of protein decomposition—histamine—was the responsible agent. Sir Thomas Lewis, the famous cardiologist, picked up this idea in England, linking it with Sir Henry Dale's studies on histamine. Lewis held that the liberation of histamine from the injured cell is an "antisocial element" within the complex of body cells. This was a beautiful metaphysical concept, postulating the living organism as composed of a society of cells and an injured cell giving forth an antisocial element comparable to histamine. Lewis called it "H-substance." Now, as we look back on it, this is as extravagant as a medieval concept but it was put forth in the early 1920's. It was in part this idea that led Davidson to propose the surface coagulation of broken-down protein substances by tannic acid.

Following the theater fire in New Haven, Connecticut, Underhill had the opportunity, as professor of pharmacology, to see many burned patients and identify the concentration of their blood. He demonstrated the rise in hematocrit and proposed the interpretation that they were suffering from concentration of their blood. He likened the burn patient to a sufferer from cholera. Cholera victims lose fluid internally from the surface of the bowel. It was Underhill who was responsible for the concept that the delayed shock following a burn was attributable to the loss of fluid from the surface of the burn. Nothing could be more obvious once one looks at a burned surface and sees the formation of blisters. When a blister ruptures, the surface keeps on exuding fluid.

Davidson and his supporters countered immediately by saying, "Even if there is no toxin and the patient is losing fluid from the surface of a burn, tannic acid will prevent the fluid loss." There was an immediate shift in the rationalization of tannic acid treatment—a continuation of the same therapy but for a different reason.

In Hartford, Connecticut, where doctors treat a great many burned patients from the local industries, Welles Standish had been an advocate of tannic acid treatment. It was called to his attention that patients treated with tannic acid were dying of necrosis of the liver. This linked the tannic acid treatment of burns with death from liver damage, showed that the absorption of tannic acid is dangerous. It was also recognized that the tannic acid coagulum concealed the surface infection under it. At this point, surgeons substituted a solution of aniline dye—a favorite one was gentian violet—to coagulate the proteins. This was supposed to act also as a bacteriostatic agent and prevent pus formation under the eschar. Aniline dyes were also damaging to the tissues. In fact, nearly every preparation available at that time which would kill bacteria would kill living cells on the surface of the body.

During the war, Roy McClure, Chief of Surgery at the Henry Ford Hospital, published in the *Annals of Surgery* an article entitled: "Tannic Acid Treatment of Burns: An Obsequy." This article appeared when I was overseas and it was of great help in eliminating tannic acid from usage in burn therapy. One of the first actions I took in the North African Theater was to publish a directive that there should be no further use of tannic acid in the treatment of burns. The Surgeon General of the Army had already taken the same position, but his decision had not reached the overseas theater. Roy McClure's action in withdrawing the recommendation of the Ford Hospital that tannic acid be used in the treatment of burns was a courageous act. He told me later that it was one of the most difficult decisions he ever had faced. I wrote to him from North Africa, telling him how much he had contributed to the treatment of burn patients there.

N.R.C. BURN COMMITTEE

One of the committee's most important jobs was to determine if highly-recommended methods of treatment were as good as the claims put forth for them. For instance, the pharmaceutical houses were pressing to secure large contracts from the Army for ointments and lotions. Each one was armed with experiments supposedly showing beyond a doubt that the proposed treatment was effective. Some of these concoctions and ointments for the treatment of burns were advocated with terrific pressure put on the Surgeon General's office. Ointments were recommended that solidified completely at a temperature that often prevailed in the battlefield, making them unfit for use. It took a great deal of vigilance and testing to try to make sure that products with flaws such as this did not slip by.

Sumner Koch served on the Burn Committee. For many years he had been determining the policy in the treatment of burns at the Cook County Hospital. His reaction to a given proposal provided a good test of realism for any blueprint that might be drawn. He accepted the loss of fluid from the surface of the burn as being important; but no one at that time had appreciated fully the loss of fluid into the tissues beneath the surface. It is not the pouring out of fluid from the surface that is important but the loss into the tissues themselves in the form of a protein-rich edema.

In the enormous Cook County Hospital of Chicago a method of treatment had to be practical, but possibly it would not be found so when used in Tunisia on a soldier burned by flaming gasoline. There, in the middle of the summer with the temperature at 110°, the application of Koch's pressure dressing might well cause the man to die of a high fever because he was unable to eliminate his body heat. In fact, instead of using pressure dressings in Tunisia, we had to strip the burned patients and employ no dressing whatsoever. An electric fan was placed to blow on the burn. This same principle was used in Texas when an oil refinery fire in Galveston injured many people. In Texas, the open air treatment of burns was essential because of the necessity for heat elimination.

It is impossible to sit in Washington and advise surgeons in Alaska and in the Malay jungle or the islands of the Pacific or in Europe. There is too vast a range of climatic and other environmental conditions. There are also, of course, many kinds of burns. They vary in depth and with the agent that has produced the burn. Any remedy, unless actually harmful in itself, is likely to be followed by a "good" result in second-degree burns. In these, only a partial thickness of the skin has been injured. Full-thickness burns create real difficulties unless they are recognized for what they are and treated in a different manner, possibly by immediate excision and skin graft.

The N.R.C. set up experimental stations in many parts of the country to work on the problem of burn treatment and to develop methods that would be practical and simple and applicable under the wide range of conditions that might be encountered in war. It took a long time to set up this program because it takes a long time to find surgeons able to assume the responsibility.

Oliver Cope took on this task at the M.G.H. and as his associate chose Bradford Cannon before he went into the service. Cope and Cannon deliberately but cautiously eliminated many erroneous concepts and arrived at methods which at least would do no harm. They recommended a skin graft as an early dressing for certain kinds of burns. They tried out recommended ointments, applying them, for instance, on the upper third of an area from which a split thickness skin graft had been taken, leaving the middle third with nothing on it and applying another remedy to the lower third. This enabled them to recognize which area healed first. A crucial question was: Does this ointment *delay* healing? By far the greater number of the preparations tried, did so. The results showed that the best a surgeon can do is to avoid putting on something that does harm. The tests with sulfa drugs were significant. Surgeons were saying: "At last we have a preparation we can put on a fresh wound or burn and it will do no harm and it kills the bacteria," but it was found that sulfa drugs did do harm by causing delay in healing.

Edwin Cohn was busy at this time rushing back and forth to Washington and holding a weekly conference with his laboratory workers. He was in a high state of excitement about blood and blood substitutes. These were being developed under another committee of the N.R.C. They were letting out projects on liquid serum and experimenting with dry serum and plasma which could be shipped as powder and reconstituted as a liquid before administration to a patient. All of this led to a situation which we were able to correct only with difficulty later on in the war. I took the position that there was no substitute for whole blood. The organization of the N.R.C. committees and the frantic efforts at secrecy, as well as the inability of the clinician to define and state his problem in terms the experimental scientist could understand, led to great gaps in preparation for the management of wounded men. It is harder to eliminate errors than to introduce new measures. To stop doing something unless it can be proven that it is positively harmful is next to impossible in the art of therapy.

Meanwhile, Harry Beecher and some of his laboratory associates were busy experimenting with chickens to try to find an effective treatment for burns. Harry soon found that a chicken anesthetized with barbiturates was less affected by a burn than a chicken without barbiturates. He then began to speculate about the actions of barbiturates in a burn. Jim Gamble at the Children's Hospital, who had spent many years studying the problem of dehydration in infants, had stimulated surgeons to think in terms of fluid loss in peritonitis and its replacement by normal salt solution. What was known as "fluid therapy" was well known in surgery. For several years we had recognized that it was essential to replace fluid loss. Peritonitis was likened to an enormous burned surface. The term "replacement therapy" came into common usage, indicating that it was necessary to replace lost fluid in kind. This meant not only salt but also other electrolytes and protein. It was necessary to recognize what had been lost and to replace whole blood or plasma or electrolytes. This is still a field for careful study and clinical investigation.

The Burn Committee wisely took the position that the simplest possible measures should be used as local treatment on the burn surface. Preferably this was to take the form of an ointment to keep the external dressing from sticking. They advised the simplest ointment that could be furnished in great quantity, such as boric ointment. Liquid petrolatum and machine oil were also considered suitable. The desired effect was largely centered on being able to change the dressing without pain. Infection was to be controlled by giving sulfa drugs by mouth to build up an effective blood level.

COCOANUT GROVE FIRE

The Committee on Burns was invited to come to Boston the night of the Cocoanut Grove fire. They examined the patients in the hospitals and were in a position to see the immediate and, later, the subsequent results of various forms of local treatment as well as the management of the patients with plasma.

The chairman of the Burn Committee was Dr. Allen Whipple. As soon as I realized the magnitude of the Cocoanut Grove disaster, I called Allen, who was in New York. This was about 1:30 in the morning. I told him the situation, that the M.G.H. and the Boston City Hospital were full of casualties. He got out of bed and caught a five o'clock train, so he started for Boston before the early edition of the newspapers had reached the street in New York. He was there before the last dressings were applied. He also alerted observers from the Office of the Surgeon General in Washington and they arrived early in the morning. They were on hand to see many methods of burn management applied. Allen spent a long time with the patients at both the M.G.H. and the Boston City Hospital.

The Cocoanut Grove fire had an immediate impact in official channels in Washington. One productive result was to clarify the treatment of burns in World War II. A major step was the elimination of tannic acid and the introduction of simple local applications. The pressure dressing advocated by Sumner Koch was also adopted as a comfortable means of excluding air and secondary infection.

As a result of the Cocoanut Grove fire, Nat Faxon and I became interested in disaster management, and we prepared an analysis of the administrative measures devised on the spot on the night of the fire. This, I believe, was one of the first papers on disaster management, a subject that has subsequently assumed increasing importance in national defense and industry.

During the admission of the patients and the administration of first aid at the M.G.H., I took no responsibilities for the treatment of individual patients but continued to circulate through the rooms of the emergency ward and the red brick corridor in order to keep in touch with the total situation.

DISASTER MANAGEMENT

The Cocoanut Grove Fire was followed by the appointment of a Disaster Committee organized under the N.R.C. This committee arranged to send observers to disaster areas as they might occur throughout the country. The task of the observer was to prepare a factual report. For illustration, at the time of the Worcester tornado John Raker visited the scene and wrote a long report of what actually happened. When some of his remarks appeared in the daily press, they aroused bitter criticism in the Worcester area and led to some scathing editorials in the Worcester papers. What he had reported was factual and, though the Worcester medical profession was up in arms for a short time, the repercussions soon quieted down.

One of the features of the Cocoanut Grove management at the M.G.H. was the employment of staff members who ordinarily would not be identified with the treatment of burns; for example, we drew in the psychiatrist, who was of great help in calming people. Disaster management at the national level drew in social anthropologists. Disaster *management* came to be seen, basically, as dealing with a problem in human behavior. *Injury*, however, is basically a surgical concern and will remain so.

At the time of the Worcester tornado, I published a short editorial in the *Annals of Surgery* entitled "Panic in Disaster." This has been reprinted more often than anything I have written, but it brought down the wrath of Worcester physicians upon my head. I remarked in the editorial how sensitive doctors were to any implied criticism of their actions, but the word "panic" was taken in the wrong sense. As I defined panic I used the words of Wilfred Trotter who observed the behavior of the English people during the Nazi air raids. One of the manifestations of panic is sensitivity to criticism; even a strictly objective analysis is taken as a criticism. Any appraisal of the behavior of people who are trying to do their best to bring aid to victims is certain to be taken as criticism. Despite saying several times in this editorial that no criticism was implied, my remarks were taken as such.

A PAPER FROM AFRICA

Later, when I was in the Army in North Africa, I wrote a prologue for a monograph on the "Management of the Cocoanut Grove Burns at the Massachusetts General Hospital." It arrived too late to be included in the June (1943) issue of the *Annals of Surgery*, but was published in a small book sponsored by the Surgeon General. It was originally dated May 24, 1943, and reads as follows:

PROLOGUE: MANAGEMENT OF THE COCOANUT
GROVE BURNS AT THE MASSACHUSETTS
GENERAL HOSPITAL

May 24, 1943

Regarding an injury as something apart from the body itself is a fallacy that has plagued the surgeon since his craft originated. The more external the lesion the more remote from the remainder of the body it appears, and the more persistent becomes the effort to assist the natural processes of healing. Surgeons (and physicians) will apply chemical substances to the skin that they hesitate to place into a deep wound, and will apply medicaments to the wound that they would not consider harmless in the deeper recesses of body cavities. Through years of hard experience it has been learned that the peritoneum has seemingly miraculous powers of resistance to infection if spared the added insult of chemical and mechanical trauma. The same is true of muscles and of the skin itself but the learning of this lesson has been delayed, largely because violation is not attended by such immediate and catastrophic results as is the case with the peritoneum.

Again, traumatic injuries lead the surgeon into a pitfall because they are so obviously of external origin. The cause is obvious and external, so the remedy must be simple and local.

The local management of burns has for years revolved about these fallacious concepts. Fortunately, the constitutional effects of severe burns have been recognized clearly, although not understood clearly. The resultant reduction in deaths from loss of body fluids, anemia, malnutrition and infection has been an outstanding achievement of modern surgery.

As one explores the history of the local treatment of burns, many remedies are found that are purely empiric. Others, particularly those employed by reputable surgeons, are supported by a perfectly logical rationalization in terms of the prevalent doctrine of the times. Turpentine was applied because the tissues have been thrown into a violent commotion by heat,

(continued)

and this commotion must not be reversed abruptly but maintained at a high pitch for a longer time. Cerate, sweet oil, soothing balsams and later carron oil were emollients designed to reverse more quickly the agitated state of the tissues, and presumably also the agitation of the patient himself. With the advent of Listerism, carbolic acid was added to the bland and emollient oil in order to kill the germs. When patients were succumbing to the effects of traumatic toxemia, tannic acid was introduced to precipitate these toxic protein substances in situ. Later, when surgeons were paying more attention to body fluids, the virtue of tannic acid was found in the prevention of fluid loss from the weeping surface of the burn. When aniline dyes were taken from their role of staining dead tissues in the pathologic laboratory and used in the clinic on living tissues, gentian violet was found to produce an eschar similar to that formed by tannic acid but with the added virtue of killing gram-positive bacteria. Counterstains were added to take care of the gram-negative group. Now that the sulfonamides are in full voice, they are either dusted on in pure form or incorporated in ointments. And so it goes.

Since being in North Africa I have seen a great many burns—mostly accidental, as this is a petrol war. I have also seen almost as many different methods of local treatment as there are burns. In fact, a single burn may recapitulate many pages of the history of the treatment of burns, as the patient is moved about the theater of operations. I have even seen burns treated by the native population with fresh cow dung—and they healed very kindly at that. Perhaps "there is something in it"—certainly some vitamin or other biotic can be isolated from cow manure by painstaking research given a little time and the necessary grant-in-aid.

In the Army, the battalion surgeon is the important fellow. He is right down at the surgical grass roots of the war. He must get results and get them quickly, and what is more, he must work with what can be carried on his shoulder in a kit bag. Here are comments regarding the treatment of burns that can be kept in the combat area by two battalion surgeons:

Number One: We believe in covering them up quickly with a big dressing and then pouring cold water on the dressing. It is not always sterile water either, usually out of my canteen. Do I clean them off? No, I never scrub anything up there at the front. (See Chisolm's excellent Military Surgery of the Confederate Army for further description of the cold water treatment of wounds. There is something in it.)

Number Two: You know I tried all of these various treatments for burns, but the one I think works best is just boric ointment. It takes the pain right away, and they seem to do better. I don't suppose I should be using it; they say you shouldn't put grease on burns. But up there at the front you begin to wonder about a good many things you were taught in Medical School.

Events move rapidly in war, and I am glad to report a heartening trend toward sanity in an otherwise schizophrenic world. When external violence reaches epidemic proportions one is forced to think in practical and simple terms. So it has happened with burns.

Although the Cocoanut Grove disaster took place in Boston, the method used for the treatment of burns was inspired by the war already in progress some months. The nightclub patrons were cared for by a method that might be applied to soldiers and sailors of an assault force on a sea beach. It is true that frills were added and elaborate laboratory tests carried out to prove to ourselves and others that the patients were not suffering ill consequences. One worries more about simplifying treatment than elaborating it.

The essentials of the treatment are being applied daily in North Africa and it has been comforting to be able to assure the battalion surgeon that is not something he "shouldn't be doing."

It is difficult to write a prologue to a collection of papers that I have never seen even in preliminary draft. During the catastrophe and for some weeks afterward we were concerned only with observing and recounting facts. I hope my colleagues have been cautious in formulating conclusions. Even if modest, conclusions are likely to be wrong or subject to modification before the ink is dry.

Opinions and impressions are plentiful and cheap, particularly under the emotional tension of a world at war. Facts are rare and precious. Complete data are next to impossible to obtain under combat conditions. Observations are fragmentary at the best. Yet the surgeons of the United States Army are already facing a barrage of surgical opinions and impressions from our many theaters of operations.

It is essential to preserve an open mind, for what is true under one set of conditions will not hold for a different set of conditions. What may be successful in the Pacific may not be at all applicable in other hands in North Africa or in England. American surgeons are at work in India and Iceland, Brazil and the British Isles, Alaska, Australia and Africa. They are in both hemispheres, down under the Equator and within the Arctic Circle. Only when we have all returned, each with a small piece of the puzzle, will it be possible to start to fit the pieces together and see the picture as a whole. In the meantime we must be content to observe and record so that our craft may rescue something constructive from a catastrophe that in other aspects represents the acme of destruction.

CONFERENCE

Death and disability from fire and explosion are by no means, of course, problems unique to military surgery. Since World War II, fire and explosions are the second leading cause of nontransportation accidental deaths in the United States. Nonfatal injuries are suffered by more than 250,000 persons each year.

Indeed, during the war, as I mentioned in my paper, most of the burns I saw were accidental. A great many were "petrol burns." A common custom was to heat a can of C-rations over a blaze of gasoline, kept alive by tossing more gasoline onto the fire. In the bright Mediterranean sunshine the blaze was often invisible, leading to neglect of precautions.

Advances in the manufacture of flame-retardant fabrics offer a safeguard to the serviceman in the field. A conference on this subject was held at the New York Academy of Medicine, December 2 and 3, 1966, and published in the *Bulletin* of the Academy, vol. 43, no. 8, August, 1967.

Jonathan B. Lundy, Leopoldo C. Cancio, and William G. Cioffi

Dr Churchill's monograph on thermal injury summarizes the evolution of burn treatment during the first half of the 20th century. Dr Churchill's direct involvement in this evolution included placing a moratorium on the use of tannic acid in the Mediterranean theater. Tannic acid was purported to be a panacea for burns. It was initially thought to bind toxins produced by dead tissue and later to encourage eschar formation and prevent fluid loss. This harmful treatment was eventually abandoned after a report in 1944 from the Henry Ford Hospital (notably the same institution from which the reported benefits of tannic acid had originated) identified hepatic necrosis as a complication of its use. Dr Churchill's elimination of tannic acid in the Mediterranean theater represents an example of the abandonment of inherited "doctrine" in favor of empiric observation.

Churchill also witnessed care provided at the Massachusetts General Hospital to victims of the 1942 Cocoanut Grove fire in Boston, MA. This experience sparked his interest in disaster response and national defense and led to the development of a Disaster Committee within the National Research Council, a predecessor to the Disaster Research Group and future national disaster response initiatives. He comments that disaster management is a "problem in human behavior," distinct from injury, which is "basically a surgical concern." While he was deployed to the Mediterranean theater, Dr Churchill wrote the prologue for the monograph on the care of the Cocoanut Grove patients. This monograph constitutes a thorough summary of burn care in the United States at the time and presciently set the stage for the subsequent evolution of modern burn care to the present day. His key observations concerned (1) the physiologic insult induced by thermal injury, (2) the importance of fluid loss and resuscitation, (3) the correction of malnutrition, and (4) the prevention of infection. Churchill also observed that military experience during wartime and civilian experience during disasters are mutually supportive: "Although the Cocoanut Grove disaster took place in Boston, the method used for the treatment of burns was inspired by the war already in progress."

Churchill further catalogued the confusing array of historic burn treatments ranging from turpentine to cow dung. He comments that "complete data are next to impossible to obtain under combat conditions" but that "it is essential to preserve an open mind . . . to observe and record so that our craft may rescue something constructive from a catastrophe." Our recent experience in Iraq and Afghanistan indicates that it is possible to do just that. Some burn care contributions during the recent conflicts included: (1) deployment of a theater burn consultant to Iraq to oversee all burn care in that theater; (2) collection of burn and trauma data into the Joint Theater Trauma Registry; (3) description of definitive burn care in the theater of local national burn patients of all ages; (4) implementation of burn guidelines and a resuscitation flow sheet; (5) development of a simpler resuscitation formula for adults (ISR Rule of 10); (6) rapid evacuation of critically ill combat casualties from Germany to the Burn Center using the US Army Burn Flight Team; (7) development of a burn resuscitation decision support system; and (8) evaluation of continuous renal replacement therapy in the burn intensive care unit.

Future wars, which may include large-scale combat operations against peer or near-peer adversaries, will present new challenges to the surgeon who cares for burns. If these surgeons rely on the principles taught by Colonel Churchill, they will be well equipped both to meet these challenges and to continue the record of scientific progress sparked by Colonel Churchill and his contemporaries.

DISCLAIMER

The opinions or assertions contained herein are the private views of the authors and are not to be construed as official or as reflecting the views of the Department of the Army or the Department of Defense.

SUGGESTED READINGS

Chung KK, Salinas J, Renz EM, et al. Simple derivation of the initial fluid rate for the resuscitation of severely burned adult combat casualties: in silico validation of the rule of 10. *J Trauma*. 2010;69(suppl 1):S49-S54.

Ennis JL, Chung KK, Renz EM, et al. Joint theater trauma system implementation of burn resuscitation guidelines improves outcomes in severely burned military casualties. *J Trauma*. 2008;64(2 suppl):S146-S151.

Massachusetts General Hospital. *Management of the Cocoanut Grove Burns at the Massachusetts General Hospital*. J. B. Lippincott; 1943.

Renz EM, Cancio LC, Barillo DJ, et al. Long range transport of war-related burn casualties. *J Trauma*. 2008;64(2 suppl):S136-S144.

Stout LR, Jezoir JR, Melton LP, et al. Wartime burn care in Iraq: 28th Combat Support Hospital, 2003. *Mil Med*. 2007;172(11):1148-1153.

3

You're in the Army Now

When Mobilization began, there was a debate about who might leave the M.G.H. and Harvard and who was to stay at home and carry on with medical education and the care of the nonmilitary population. Who was to be classified as nonessential and thereby spared to join the military effort? The activation of the affiliated hospital units was one of the first things that took place. The M.G.H. was one of these—it had been designated Base Hospital 6 during World War I. There was also the Harvard unit, which contained some M.G.H. doctors and others from the Peter Bent Brigham Hospital. There was the Boston City Hospital unit, which again included Harvard medical personnel. These reserve units were soon called to active duty. Senior physicians and surgeons who had retired from active posts formed a group to approve any further release of staff doctors to military service. They were not involved personally, being well over age for overseas service. The ultimate authority was centered in the office of the Director of the Hospital and the Dean of the Medical School. This provided a decision making body above the staff level and doctors could not follow their personal wishes. This disinterested group removed the responsibility from the chiefs of services, and I was spared any decisions as to whether this or that surgeon could depart. I was labeled as "essential" by this higher committee because I held the post of Professor and Head of the Surgical Service at the M.G.H. Both Harvard and the M.G.H. labeled me as essential. This meant that if I did not volunteer for active service, I was in no way under pressure to do so. If I decided to go, all I had to do was say that I didn't consider myself essential because my teaching and hospital duties could be handled by others.

REASONS FOR VOLUNTEERING

It is hard to identify one's motives in wanting to participate. Perhaps I had always had a slight feeling of guilt for not having taken part in World War I, whereas some of my friends and contemporaries had seen active service. I was protected from the draft by my status as a medical student. Neither of my two brothers had been on active service in World War I; Clarence was doing essential work in running the Indiana farm and Frank was over age, with family responsibilities. I recall discussing it with one of my brothers and his saying: "Our family does not have a very distinguished military record." One is aware that these and other emotions are working below the surface.

I was able to talk frankly to the medical students at Harvard, and was able to contribute my personal experience when discussing the problem at Vanderbilt Hall with the incoming class. I explained what it meant to be in medical school, out of uniform, in time of war. I told them that in the First World War, I was a student at the Harvard Medical School. We students were given a bronze button—a caduceus—to wear on our lapel. I recalled going to the theater one evening with one or two classmates, sitting in the gallery and having people in the audience hiss as we clambered up the aisle during the intermission. Young men who are not on active service, I emphasized, are exposed to intense emotional pressures.

As I try to sift my reasons for volunteering for active service in World War II, one of the compelling ones was the departure of many young interns and residents from my own hospital staff. It moved me deeply to have these young fellows come into my office and say good-bye as they went off into the unknown. In a professional sense I played the role of a parent to these young surgeons and I wanted to join them and help take care of them.

I also foresaw that a situation was developing which might, when the war was over, split the hospital staff into two factions—those who served with the military and those who did not. I could see that my usefulness as a teacher and a member of the M.G.H. staff might be finished if I could not share this experience with the youth of the country. Furthermore, I strongly agree with something Theodore Roosevelt said, ". . .my power for good whatever it may be, would be gone if I didn't try to live up to the doctrine that I have tried to preach." These are subtle considerations, but I feel certain that after the war my contacts, both with the older men on the staff and with the residents and interns, were far closer than they would have been if I had remained at home.

I preserved bonds with the oncoming generations and these boys have been a great help to me and to the hospital in the postwar years. It is my firm conviction that the medical profession vitally needs to reestablish such bonds and to strengthen those that may lead to a better mutual understanding of other activities and professions. Doctors need to learn to be more a part of the world outside of medicine. All these were reasons that led me to consider ways I could serve.

ARMY OR NAVY

I did not join the M.G.H. unit, which was to be the 6th Hospital during World War II, because there were plenty of men on the staff who wanted to organize it and who were well-qualified to occupy the important positions. These were largely men who had some experience in World War I or who were in the reserve. Also, I wasn't attracted to working in one particular hospital unit.

I talked several times with the Surgeon General of the Army and also with senior officers in the Navy. The latter I knew through my contacts in the N.R.C. In particular, I talked with Admiral Stevenson, a dynamic, understanding man who had the experimental point of view.

I recall saying, "Steve, as soon as the Navy gets to the point where it wants a small group of troubleshooters to get into uniform and identify and find solutions for surgical problems that crop up in the field, let me know. Nothing would please me better than to participate in such a group."

I didn't imply that I wanted to lead it or enjoy a high rank, but that I was ready to volunteer for active duty. I thought this would be my best contribution. Steve was quite intrigued by the idea and talked it over at the Navy Medical Bureau.

He knew the Navy far better than I and finally told me, "Pete, the Navy won't get into this kind of business," and it didn't. The Navy is a unique organization, more centrally directed and coordinated than the Army. It is also a closely-knit organization, extremely sensitive, almost intuitive in its actions. If the Chief of Naval Operations in Washington changes his mind about something, there's an excellent chance that even a junior officer in the Boston Navy Yard knows it before the change is recorded on paper. It reminds me of how a school of fish or a flock of birds will suddenly turn and take off in a different direction. No one knows what the mechanism of their communication may be.

The Navy itself is patterned after the model of a ship. All activities on a ship are integrated, not unlike the integration that binds together the vital activities of any living organism. The medical officer on a ship has no logistic problem in obtaining supplies, food, or of moving independently. He has assigned to him a certain cubic footage and everything he needs must be packed into it like the equipment of a space capsule. His space requirements are determined and allotted with precision, just as are the space requirements for every fire extinguisher or other piece of equipment aboard. Wherever the ship goes, the fire extinguisher and the sick bay with the doctors in it travel as integral bits of the ship organism. When an Army moves, in contrast, the doctors traipse along like gypsies with their equipment, tentage and supplies.

After I heard from Admiral Stevenson that the Navy would have no use for a consultant in the field, I turned to the Army and talked with Frederick W. Rankin. Fred was a surgeon, originally of the Mayo Clinic, and then of Lexington, Kentucky. He had entered active service as a consultant to the Surgeon General. A diminutive bantam rooster, greatly respected as a practical surgeon, he had been in and out of the Mayo Clinic organization but it was recognized generally that he was too much of a fighter to become a good "clinic man." He was commissioned first as colonel and soon promoted to brigadier general. I called on him in Washington early in July, 1942, and told him that any time he could use me I was ready to enter the Army. I was introduced to General Hillman, Chief of Professional Services, a Medical Corps officer in the regular Army.

Hillman remarked that he was glad to know I was available, then said: "You haven't got one of those little inguinal hernias that men of our age are likely to have?" I replied, "Oh, no," but this query focused my attention on my inguinal canals and, sure enough, I soon detected the symptoms and physical signs of a hernia and quickly went into the Phillips House and had it repaired. I had not been aware of it until I was asked that question. It was a shrewd remark on the part of General Hillman, probably based on having a number of middle-aged volunteer doctors.

Although I had made my intention known, I still had to wait six months for events to clarify a position for me.

Elliott C. Cutler, Surgical Consultant for Allied Headquarters in London, took off to England. The North African area was not to be set apart from this command until February 6, 1943, after the North African invasion. I suppose the plan to divide the theater of war was known or anticipated in Washington. It's now obvious that the Surgeon General of the Army could not appoint a second consultant in the European area until a second theater of war had been announced officially. Consequently, Torch Operation—the landing of the forces from the United Kingdom and the coming in of the Western Task Force under General George Patton—were all under the European headquarters in London. General Paul Hawley and his staff carried responsibility for the casualties of the North African forces up to the time of the formation of the new theater.

It was in December, 1942, that I was informed through Rankin's office that they were ready to have me volunteer and enter the Army on active duty. Rankin insisted that I be commissioned as a full colonel, although the Army tried to settle for a lieutenant colonel. He pushed this through and I was given the initial commission of colonel, which I held throughout the war.

A PERIOD OF WAITING

A moist January snow was falling on Belmont Hill the evening I left there for Washington on the Federal. I was sworn in at Washington and remained there for a short period in the Surgeon General's Office.

I received my orders for North Africa early in January. They were secret. In fact, I was not told directly *where* I was going to be assigned because the North African Theater had not yet been formed, even after the landing on November 8, 1942. The magnitude of the operation was a secret. It wasn't until I was ready to depart that I was informed that I was to travel to Allied Force Headquarters in Algiers.

Meanwhile, I was like a pitcher warming up in the bull pen, ready to be moved to North Africa the moment it became a separate theater. My assignment as Surgical Consultant to the North African Theater might have upset Cutler, Loyal Davis and others in England because they had the understanding that they were the consultants for all activities of American forces in the Atlantic area and had not anticipated the breaking off of a North African and subsequently a Mediterranean area as separate commands. It was made more confusing to them by General Eisenhower's moving from London to become Commanding General of the North African Theater with General Howard Alexander, the British Commander-in-Chief in the Middle East, as the Chief of the Ground Forces. So my "warming up" period continued until these operational plans were clear.

There was little for me to do in the Surgeon General's Office except to try to get hold of every document I could about North Africa. I wanted information about the terrain and the endemic diseases, so I looked around the Preventive Medicine Section and dipped into its file of military intelligence (very secret) only to learn about the obstetric practices of the desert nomads in southern Algeria. Such data were filed away and guarded carefully.

I spent several afternoons in the Division of Experimental Medicine trying to find what the climatic conditions were. So far as U.S. Army hospital work was concerned, there was little beyond the tables of organization and the number and rank of medical officers authorized.

There was no intellectual preparation for entering upon the tasks with which World War II was to confront the medical profession. The writings from World War I had been put together in a haphazard manner. Consequently, on departure for overseas I received no instructions in the management of the wounded and there was no guide to the buried periodical literature of 1918. The Surgeon General's *History of World War I* was inadequate as far as casualty care was concerned. In fact, the *History* was not even included in the library list available to overseas hospitals. Finally I requisitioned a copy for the Theater Surgeon's Office. In the hospital libraries there were, of course, current medical journals and other books on surgical diagnosis and techniques. The Surgeon General's *History of World War I* probably was stacked by the thousands somewhere in warehouses.

UNDEFINED DUTIES

There was absolutely no conception of the duties of a consultant or what responsibilities he might be assigned in an overseas theater. The consultants had no command status whatsoever. Rankin's task was to establish the value of consultants. As background, Hawley once told me that when he went to England his confreres of the regular Army who had had experience in World War I told him that there were two things that were likely to cause him trouble: affiliated hospital units and consultants. He said, "I soon found that I could not get along without either." I started with a complete lack of definition and understanding of what the post of Surgical Consultant to a Theater Surgeon really meant. The table of organization (T/O) called for one consultant in surgery, one in medicine and one in psychiatry. The Professional Services Division of the Surgeon General's Office was doing its best to get posts of consultants inserted into the new T/O of headquarters organizations. A headquarters, of course, has a table of organization as does a hospital unit, and the Theater Surgeon can assemble a staff within its frame until he receives authorization from his commanding general to add additional personnel. A change has to be defended through the General Staff and the Chief of Staff. The commanding general may authorize a change or authorize it only on a temporary basis.

It proved to be a great advantage in World War II to take up a position for which the duties were not defined. Although in World War I, Dr. John T. Finney of Baltimore was the Consulting Surgeon for the A.E.F., the expeditionary force fought in Europe for only a short time and there was little time to define a role for Consulting Surgeons. One reason the consultants achieved a bad reputation with regular army officers in World War I was that some of them acted unwisely. Dr. Harvey Cushing went over with a general hospital, the story of which is in his published diary. He served with the British in France before the A.E.F. arrived. Consequently, Cushing felt that he had more actual war experience than the regular Army officers when they came over in administrative posts. Cushing on more than one occasion narrowly escaped court-martial for defying the orders of superior officers of the A.E.F. Doctors who behaved as Dr. Cushing did were viewed by the regular Army officers as headstrong and undisciplined civilian volunteers who had no knowledge or respect for military orthodoxy and would defy commands in order to accomplish some professional purpose. In Cushing's diary it is obvious that he believed it was best to set up special centers to handle head injuries and wounds, so he went about doing so. He may have been right from a surgical standpoint but in error within a military context. Cushing described how he set up such a center and personally went along the road posting signs which directed ambulances to take head wounds to his particular station. From what can be gathered from the surgical records of the A.E.F. in 1918 there was a state of confusion but the competent, wise consultant in the person of Dr. Finney was doing his best to straighten things out; but he was handicapped by civilian officers dashing here and there and causing friction with the regulars who were both inexperienced and at times agonizingly stupid. The war was over before a well-organized medical service was achieved.

Perhaps this is why one of my friends in the regular Army—General Morrison C. Stayer—was accustomed to say that the most important assignment for a young medical officer was duty at Fort Benning where infantry officers were being trained. Stayer believed that the Surgeon General should pick out his best medical officers to be assigned to Fort Benning so that they could become acquainted with infantry officers as personal friends. An ever-present problem in Army medicine is that it cannot be understood by commanders and that they must trust their medical officers. If a gap exists, not only medicine suffers but the wounded soldier is right in the middle.

Neither General Hillman, Rankin, nor anyone else had definite ideas about the scope of an overseas consultant's job. They did know that somebody was needed who might know something about wounds and wounded men, and that someone was desired with sufficient professional prestige to speak for and represent American surgery. With few exceptions, the names of the high-ranking officers of the regular Medical Corps were unknown outside Army circles, and the Army had to cloak itself with civilian professional prestige. Many frankly recognized the need for help. Looking at the situation from their point of view, one must remember that they are responsible to their commanders and this responsibility extends to the behavior of the civilians they bring into staff positions. It is a heavy responsibility to accept a man who is known only through his civilian reputation and put him into a staff position in theater headquarters. My experience with the regular Army officers was not at all difficult. Some of my colleagues, however, had serious problems.

When I finally left Washington for North Africa, my ignorance of the Army was still so great that I would not have been surprised to have found General Eisenhower meeting me on arrival in Algiers; I was that impressed by the importance of my mission as I saw it and with my exalted rank of "chicken colonel."

My description of the haphazard circumstances that surrounded my departure may seem overdrawn. The confusion in Washington and the general excitement was indeed like that of the "sound of a going" when birds take off from a mulberry tree. I paid a brief courtesy call on the Surgeon General whom I saw once or twice. Everyone in Washington was irritable and frantically busy. As to plans for communication, someone, it may have been Hillman, said: "If there's any important message that you want to get back, it can be inserted in paragraph 'C' of the Sanitary Report."

The Sanitary Report was a document by which a medical officer could bypass line officers. A line officer could comment on its contents or express nonconcurrence, but he had no authority to delete or otherwise divert it from the channel to higher headquarters. The humblest medical officer could say that his battalion was being exposed to the dangers of dysentery by improper preparation of food or exposed to the hazard of malaria by bivouac in a swamp, and no one from his company commander on up could keep that message from going through to the Chief Medical Adviser of the Commander-in-Chief. Hillman informed me of this, but for many months there was no Sanitary Report that I had anything to do with, so there was no way that I could get any message back.

I received no briefing in military etiquette. Being commissioned as a colonel on temporary assignment to the Office of the Surgeon General in Washington, I escaped what my confreres in the 6th General Hospital had been getting for months—namely, drill, etiquette and unit organization regulations. They were "browned off" with their experience at Camp Blanding. Nothing would have been gained by drilling me several hours a day. It is now recognized that an expert need not be called into active duty until there is need for him. He is then sent immediately to the place where he is needed without going through disciplinary instruction on military etiquette. I was one of the few examples in World War II of a doctor being treated intelligently by the Army.

You're in the Army Now
COMMENTARY

Eric H. Twerdahl, Matthew J. Eckert, and Keith D. Lillemoe

Churchill explores two broad themes in the book's third chapter, *You're in the Army Now*, no doubt a reference to the 1941 comedic film of the same name. The movie features two vacuum cleaner salesmen who accidentally join the Army, but there is nothing accidental about Churchill's military service. The first theme he explores is volunteerism, informed by his own personal reasons for volunteering. He alludes to a sense of regret—guilt even—at having been "out of uniform" during the First World War, and he describes his desire during the Second World War to serve in solidarity with the younger generation of Massachusetts General Hospital (MGH) surgeons and surgical trainees. Also explicit among his reasons for volunteering is the power—indeed, the necessity—of fostering strong civilian-military bonds in medicine, captured by the statement that "Doctors need to learn to be more a part of the world outside of medicine." Indeed, just as the care of the injured soldier has been advanced by discoveries made far from the field of battle, so too has civilian medicine benefited from lessons learned only in war.

The second theme Churchill explores is more nuanced, related to the often confused intersection between the *profession* of medicine and the *profession* of military service. Speaking to an annual meeting of the Massachusetts Medical Society in 1949, Roscoe Pound, University Professor *Emeritus* and former dean of the Law School of Harvard University, defined a profession as an "organized calling in which men pursue a learned art and are united in the pursuit of it as a public service." Beyond that definition, the professions of medicine and military service are further characterized by distinct moral codes, requiring the physician in uniform to straddle two distinct professional worlds. In most circumstances, those two worlds overlap completely. However, any tension between them is thrown into sharp relief in times of war or other crises, when the military physician is called upon to subjugate the obligations of one profession to the obligations of the other—to prioritize the success of the mission over the care of the patient. In such an instance, Churchill writes, "the wounded soldier is right in the middle."

Churchill further illustrates this point through the example of Harvey Cushing, who led the Harvard Unit of the *Ambulance Américaine* and later the Harvard University Base Hospital Unit during the First World War. Cushing was not shy in voicing his disdain for military leadership—both British and American—whom he thought had no business interfering in medical matters. Despite *Doctor* Cushing's unassailable expertise in the management of head injuries, it is clear from Churchill's description that *Lieutenant Colonel* Cushing's effectiveness as a military physician was likely diminished by his weakness as a military officer. Churchill writes that "Doctors who behaved as Dr Cushing did were viewed by the regular Army officers as headstrong and undisciplined civilian volunteers who had no knowledge or respect for military orthodoxy and would defy commands in order to accomplish some professional purpose." Accordingly, Colonel Churchill would take a more tempered approach in his role as consulting surgeon, realizing that he could have a far greater medical impact working from within the "military context" than from outside of it. It is a perspective that should be of interest and utility to all physicians, especially those in uniform.

SUGGESTED READINGS

Bliss M. *Harvey Cushing: A Life in Surgery*. Oxford University Press; 2005.

Cushing H. *From a Surgeon's Journal, 1915-1918*. Little, Brown & Company; 1936.

Huntington SP. *The Soldier and the State: The Theory and Politics of Civil-Military Relations*. Harvard University Press; 1957.

Pound R. The professions in the society of today. *N Engl J Med*. 1949;241(10):351-357.

Spencer FC. Historical vignette: the introduction of arterial repair into the US Marine Corps, US Naval Hospital in July-August 1952. *J Trauma*. 2006;60(4):906-909.

4

Wound Shock and Blood Transfusion[1]

In This Chapter and the following one, I am going to skip ahead—as well as back—in time, in order to present a picture of some of the medical problems that were being encountered in the field.

During trips which I was to take, later, through southern Tunisia (see Chapter 6, Arrival in Algiers), I pursued the subject of the need for whole blood transfusion with both British and American medical officers. In the British forward hospitals it was estimated that 10 per cent of all patients coming to operation required resuscitation and that of the 10 per cent, one out of five required whole blood.

"If treated with plasma alone," I was told at No. 1 Casualty Clearing Station (C.C.S.), "the blood pressure can be brought back but falls again with operation and does not come back a second time. Patients treated with plasma remain pale, the pulse is rapid and the labile blood pressure is very sensitive to further operative procedures."

A Colonel Beckwith had sustained a laceration of the knee joint and compound fracture of both bones of the lower leg. He was treated for three hours in the main dressing station and received 1,500 cc. of plasma. His blood pressure remained at 60/0 with a pulse rate of 120. He was then given two pints of blood and his pressure rose to 90/ in three hours. Another pint of blood brought his pressure to 120/. His red blood cell count was 2,000,000 and the hemoglobin 30 to 35 per cent.

Colonel Frank Berry, at the U.S. 9th Evacuation Hospital, told of a soldier with bilateral injury to the feet from a land mine. The injury was not compounded but "*bleeding into the tissues* caused the red cell count to fall to 1.5 million."

In Beja, one of the forward main dressing stations had a field surgical unit (F.S.U.) attached. Here I stayed by the stretcher of a severely wounded British soldier. It was a pathetic sight. He was showing the mental anguish

---

[1]Part of this chapter first appeared as the Introduction to *The Physiologic Effects of Wounds*, published by the Office of the Surgeon General of the Army in 1952.

and restlessness of a patient dying of hemorrhage. He also had dysentery. He was screaming: "I need to shit! I need to shit!"

My notes made on this trip contain this comment: "The goal of resuscitation . . . is not solely to save life but to prepare for necessary surgery. This will in turn be accompanied by further loss of blood."

The surgeons in the field were acutely aware of the problem before I came to North Africa. In his diary dated February 2, 1943, Kenneth Lowry gave vivid descriptions of wounded American soldiers. (See Chapter 8, Diary and Letters of a Forward Surgeon.)

In her book *G.I. Nightingale. The Story of An American Army Nurse* (W. W. Norton, 1945), Captain Theresa Archard, writing of her experience in the 48th Surgical Hospital, gave the following description:

> The corpsmen had donated all the blood they could spare. Nurses offered but were refused. The doctors couldn't afford to give blood—they had to keep going, all of them. Colonel Wiley hit upon a solution. He got in contact with Ordnance and Quartermasters and asked them for blood donors. Within two hours thirty men had been sent to our area. They were to rest in an empty tent, and as blood was needed they were called. The blood given the patients was of the same type but we cross-matched it, too. We could take no chances on their getting chills—they were too sick to stand any more than they had to.

An official report written from II Corps in mid-February records that "plasma is being used generously and successfully. Blood transfusions, using unmatched donors, but ones of the right blood group have been attempted. Sometimes they go off without an incident, at other times they have had to be abandoned because of reactions. . . . Patients are treated for shock in clearing stations, for as long as twenty-four hours before definitive surgical therapy is attempted."

The logical question is, why was the Army sent to North Africa with plasma and no methods of obtaining whole blood that was so clearly needed? Part of the answer is found in the general lack of preparedness the country faced. But the decision to use plasma in fighting the war had many roots, not the least of which was a faulty conception of the nature of shock itself. Because the myriad of theories on the nature of shock were in part responsible for the lack of whole blood, I am going to trace the development of ideas in World War I when wound surgeons began to analyze how and why soldiers died.

BACKGROUND

World War I revealed wound shock was a complex problem. Sufficient observational data were not accumulated to permit clear identification and subsequent analysis. Certain preexisting hypotheses (vasomotor exhaustion, acapnia, adrenal exhaustion) were discredited, but other concepts inadequately supported by facts (traumatic toxemia, the distinction between shock and hemorrhage) were substituted. These concepts centered on wound shock as an entity not accounted for by hemorrhage, infection, brain injury, blast, asphyxia of cardiorespiratory origin, fat embolism, or any other clearly demonstrable effect of trauma. World War I thus recognized a problem of shock but left it wrapped in mystery.

At the end of World War I the so-called shock problem was transferred to the experimental laboratories of medical science. Attempts were made to resolve it by physiologic and chemical techniques under a wide variety of experimentally induced circumstances. As the methods of initiating experimental shock multiplied, the term itself became broadened, so that it included a number of processes that appeared to have one feature in common—a reduced effective volume flow of blood with inadequacy of the peripheral circulation and resulting tissue asphyxia. In the clinic as well as the laboratory, shock became separated from wounds, and "medical shock," "obstetrical shock," "burn shock," "shock due to infection," and other types were described as entities. So-called shock became synonymous with the process of dying from almost any cause unless death was practically instantaneous or, as Henderson stated, "unless one is burned alive." The phrase, "the problems of shock," was used by Mann to describe this confusion of definition.

In the welter of animal experimentation during and after World War I, there were certain findings pertinent to the original problem. Bayliss and Cannon had imitated wound shock by crushing and lacerating the thigh muscles of anesthetized animals. This was supposed to produce a destruction of tissue but not a very great extravasation of blood. Failure to measure the factor of blood and fluid loss in the local area of trauma (and, as shown later, failure to recognize the superimposed clostridial infection) enabled Cannon and other experimenters to propose that toxic products of tissue disintegration were absorbed into the general circulation, causing what was termed traumatic toxemia. Parsons, Parsons and Phemister, and Blalock measured the local blood and fluid loss in traumatized legs by precise methods and showed that it was far greater than had been suspected and quite sufficient to account for the reduction in blood volume observed.

It was thus made clear that estimation of the amount of hemorrhage in an injured man must include the blood extravasated into the tissues as well as that poured on the ground or caught by the dressings. It was also found necessary to consider the blood volume that remained in circulation in terms of plasma and red cells, for the proportionate loss of these elements varied under different circumstances. The phenomena of hemoconcentration and hemodilution were thus made understandable. Nevertheless, certain investigators insisted on using the physical state of the blood to define shock as an entity, and confusion was introduced by proponents of the thesis that shock could not exist unless hemoconcentration was present.

In a critical review of the shock problem in 1942, Wiggers commented that contributions to the literature on shock appeared to be directed toward the support of one or another favored theory. Experimental conditions, he stated, had not been carefully evaluated and conclusions, rather than facts, were emphasized. "Beneficial effects," Wiggers said, "are claimed for various forms of therapy in instances in which it was never shown that the subjects were in a state of shock which would have proved fatal without treatment."

"Apparently," as Wiggers wrote, "at a certain stage an adequate circulation cannot be restored by merely filling the system as one does an automobile radiator." The same writer expressed his surprise at "how well tissues or organs withstand a very low rate of blood flow before they cease to function or are unable to revive."

Thus the assumption was made that at one moment restoration of blood volume could stay the progress of death, but in the next moment it would be unable to do so. It seemed reasonable to believe that if this phase-line could be identified by experiment and an analysis be made of the physiologic processes then in motion, corrective measures might suggest themselves. But even under precisely controlled laboratory experimentation, minor variations in conditions may determine whether the animal lives or dies. Subtle differences in environmental temperature, anesthetic agents, age, and previous nutritional state of the subject, as well as other conditioning factors make it difficult to halt the cinema of life at a particular frame where one may say: "Up to this point, continuing life is possible—beyond this, death is inevitable." If difficult in precise experimentation, identification of the onset of irreversible shock becomes impossible when one is confronted by the results of the random trauma sustained by soldiers under combat conditions. Although the diagnosis of "irreversible shock" appeared with some frequency on the clinical records in World War II, it was merely a pretentious way of indicating that the man had died of a lethal wound.

This, then, was the background of our knowledge of wound shock when World War II began. The war was entered with the concept that (1) plasma to restore the bulk of the blood in the intravascular space and (2) sodium chloride solution for dehydration and electrolyte depletion of the interstitial space were therapeutic measures adequate to the purpose of adjusting homeostasis in a wounded man. As the war progressed, this concept changed. It soon became clear that much precise information about the physiologic state of a wounded man was wanting, and efforts toward this end culminated in the establishment of the Board for the Study of the Severely Wounded in the Mediterranean Theater of Operations (see Chapter 31, The Board for the Study of the Severely Wounded).

PLANNING FOR TREATMENT OF SHOCK IN WORLD WAR II

The initial decision to rely on plasma rather than blood transfusion for the resuscitation of the wounded appears to have been based in part on the view held in the Office of the Surgeon General of the Army, and in part on the opinion of the eminent civilian investigators summoned by the N.R.C. to act as advisors to the Armed Forces. The Committee on Transfusions first met on May 31, 1940. The Army representative made the following statement: "If the theaters of operations are mostly outside the United States . . . the Army would likely discourage the use of blood banks. If war should come closer they might want to use blood that could be transported by airplane or specially devised refrigeration. In more distant places where blood could not be collected locally, plasma, either plain or dried, would have to be used." The representative of the Navy also favored "dried blood" (plasma).

The following is quoted from a report of the meeting submitted to the chairman of the Committee on Surgery, N.R.C., dated July 24, 1940:

E.D.C. Comment: The greater part of the day was devoted to a consideration of whole blood and blood plasma and blood serum transfusions. The consensus of opinion was that the greatest emphasis should be placed on the use of blood plasma for the following reasons: (1) Most instances of shock are associated with hemoconcentration and a given quantity of plasma is more effective than an equal quantity of whole blood in treatment; (2) blood plasma is approximately as effective in the treatment of hemorrhage as is whole blood; (3) the difficulties of preservability and transportability of plasma are considerably less than those of whole blood; and (4) matching and typing are not necessary when pooled plasma (suppression of isoagglutinins) is used.

The last two reasons given may have been concessions to the position taken by the representatives of the Army and Navy; the first two, however, appear to reflect the prevailing concept of wound shock held by experts at that time. The efficiency of blood in the treatment of hemorrhage had been established in World War I. In small quantities it had been preserved and transported considerable distances, even up to regimental aid posts. It had been recorded that "in cases of profound shock accompanied by loss of blood, excellent results are obtained from direct blood transfusion." Robertson had cast doubt on the efficacy of various fluids used as "substitutes" for blood in World War I (gum acacia, gelatin) and called attention to the fact that their beneficial effects were often slight. "The only means available of increasing the oxygen-carrying power of the blood is the addition of new red blood cells" he had said. "This constitutes the unique value of blood transfusion." Whole blood transfusion also had become universally employed in surgery in civil life.

It is of real interest, therefore, to inquire into the process of reasoning that led the Committee on Transfusions of the N.R.C. to take the position that "most instances of shock are associated with hemoconcentration and a given quantity of plasma is more effective than an equal quantity of whole blood in treatment." This concept can be traced back to observations on the wounded made in World War I by Cannon, Fraser, and Hooper who reported that counts of red cells in blood taken from the capillary bed were high, particularly when compared with those of venous blood. This also was a keynote in the establishment of shock as an entity distinct from hemorrhage and led to the widely accepted hypothesis of a generalized increase in capillary permeability. "Hemoconcentration was found to furnish a practical means for differentiating shock from hemorrhage, but the enormous potential value of this sign was not comprehended by the members of the Special Committee on Wound Shock nor has it been sensed by physicians during the 20 years since that time," wrote Moon in 1938. The manual on shock (1943), prepared under the auspices of the Committee on Surgery of the Division of Medical Sciences of the N.R.C., also set forth this erroneous concept.

The advantage of the use of whole blood in the treatment of shock is that it contains red cells, which is of great importance when severe anemia is present. This advantage, however, is more than balanced by many disadvantages, three of which are: (1) An interval of time is necessary to make whole blood available for transfusion, unless universal donor's blood is employed. (2) Preservation can be for a relatively short period and transportation is difficult because of the need of bulky and heavy apparatus for proper refrigeration. (3) The addition of red cells to the blood stream is often undesirable, especially when large quantities of blood are necessary (1,000 cc. or more) or when hemoconcentration already exists. Even if hemoconcentration is initially not severe, addition of 2,000 or 3,000 cc. of whole blood would not be tolerated in the majority of cases, unless loss of blood had been severe.

The first and second objections are technical, and would be particularly operative in emergencies on the field. The third is one that is of especial importance in cases of late, severe shock and in the presence of burns.

The statement of the Committee on Transfusions, namely, that "blood plasma is approximately as effective in the treatment of hemorrhage as is whole blood," appears to have found origin in conclusions drawn from laboratory experiments that were purposely designed so that the number of variables could be rigidly limited. Transference of these conclusions to a situation that introduced a number of additional variables was an error of human reasoning. An example may be found in the widely-quoted experiments of Rous and Wilson (1918). These authors made a precise determination of the limits within which plasma may replace the loss of whole blood in acute hemorrhage induced in rabbits. In summarizing the results of their experiments these authors stated that "however desirable transfusion may be, it is not essential to recovery from even the severest *acute* hemorrhage, if only the blood bulk can be restored in other ways." The conclusion drawn from this and subsequent observations by others led to formulation of the statement by the Committee on Transfusions. The brief description of a rabbit in which up to three-fourths of the blood volume, as measured by the hemoglobin depletion, had been withdrawn and replaced by plasma contains one phrase that is significant: "The least exertion would cause the animal to pant heavily."

Presumably the rabbit had no semblance of a wound other than the needle puncture. Substitute for the rabbit housed quietly in its cage a wounded soldier picked up by litter bearers and transported by ambulance, who has an extensive and painful wound with continuing extravasation of blood and plasma into adjacent tissues. Then add sedation, roentgenographic examination, anesthesia, and surgical operation with a further loss of blood. It is obvious that the introduction of these and other variables, purposely and of necessity excluded from the original experiments, may completely negate the conclusion. Both errors, the association of wound shock with hemoconcentration and the estimation regarding the effectiveness of blood plasma, are undesirable in view of the paucity of observations made in World War I concerning the disturbed physiology of wounded men.

Restoration of the blood bulk in the intravascular space by infusion of a colloid solution that might be expected to stay within the confines of the semipermeable membrane of the capillary walls was envisioned during World War I. This was a projection of the Starling concept elaborated by Scott in 1916. Tests were made of the properties of soluble starch, dextrin, gelatin, and gum arabic, and preparations of the latter were given extensive field tests, particularly by the British, guided by the basic experiments of Bayliss.

An editorial in the *Journal of the American Medical Association* (January 7, 1933), entitled "Shock," repeated the World War I theme of traumatic toxemia[2]:

> Until recently, traumatic or surgical shock was the basis for numerous theories. . . . The mechanism of traumatic toxemia, reported by the Special Research Committee and further elaborated by Cannon and others explains all the characteristic features

(continued)

> of shock. . . . Injurious products of tissue autolysis, arising in areas of extensive trauma, are absorbed into the circulation. These products affect the circulation in a manner similar to histamine, causing injury to the capillary walls resulting in increased permeability and dilatation. Extensive capillary dilatation results in the withdrawal of blood from currency as effectively as if by external hemorrhage. The individual is bled to death into his own capillaries.

Reference was made to Blalock's work and an extensive bibliography was provided. The advent of human plasma, as a result of the development of methods that enabled it to be preserved and packaged in desiccated form, appeared to provide a final answer to the problem of the restoration of blood bulk by infusion. The treatment of shock and hemorrhage was thus reduced to the simple terms of the exchange of fluid between the intravascular space and the interstitial space under clearly defined physicochemical laws. Extension of this same reasoning led to the proposal that because the serum albumin fraction of the blood as prepared by Cohn packaged a high proportion of the total colloid osmotic activity of the serum in small liquid volume, it was peculiarly appropriate to military needs. It was postulated that the interstitial fluid compartment would provide the necessary diluent unless the patient were badly dehydrated.

This oversimplified physicochemical approach, which was an extension of the World War I quest of Bayliss aided by the availability of refined and human-derived preparations, not only failed to take into account the variables described, but also placed undue emphasis on a single physicochemical property of the blood; namely, the osmotic activity of the plasma proteins. Not only was the important function of the red cells as oxygen carriers ignored, but also their contribution to the total blood mass under abnormal circumstances. Both the magnitude of the initial loss of whole blood occasioned by wounding and the significance of a continuing seepage of blood and its fluid components into the tissue spaces were underestimated. And, finally, an effort to restore and maintain blood bulk based on colloid preparations, either derived from human proteins or otherwise, presupposes a space bounded by a semipermeable membrane—not one in which large areas of the membranes may have been rendered freely permeable by the direct effects of trauma.

Perrin Long and I. S. Ravdin, in *Reports from Pearl Harbor*, described an experience that should have been a warning to those who were making the decisions.

> During the period prior to operation, an attempt was made to treat all cases of apparent shock by means of warmth, the administration of morphine and liquid

plasma, large supplies of which were obtained from the Civilian Plasma Bank in Honolulu. Despite all attempts to combat shock, some of the patients had to be operated upon at a time when they were still in a state of severe shock.

While I had been in Washington, D.C., awaiting my orders for North Africa, I had visited the Walter Reed Hematology Laboratory and the Army Medical Center and talked with the staff. My notes on the subject of transfusion, dated January 26, 1943, follow:

E.D.C. Comment: Conversation with Lt. Col. Douglas B. Kendrick of the Army Medical School. . . . Plans to have plasma available as far forward as Battalion collection station. Supplies are in prospect which will permit liberal use. Use too much rather than too little. Information desired on average number of units used *per man.* Now packaged in 250 unit containers. Plan under consideration to increase this to 500 units with belief that if casualty needs plasma at all he will need 500 units. Discussed probable need for setting up blood banks in large hospitals. Kendrick would like to know if this need becomes apparent so proper supplies can be sent.

Hospitals are provided only with Erlenmeyer flasks. Should be equipped for closed system collection. Maximum storage time for whole blood in refrigerator is 7 days. Fresh whole blood may be kept 48 hours at 70°-80°. Preserved blood (added dextrose, citric acid, citrate) may be stored in refrigerator for 30 days. For whole blood transfusions use military personnel as donors. The Hinton test for syphilis advisable except in urgent situations. Do not depend on dog tag typing for transfusions but always cross match. A 10% - 25% error in typing recorded on tag may be anticipated. Due to use of inactive rabbit serum and inexperienced laboratory technicians. Can administer 3,000 cc. plasma in 24 hours without fear of citrate toxicity. This contains 300 cc. of 4% citrate. Speed of administration as well as total dosage determine toxicity of citrate. Causes depression of the vasocenter and asphyxial death. *Filters* are essential. Rh factor antigen in repeated whole blood transfusion of no military significance. Cautions on use of albumin in presence of concealed hemorrhage from large vessels. Possibly speed at which normal blood volume and pressure are restored before adequate clotting takes place is danger factor.

There is another note in my diary jotted down while I was in Washington, dated February 9, 1943. The episode shows some of the activity behind the campaign to get the public to donate blood—blood that would be processed into plasma.

> *E.D.C. Comment:* A new bleeding center was established yesterday in the Pentagon Building. Publicity was arranged for by having Patterson, the Undersecretary of War, and the Surgeon General (McGee) be the first to donate their blood. Unfortunately the Surgeon General showed up with a large breakfast aboard containing eggs and other things he shouldn't have eaten.
>
> Dr. Canby Robinson (then in charge of the Red Cross Blood Procurement Program) had been greatly distressed about bleeding him because he was a month or so beyond the age which had been set as the maximum limit. Judge Patterson was the center of the show. At the last moment someone had the bright idea of photographing the Surgeon General in the act of bleeding Patterson. Strenuous objections were raised by the Undersecretary about having the Surgeon General put a needle in his vein. Somebody else did it.

Blood procurement centers were established in sizable cities throughout the nation. By January, 1944, there were thirty-five of them. The success of the program was achieved by press and radio publicity featuring the almost incredible effects of plasma in wounded soldiers. A central agency was set up for the dissemination of material designed to spur the enthusiasm of prospective blood donors. By December, 1943, 5,652,351 bleedings had been recorded. Of these, 5,472,797 had been processed into dried plasma and serum albumin, the remainder into liquid plasma.

On February 15, 1943, at the Army Medical Center, Reichal, Elliot and other workers in the Hematology Laboratory, all plasma experts, vigorously urged provision for whole blood transfusions. "Walter Reed Hospital uses as much whole blood as plasma or more," I noted in my diary. "No provisions for whole blood transfusions overseas except by the old citrate method. Storage requires drawing with closed systems. The need for whole blood transfusions should be checked immediately in terms of life and loss of effective days."

The group of officers in the Army Hematology Laboratory knew what was going on and knew from the clinical experience in Walter Reed Hospital that whole blood was essential, but their opinion was not accepted. I returned to the Surgeon General's office and said to B. Noland Carter, who was with Rankin in the Consultant's Division: "Nick, we're totally unprepared to give transfusions overseas, aren't we?"

He replied: "Yes, but you must not say anything about it outside of this office. We know that we're behind but we can do nothing about it. We meet a stone wall everywhere we go."

At that time, Norman Kirk, soon to become Surgeon General of the Army, was chief surgeon at Walter Reed. Norman Kirk was a straightforward, experienced surgeon—I have a lasting respect for his integrity. Kirk told me after the war that he assumed all responsibility for not having whole blood ready for World War II; but no one individual can assume that responsibility. Civilians were busy helping with the war effort and many had their prestige at stake in the publicity launched to provide plasma for the wounded. The Red Cross as well as the N.R.C. was behind it. Edwin Cohn was working to improve plasma and was trying to get an albumin solution into production particularly for the Navy. A huge vested interest had been built up starting from assumptions and erroneous thinking.

NORTH AFRICA BREAKS THE BOTTLENECK

A study by Lieutenant Colonel Wilson, later Professor of Surgery at Aberdeen, came to me through British channels. He had set up a laboratory in a casualty clearing station where he reviewed the condition of the wounded from the battle of El Alamein. Wilson set forth the need for a strict wartime definition of the term "shock."

Wilson's study had been focused on a selected point in the stream of evacuation—a C.C.S.—so I undertook a study from patient's records, aided by personal observations. This I sent to the Surgeon General and gave as a conclusion that the "problem of shock," as observed in the Tunisian campaign, centered in the application of accepted means of treatment rather than in the need for additional methods of management. From the perspective of Tunisia, it appeared that everyone in the United States was going haywire with the belief that some mysterious entity caused shock.

I was not popular when I said that *wound shock is blood volume loss. It is identical with hemorrhage.* The wounded require replacement of the blood loss. We were soon able to say that there was no hemoconcentration. There was *hemodilution* unless peritonitis or infection was present. We brushed away the cobwebs from "shock" so that we could get proper means of treatment.

The reports I wrote when I returned from the early consulting trips included a plea to get a Baxter Laboratory for the theater so that we could obtain closed system transfusion equipment and blood refrigeration.

The Theater Surgeon, General Frederick Blesse, was placed in a difficult situation. I was a new consultant whom he had never seen before and who said: "We must have blood." The Surgeon General had said that we must fight the war on plasma. It was too late to obtain equipment to set up a distribution system in Tunisia. That battle was going to be over very shortly.

My report was politely received. Soon the Deputy Surgeon, Colonel Earle Standlee, said that he and Perrin Long were going to northern Tunisia and they would look over what the British were doing because they were using whole blood transfusion. El Alamein was the first battle in which blood was in supply, but the British in the field were not receiving support from their War Office. There was a report on blood transfusion arrangements during El Alamein, dated February 26, 1943, which had been issued by No. 1 Base Transfusion Unit in Cairo. The heavy engagement of the infantry greatly increased the need for blood transfusion. It seemed likely that the need would always occur when a strongly defended line was attacked. For the period of October 1 to November 1, 1942, 3,225 bottles of blood, 300,267 bottles of plasma or serum, and 3,527 bottles of saline had been issued to the Eighth Army. The number of wounded in the Eighth Army from October 4 to November 28 was 17,572. If it is assumed that medical units carried an equal supply both before and after the battle, it appears that for each 100 casualties, 18 bottles of blood, 19 bottles of serum or plasma, and 20 bottles of saline were used.

These figures showed that the needs of battle casualties in the field differed from the experience in air raids, which was the only previous large scale effort to supply blood. Resuscitation of battle casualties often was delayed from eight to 48 hours, whereas air raid casualties could be cared for more rapidly. Also, battle casualties required transportation up to 100 miles before resuscitation. It seemed likely that the first group suffered more hemorrhage than the second because, in many cases, first aid could not be applied during a battle.

The British had a good system of blood distribution but it was an improvised one. They were very short of supplies and had no closed system for drawing blood. A closed system requires a vacuum bottle, sealed and connected by tubing to the donor's vein. The blood flows in by vacuum and is never exposed to the air. When I visited the British base transfusion unit in Cairo that had supplied blood to the battle of El Alamein, Major Buttle, who was running this unit, told me that he had to send his men out into the streets of Cairo to pick up old beer bottles. These were washed and sterilized and used to ship blood to the front line. (See Chapter 21, To Cairo.) On a visit to this transfusion unit after the Sicilian campaign, I saw Egyptian civilians sitting on the floor, placing bottles of blood into containers and packing straw around them. It seemed unbelievably primitive and yet, in the opinion of the doctors who needed this blood, Buttle's accomplishments warranted the Victoria Cross. To supply an army with a large quantity of blood in such a manner invited difficulties with putrefaction and infection.

Major Buttle was aware of the limitations of the use of blood that were imposed by the conditions under which it was drawn and stored. He pointed out that they were not able to use the massive transfusions that were used later in Italy by the U.S. Army with the closed system of bleeding and better refrigeration in storage and shipping.

The British experience confirmed my thoughts on the need for transfusion. There was the pertinent definition of wound shock phrased by Wilson, which coincided with my thinking. But I could get no action. I had been asked by the Theater Surgeon not to send personal communications back to Washington. Every communication had to go through "channels." My only recourse was to talk to a *New York Times* reporter and say: "You must break the story that plasma is not adequate for the treatment of wounded soldiers." He did. *The New York Times* (August 26, 1943)[3] quoted me as saying that whole blood was urgently needed and that plasma was inadequate.

PLASMA ALONE NOT SUFFICIENT

Col. Edward D. Churchill of Boston, Professor of Surgery at Harvard, and now consulting surgeon for troops here, has pioneered in setting up blood banks similar to the Red Cross blood deposits in the United States.

In a report to the surgeon's office Colonel Churchill declared:

"There is need for whole blood transfusions in the treatment of a significant proportion of wounded. Plasma is not an adequate substitute in these cases."

The outgrowth of Colonel Churchill's report was the setting up of a far-flung system of blood banks in the rear echelons of medical support. The blood bank method—result of an extensive survey among units that were in combat in North Africa—will be another rung in the ladder of curative medical science.

Approval of the blood-storage program was announced by the Surgeon's Office of the North African Theater of Operations after four months of research and questioning of medical officers in the combat areas.

As "live blood" transfusions are difficult to safeguard in front-line medical service, adequate blood banks are being set up in evacuation and general hospital areas, some of which are as close as three or four miles to the combat zone.

Functioning much the same as the Red Cross collection agencies' blood bank teams in the United States, the Army's evacuation and general hospitals will collect in bottles live blood from volunteer donors. Donors, the Surgeon's Office reported, will come from noncombatant troops, convalescent and mildly wounded patients and soldiers from medical detachments.

---

[3]Excerpt from "Plasma Alone is Not Sufficient", published by *The New York Times*, August 26, 1943.

The initial breakthrough thus came with upsetting the balance of power in Washington through *The New York Times* and making people in the States begin to think reasonably about the need to transfuse the wounded and realize that World War II could not be fought on plasma, "dried blood" or salt solution.

My report began to break the bottleneck in North Africa. Soon we were able to get refrigerators for the mobile hospitals. For a long time they had to draw their own blood, but they could draw it in advance of a pressing need. They took a chance on transmitting malaria and syphilis. It was a makeshift arrangement but at least blood could be stored in a refrigerator until needed. But our theater still did not have a distribution system to take blood forward from the rear areas.

AFTER NORTH AFRICA

Later, in Sicily, erroneous beliefs continued to haunt us. A II Corps Circular Letter, No. 3, dated August 7, 1943, still made a distinction between shock and hemorrhage. The former was treated by plasma, the latter by blood transfusion.

I urged the setting up of a central laboratory for collection and distribution, but there again ran into difficulty. The Theater Surgeon went to Sicily and talked to some of his friends who were in command of hospitals. "We're getting along all right. We don't need much blood. Plasma is wonderful." The idea of a *substitute* for blood still haunted all efforts. Then the Fifth Army landed at Salerno and Howard E. Snyder became its Surgical Consultant. Snyder persuaded Joseph Martin, the Surgeon of the Fifth Army, to interest himself in the problem.

Snyder saw the problem clearly. At an AMA symposium in 1946, he said the following:

> The laboratory findings and the clinical observations allow the following conclusions to be drawn:
>
> One. Lowered blood volume in the shock of battle casualties is due entirely to loss of whole blood and not to plasma loss except in those cases in which there is gross peritoneal or pleural contamination, beginning sepsis, gas gangrene, a burn or a crush injury.
>
> Two. When whole blood has been lost, whole blood is the replacement medium of choice, particularly when the loss has been large . . .
>
> Blood replacement therapy must be integrated in a program dealing with all etiological factors in shock. Surgery is an essential part of this program. Frequently it must be performed before the individual is completely resuscitated from shock, and as a part of the resuscitative program.

The second breakthrough came with the tactical situation of Anzio. We already had fairly adequate supplies in the stationary position of the Fifth

Army behind the winter line south of Cassino, but it was difficult to get enough blood even there.

At Anzio, Martin and Snyder further forced the hand of the Theater Surgeon by saying that if the base was not to supply blood, Army would not permit the use of service troops as donors. Therefore, theater must ship blood to the beachhead. This ultimatum made it necessary to set up a blood bank center in Naples, which then supplied the theater for the remainder of the war.

Then when the Fifth Army jumped into Anzio with the only supply line via LSTs, the Army Surgeon said: "In this tactical situation we must have blood shipped in large quantities to the beachhead. If you don't give it to us, we'll get it from the British." The British couldn't supply us. They also were vociferous in their demands for blood.

Major Eugene R. Sullivan, laboratory Officer in the 6th General Hospital, who had made a survey of the needs for blood in the hospitals in North Africa, was then placed on temporary duty with the 15th General Medical Laboratory in Naples. Sullivan sparked the organization of a blood bank which was put into operation in Naples to supply the Fifth Army. This was in operation shortly after the Anzio beachhead was established. This bank later had branches in southern France because the Mediterranean Theater never received blood from the United States.

SUMMARY

In view of the present liberal use of whole blood, it is amazing to recall that World War II was started with the concept that plasma for the intravascular space and sodium chloride solution for the interstitial space were therapeutic measures adequate to reestablish equilibrium in a wounded man. Experience in North Africa immediately demonstrated the inadequacy of this program and showed the necessity for whole blood. As soon as equipment could be obtained, a blood bank, organized by the theater, with service troops as donors, supplied the full needs of the Mediterranean forces to the end of the war.

The loss of whole blood following wounding far surpassed that estimated at the beginning of the war, and the degree of shock closely paralleled the amount of blood lost. The obvious explanation of why whole blood is needed rather than plasma is that replenishment of red cells maintains the required oxygen-carrying capacity. Future investigation will test the validity of certain less obvious explanations. Red cells form an appreciable portion of the *mass* of blood and a portion that cannot be lost into an area of injured tissues without actual disruption of vessel walls. The physical action of cells as a "filler" for the intravascular space may be significant, because it is not clear how long plasma remains in circulation.

Again, there is the problem of the electrolytes. Potassium appears in considerable concentration in the urine following hemorrhage. From what cells it is lost and by what mechanism is not clear. The specific effects of the departure of the potassium ion from cells on recovery from shock or recovery from other effects of the wound remain to be explored. Suffice it to say that potassium and also phosphorus are virtually lacking in plasma but present in large quantity in red cells.

Other considerations have led the attention of the surgeon beyond the capillary wall, across the interstitial compartment to the cell. The term *irreversible* was borrowed from elementary chemistry. The issue is kept clear only if its use is restricted to the effects of shock and not extended to the condition of shock itself. Shock, defined as reduced blood volume flow, is reversed by replacement of blood volume. Selective death of organs or tissues brought about in whole or in part by shock is not reversible. It is probable that each tissue and organ has a different threshold at which it succumbs to asphyxia. Functional impairment or complete suppression of function may appear in certain organs, for example the kidneys, and delayed death of the entire body ensues, despite the fact that other organs have been "resuscitated" and the direct effects of the missile that caused the wound have been repaired. In this sense, the effects of the wounding as reflected on the kidney in many cases have been irreversible—at least with our presently available modes of treatment.

In World War II, replacement of lost blood reached an extraordinarily high level of effectiveness. It is certain that hundreds of injured men survived the immediate effects of wounds that under slightly less favorable circumstances would have proved fatal. Irreversible shock as such was not encountered. An appreciable number of the wounded survived, however, only to die about the tenth day with complete anuria. A chain is as strong as its weakest link. When links are strengthened where the chain has broken previously, new weak spots appear simply because the chain holds to test them. The obvious weak link in the severely wounded in this war was the kidney.

PERTINENT COMMENTARIES

Extract

So the stream of military medicine that will naturally flow into civilian practice, steadily grows. Unusual interest stems from the remarkable progress in studies of the blood and blood processing for transfusion in the Armed Forces. Basic studies (Army) have been directed to the genetics of the erythrocytes and iron metabolism. The life span of the platelets has been fixed to 2.2 days. Under Army contract, workers at Michael Reese Hospital (Chicago) have conducted an experiment of unusual promise. The removal of the stroma of the erythrocytes abolishes their antigenic properties. As a hemoglobin concentrate, such a preparation affords a ready transport and exchange for oxygen without disturbance of the oncotic pressure of the plasma. Fort Knox studies have established a prolongation of the erythrocyte survival period from 21 to 42 days upon the addition of adenine. The Naval Blood Research Laboratory, Chelsea, has continued its program of frozen blood. In Vietnam, a wounded Marine, who received 93 units of blood, 41 of them frozen, survived without adverse reactions. The frozen blood is still held as a reserve for the normal supply of acid citrate dextrose blood. One of the most impressive medical lessons of the current hostilities is the advantage of the prompt delivery of skilled attention to the wounded combatants. Early evacuation by helicopter facilitates the prompt correction of shock. The Military Blood Program Agency (July, 1962) coordinates the plans, policies and procedures of this effort in the Army, Navy and Air Force under the Surgeon General of the Army. In a national emergency, this Agency would assume immediate responsibility for the procurement, processing and distribution of blood for civilian as well as military requirements. Another healthy sign of the times is the close coordination of far-flung laboratories over the world with the parent laboratories in the United States. For example, the interchange between a field laboratory at Da Nang, Vietnam, and the key laboratories at Bethesda and Chelsea is paying large dividends. Schooled in the shock units of World War II, the sophistication of the present day treatment of traumatic shock in the forward areas, with continuous or repetitive checks on many physiological parameters, is a miracle of modern medicine.[4]

Operational Lessons Learned

The Supply of Blood in Forward Areas

A blood producing and distributing unit has been demonstrated as an essential part of the field medical service. Such a unit was organized provisionally in the theater, and functioned until the conclusion of the campaign. In addition to the

(continued)

---

[4]Reproduced by permission of Oxford University Press. From Middleton WS. Military medicine: its role in world health. *Mil Med*. 1968;133(4):257-264

base blood bank, a bank capable of drawing and processing 150 pints of blood daily was established in the forward area by the Army medical laboratory. Blood was transported by C-47 aircraft from base to army, and by truck, or on occasion L-5 aircraft, to field and evacuation hospitals. Blood used during the campaign averaged 2.5 units (1,250 cc.) per patient transfused and 0.7 units (350 cc.) per battle casualty admitted to hospital.[5]

*   *   *

Abstract

More liberal use of a plasma expander in the treatment of operative traumatic blood loss, with transfusions given only when the hematocrit was less than 30 per cent, reduced the amount of blood distributed by our blood bank. Blood consumed per patient admission dropped 35 per cent, and blood used by the surgical service decreased 320 ml per patient operated on; relative use of single unit transfusions decreased 47 per cent and relative use of plasma fell 50 per cent. Calculated amounts of blood saved in the past year was 3,863 units, and transfusion reactions avoided were 81.

A plasma expander can be employed in properly limited amounts in patients suffering acute blood loss without detriment to the patient's clinical state and with a diminished need for whole blood.[6]

[5]Martin, J. I., Brig. General, Fifth Army Surgeon, U.S.A.: "Medical Experience in the Italian Campaign," July 1, 1945.
[6]From Rush BF Jr, Stewart RA. More liberal use of a plasma expander. Impact on a hospital blood bank. *N Engl J Med.* 1969;280(22):1202-1205. Copyright © 1969 Massachusetts Medical Society. Reprinted with permission from Massachusetts Medical Society.

Christopher D. Barrett, Andrew Neil Beckett, and John B. Holcomb

Much like John Hunter's treatise on blood in the Seven Years' War, if there were no timestamp or reference to World War II, one may walk away from reading this chapter thinking Churchill is a visionary articulating best practice in 21st-century trauma surgery and combat casualty care. With trials over the last several decades evaluating starch-based colloids (the CHEST trial) and plasma-first resuscitation (the COMBAT and PAMPer trials), we have truly come full circle having now validated insights from World War I and before, including the benefits of whole blood over saline. Other old concepts we have recently "rediscovered" include "traumatic toxemia" from tissue destruction that foretold the discovery of danger signaling responses and damage-associated molecular patterns (DAMPs) in trauma by Drs. Carl Hauser, Polly Matzinger, and others; transfusion-associated circulatory overload (TACO) when giving red cell–containing products to nonhemorrhagic ("late") shock; and the danger of nonblood products as a primary resuscitative fluid in trauma that was relearned in Vietnam through sequelae like "Da Nang lung" (i.e., acute respiratory distress syndrome, ARDS) as described by Lewin and colleagues in 1971. Even damage control resuscitation was conceptually known, as made clear through the advice of LTC Kendrick to Churchill that the "speed at which normal blood volume and pressure are restored before adequate clotting takes place is danger factor," an observation that was also apparent to Dr. Walter B. Cannon in World War I and Dr. Churchill's longtime anesthesia colleague, Dr. Henry Beecher.

This chapter serves as an important critique of the erroneous logic underpinning the plasma-based resuscitation strategy used by the United States early in World War II. Although others came to recognize the benefits of whole blood resuscitation, for myriad unacceptable reasons, no effort was made to adjust our approach. One particularly prominent reason was to spare public embarrassment of prominent civilians who had participated in the public appeals to donate blood for dried plasma production for the war effort. After significant efforts to relay his concerns through the chain of command to no avail, Dr. Churchill bypassed the North African Theater Surgeon by contacting a reporter at the *New York Times* to disseminate his message that "World War II could not be fought on plasma, 'dried blood,' or salt solution" to both Washington, DC and the American public. This desperate approach ultimately proved effective, leading directly to the Surgeon

General approving whole blood banking in the North African theater with provision of refrigeration systems to the mobile hospitals. This transition unquestionably saved the lives of thousands of warfighters. This also led, strangely, to a reminder about the importance of a fundamental tenet of the modern democracies that have proliferated following World War II—freedom of the press, without which World War II may have continued to be "fought on plasma" and countless more lives would have been lost.

In the end, this essential chapter embodies a requisite trait of combat surgical leaders: candor. Doing the right thing at the right time, even if it makes one unpopular, was clearly Dr. Churchill's guiding ethos. Objectivity in the pursuit and acquisition of medical and scientific knowledge is similarly critical. Too much focus on conclusions that support a particular notion or bias without appropriate focus on the methods and results creates a dangerous echo chamber. While this chapter and its prescriptions were written on the topic of shock and blood transfusion, the underlying messages contain universal truths with broad applicability to modern military and civilian surgeons alike.

SUGGESTED READINGS

Holcomb JB, Jenkins D, Rhee P, et al. Damage control resuscitation: directly addressing the early coagulopathy of trauma. *J Trauma*. 2007 Feb;62(2):307-310.

Hunter J, Home E. *A Treatise on the Blood, Inflammation, and Gun-Shot Wounds*. Thomas Bradford, Printer, *Book-Seller & Stationer*; 1796.

Lewin I, Weil MH, Shubin H, Sherwin R. Pulmonary failure associated with clinical shock states. *J Trauma*. 1971 Jan;11(1):22-35.

Matzinger P. The danger model: a renewed sense of self. *Science*. 2002 Apr 12;296(5566):301-305.

Stansbury LG, Hess JR. Blood transfusion in world war I: the roles of Lawrence Bruce Robertson and Oswald Hope Robertson in the "most important medical advance of the war". *Transfus Med Rev*. 2009 Jul;23(3):232-236.

5

The New Sulfa Drug Era of Surgery

DURING MY FIRST trips in the theater, talks and personal associations with American surgeons who had participated in the care of the wounded since the landing in North Africa helped me identify many problems. Of these men, the one who was the most helpful was Colonel Frank Berry, whom I referred to briefly in the last chapter. He was, at that time, Chief of Surgery at the 9th Evacuation Hospital, which was then situated at Youks les Bains, supporting the southern Tunisia front. Among the problems that were identified, perhaps the most urgent one was that of resuscitation for the seriously wounded soldier.

The second major problem that caught my eye was wound infection and suppuration. It was obvious that many of the débridements were inadequate. Fortunately, gas gangrene was relatively rare and the inadequate débridements were being corrected by a second operation at a closely supporting hospital. The 48th Surgical Hospital was operating at the apex of the American medical support and was doing incomplete wound excisions. As a result, the two large Evacuation Hospitals, the 9th and the 77th, were x-raying and reoperating on a considerable number of their patients, particularly to remove some metallic foreign body with the dead and devitalized tissue which surrounded it.

I was distressed also by the careless techniques used in the protection of wounds after the initial débridement had been accomplished and I saw the inevitability of superimposed contamination. As an ambulance unloaded wounded men, the admitting Officers in the hospitals would peek under the dressing by raising it with their fingers in order to see the condition of the wound. In my first circular letter dealing with wounds, I called attention to this custom and pointed out that carelessness in the technique of dressings would make it impossible to develop a program of secondary wound closure in the rear echelon. Wound infection and suppuration emerged as one of the major considerations as it has been in every war since the dawn of history.

Just before the outbreak of World War II, a group of compounds that were selective in their actions on bacteria became available. These were the sulfonamides. There were several of these "sulfa drugs," closely allied in their chemical structure—sulfanilamide, sulfathiazole and sulfadiazine were the most widely used. These compounds were not bacteriocidal but were *bacteriostatic.*

The therapeutic values of sulfanilamide were confirmed in the United States largely by the efforts of Perrin H. Long, E. A. Bliss and E. K. Marshall. And the experiences and reports of surgeons at Dunkirk and Pearl Harbor led to the conclusion that sulfa was a "cure-all" for wounds. In fact, it took the experience of North Africa to convince many surgeons that adequate excision of the wound was of equal or greater importance.

DUNKIRK, 1940

Major J. S. Jeffrey, R.A.M.C., writing of the British Expeditionary Force's (B.E.F.) experiences through the withdrawal at Dunkirk, observed that there would be little doubt that the sulfonamides had proven to be invaluable. The surgeons of the B.E.F., he wrote, were particularly intrigued by the local application of sulfonamide. Reference was made to the success obtained by Jenson in the treatment of compound fractures with sulfonamide powder; also, to the experimental work of Legroux at the Paris Pasteur Institute. This work had been interpreted as showing that oral administration could not produce a concentration of the drug in the blood sufficiently high to combat the local infection, whereas the sulfonamide powder allowed a direct attack on the organism (hemolytic streptococci).

The great majority of the wounds we had to deal with, "wrote Jeffrey," *were septic, and culture showed a mixed growth of staphylococci, streptococci, B. coli and anaerobic organisms. If there was an entrance and an exit wound our practice was simply to open up the track by cutting through the tissue between the two openings, performing a toilet on the wound—that is cleaning out any loose tissue or foreign body, and gently scrubbing it clean—and then packing the wound with sulfonamide powder . . . or to enlarge each end of the track and insert sulfonamide powder and a rubber drainage tube. Compound fractures were confidently encased in plaster if the toilet of the wound had been satisfactory, and especially when local sulfonamide had been used.*

PEARL HARBOR, 1941

Fortunately, in the spring and summer, surgical teams had been organized by the Honolulu County Medical Society and were prepared to provide emergency care to the injured. On December 7, 1941, the station hospital at Hickam Field was immediately overwhelmed with casualties and many improvisations were made. The station hospital functioned as a divisional clearing station and evacuated by ambulances and trucks to the Tripler General Hospital. Wounds had been caused by high-explosive (H.E.) fragments, machine gun bullets and secondary missiles.

Many patients (especially in those instances when an operation had to be postponed) had ample amounts of crystalline sulfanilamide packed in their wounds as a prophylaxis against infection at the time their injuries were inspected in the receiving wards.

Sulfanilamide was placed in pleural and abdominal cavities, amputation stumps and other wounds. Sulfathiazole was given by mouth usually in 4.0 gm. per day dosage. Soft tissue injuries came to débridement twenty-four or more hours after injury. It was noted and commented upon by the surgeons that the wounds were in good condition, that there were no signs of infection. Following débridement, the wounds were sprinkled with crystalline sulfanilamide and in most instances were left open.

Through joint action of the Committee on Medical Research and the N.R.C. and Surgeon General James C. Magee, Professors I. S. Ravdin, of the University of Pennsylvania, and Perrin Long, of Johns Hopkins, were flown to Hawaii for the period December 17-22, 1941. The primary purpose of the trip was to obtain information concerning the treatment of Pearl Harbor casualties.

> *We have been impressed again and again,* they stated, *with the incalculable value of sulfonamide therapy. We believe that it is highly important that physicians—both civilian and military—become familiar with the general and specific considerations which govern the oral and local use of the sulfonamides in the treatment of wounds and burns.*
>
> *Finally, there can be little doubt that the local and oral use of the sulfonamide drugs contributed markedly to the splendid condition of the wounds and the absence of infection in these patients, which has been noted and remarked upon by all who have seen them....in every instance when wounds are dressed they should be sprinkled with crystalline sulfanilamide until final healing has taken place.*

Ravdin wrote a follow-up report to Surgeon General Magee, February 7, 1942, on the status of battle casualties arriving from Honolulu at Letterman General Hospital, San Francisco:

REPORT TO SURGEON GENERAL JAMES C. MAGEE
FROM PROFESSORS I. S. RAVDIN

February 7, 1942

There were no septic temperatures and no serious infections. The wounds were in nearly every instance clean. General Dewitt, Colonel Emerson and Lieutenant Colonel Bolibaugh voluntarily declared that they had never observed a group of men with such severe injuries who looked so well and who were doing so well . . . we are able to fully concur in the opinion of the medical officers. . .

(continued)

Compound Fractures. . . . In many instances the local wounds which were clean on admission were being treated with B.I.P.P. gauze or pads. The wounds remained clean but this compound interfered with subsequent x-ray examinations. It should not be assumed from this experience that had B.I.P.P. been used from the beginning the results in these patients would have been as satisfactory. There is in fact every reason to believe that such would not have been the case, for B.I.P.P. was used during the First World War and has found no general acceptance in the intervening years.

Some masses of sulfonamides were found in a few of the wounds when the casts were removed. It was supposed that these were masses of sulfanilamide but we are convinced that they consisted of sulfathiazole.

Amputations . . . the guillotine amputations had been revised and excellent plastic closure had been obtained. These patients had oral sulfathiazole before and after operation, and about one-half of them had sulfanilamide locally. To have obtained these results . . . within seven weeks of injury we believe is unequalled in previous military experience. Col. Emerson and Lieut. Col. Bolibaugh expressed the opinion that under the older, more traditional methods of care it would have been considered satisfactory had the stumps been closed within one year.

Soft Part Wounds . . . Many had been skin grafted. The grafts looked very healthy. This was possible in most instances without subsequent infection, excellent testimony of the value of sulfonamide therapy in preventing infection.

Despite this initial enthusiasm, more cautious voices were heard. In a review article on "Local Sulfonamide Therapy" prepared in 1941 for International Abstracts of Surgery, Champ Lyons concluded that "The enthusiastic clinical adoption of local sulfonamide therapy has failed to provide factual data for analysis of the extent to which such treatment has prevented the growth of bacteria in wounds." The review covered 111 references.

NORTH AFRICA, 1943

When I arrived in North Africa the oral and local use of sulfonamides was officially urged and enthusiastically pursued. Heneage Ogilvie (Sir William Heneage Ogilvie) had written from the Middle East:

"The sulfonamides have so modified the outlook in contaminated wounds in favor of tissue defenses, that the place of surgery as a primary treatment must be reconsidered. . . . the débridement of 1918 can be justified only by extreme necessity. If the sulfonamides can arrest the multiplication of bacteria sufficiently long for the defense mechanism of the body to establish an ascendency, something much simpler will be adequate." Such confidence in the sulfonamides gave rise to "wound trimming," a less radical elimination of dead tissue than was necessary in the muddy trenches of World War I.

A mimeographed "Memoranda on Surgery" written by John M. Weddell, British Consulting Surgeon, A.F.H.Q., made the same optimistic appraisal of battle casualties seen in January, 1943.

> *"Generally speaking the condition of wounded received from the Forward Area has been satisfactory. Sulfanilamide powder and surgical gauze dressings have been used extensively and the results appear to justify this method of treatment. In some cases unnecessarily large quantities of sulfanilamide powder have been used. It is sufficient to 'frost' the wound surface with the powder either with an insufflator or a pepper pot dredger. As a rule not more than 10 grammes of sulfanilamide (a level tablespoonful) should be used as a local application."*

Not all surgeons were this enthusiastic. The 77th Evacuation Hospital (University of Kansas) had entered Oran on December 11 and 12, 1942. The surgical staff under the leadership of Lieutenant Colonel James B. Weaver took over the treatment of American wounded who had been cared for by the French. Wounds had been excised widely with very liberal implantation of sulfanilamide and a tight gauze packing.

> *"Practically all wounds,"* Weaver stated in his report, *"were impregnated with sulfanilamide powder and, as nearly as could be learned, most wounded took sulfanilamide by mouth. However, for practical purposes practically all open wounds were infected. About 40% of these enough so as to require hot packs, drainage, etc. Not over 50% of the puncture type of wound caused by rifle bullets and an occasional piece of H.E. . . . were infected. In instances where these wounds were excised, sulfanilamide implanted, and gauze packs inserted, the reverse was true."*

In the first few days with no antiseptics available, sulfanilamide was dusted into the wounds at change of dressings. This had a definite harmful effect . . . On first dressing, cakes of undissolved sulfanilamide were frequently found in the wound, and obviously did not add to the comfort of the patient. One patient probably died from the toxemia of wound infection.

> *Secondary closures were done on 26 patients. Wounds looked clean at the time and sulfanilamide was dusted into the wounds. This was not successful. Many of these wounds broke down and several of these patients had high fever and pain necessitating removal of sutures and the institution of hot packs. From the foregoing it would seem that sulfanilamide is of little, if any, value in the treatment of wounds . . . But it must be pointed out that in most cases, treatment of these wounds had been delayed and improperly done.*

My own notes record a wounded soldier seen at the 77th Evacuation Hospital.

E.D.C. Comment: Sulfonamide was taken right after wounding—the contents of his little box. It was continued that night and subsequently. Powder was put on his wound by the aide and reapplied both at the aid station and at the collecting battalion. At the hospital he had fever and obvious infection. With wide drainage an H.E. fragment was removed and his course has been satisfactory.

With reference to these and other wounded seen in southern Tunisia I noted: "The timing factor (interval between wounding and operation) in soft tissue damage is still important despite sulfonamide."

A memorandum from Perrin Long, dated February 18, 1943, was accompanied by a proposed "Circular Letter No. 1." My copy is unsigned and carried no dateline. Whether it was distributed to the medical Officers of the theater, I do not know. However, I became responsible for Circular Letter No. 1 (March 18, 1943) properly signed by Colonel Earle Standlee, Deputy Surgeon. This carried a somewhat different emphasis particularly with respect to the local application. The effects of topically applied sulfonamides are not purely local, as absorption of the drug is often as rapid as if given by mouth.

EXCERPT FROM CIRCULAR
LETTER NO. 1

March 18, 1943

Because of rapid absorption, topical applications must be regarded in terms of total dosage. If the man is receiving systemic drug, the amount applied to a raw surface is correspondingly reduced.

Dead tissues and pus contain substances that inhibit the action of sulfonamides. Local application is not a substitute for adequate surgery. Even if the prophylactic value of local application be questioned, the fact must not be overlooked that it is a rapid method of establishing a blood concentration at a time when it may be difficult to assure regular peroral dosage under the exigencies of military action.

"Subsequent local sulfonamide therapy will depend on the dressing employed. In general, it will be found preferable to minimize the frequency of dressings and rely on systemic administration, than to take down dressings at frequent intervals in order to apply the drug locally. The disadvantages of a window in a plaster cast appear to outweigh any benefits that might be derived from repeated local application.

The following is a case history of a patient seen at the 12th General Hospital in Oran, Algeria, on April 20, 1943:

> On February 1 gasoline spilled on his trousers became ignited. This happened near Rabat and he was treated at his organizational dispensary with sulfa ointment. Sulfa powder was sprinkled on top of the ointment. This dressing was repeated daily for 3 days, then applied on every third day. At the end of the month he was sent to the Constantine area and was on a train for 6 days. More sulfa was put on during the trip. He then went to the medic in Ordnance where the same treatment was continued. At a replacement center near Tebessa sulfa treatment was continued.
>
> A rash had appeared on his hands, face and body early in February, in fact only about 4 days after he was burned. This itched and troubled him a great deal. The doctor told him it was because he was dirty.
>
> On March 17, at the 1st Armored Division Dispensary, a diagnosis was made of "Psoriasis, acute, moderately severe, generalized. Burn of left leg." Sulfadiazine ointment was applied and he was evacuated to the 77th Evacuation Hospital. He remained there 3 days and more sulfa ointment was applied to the burn.
>
> On March 20, he was received at the 38th Evacuation Hospital. The note read: "Irregular rash over body and legs, extensor surfaces and arms above elbows. Vesicular rash thenar prominence of hands. Does not flake like psoriasis. Diagnosis: Dermatitis medicamentosa from sulfa ointment." The drug was stopped and the rash cleared quite rapidly.
>
> He was evacuated to the 12th General Hospital. Here he had a flare-up of infection starting with lymphangitis starting in a crack of his skin. On April 7 he was given 20 mg. of sulfadiazine and three subsequent doses totalling 80 gm. The rash and itching reappeared. When the drug was stopped the rash faded and on April 20 it was gone.
>
> This man had taken no sulfa drug by mouth. To the best of his knowledge he never had taken chemotherapy previously and had never been treated for gonorrhea. His burn, which was a chemically irritated second degree lesion, is now almost healed.

"The sulfadiazine ointment that has been applied forward is not satisfactory," I recorded in my diary. "It drys and cakes, forming a shell that closes in infection. I saw two or three instances of difficulties with it, particularly when applied on the face. It also dries under bandaging."

And the following is an appraisal by a battalion surgeon, made on April 28, 1943: "As to sulfadiazine ointment—I could find nothing it was good for. I tried it on impetigo, open sores, athlete's foot and other things, but it didn't seem to work."

The foregoing account of the usage of the sulfonamides can best be summarized by a phrase from a "Preliminary Report to the War Office and the Medical Research Council on Investigations Concerning the Use of

Penicillin in War Wounds," under the dateline of October 13, 1943: "…after four years of war there are still no conclusive observations of the effect of sulphonamides on the prevention and treatment of wound sepsis."

The sulfa drug era of wound surgery was over.

Why was the sulfonamide era of relatively short duration? There were two major reasons: (1) Bacteria rapidly develop their own "immunity" to chemotherapeutic agents; (2) the discovery of penicillin and other antibiotics.

To these reasons must be added both the unfamiliarity of surgeons with the healing of gunshot wounds and the tendency to see what one is looking for. The compelling desire to put some medicament on a burn or into a wound is as old as surgery itself.

COMMITTEE REPORT

The seventeenth meeting of the Committee on Surgery was held on May 8 and 9, 1944, in Washington, D.C. The first order of business was Reports from Surgical Subcommittees. Dr. Allen O. Whipple reported, for the Subcommittee on Infected Wounds and Burns, that Drs. Hall and Meleney were completing their studies on the use of sulfonamides locally and systemically in contaminated and infected wounds. "The experience in the local use of the sulfonamides is being corroborated in a number of the Army units, as reported by the consulting surgeons, especially Churchill and Cutler . . . It is already becoming obvious that, as in the sulfonamides, penicillin is only an adjunct to sound surgery."

Tamara J. Worlton, Benjamin K. Potter, and Peter A. Learn

This treatise addresses the core principle of surgical wound therapy in war: adequate irrigation and debridement. Churchill noted poorly explored wounds, retained foreign bodies, inadequate removal of devitalized tissue, and even frank pus. Through this chapter we also see early evidence of attempts at performance improvement (PI) with information flowing bidirectionally between the front lines and the "Committee on Surgery" in Washington, DC. In fact, several times in the chapter, Churchill mentions "circular letters." These letters were distributed within a theater of operations to address specific treatments, general guidelines, and tallies of consumables like blood or antibiotics. Original circular letters from World War II can be seen at the National Library of Medicine and their contents are also recorded at the AMEDD Center of History & Heritage. Lessons now (re) learned can be found in their contents, such as one from August 7, 1943, where the instruction was "whole blood was to be used" in cases of hemorrhagic shock. Ultimately, just over 60 years later, the Joint Trauma System (JTS) was established to systematically coordinate combat casualty PI on a grand scale. Rapid feedback to far forward surgeons about missed injuries, avoidable complications, and eventual patient outcomes is critical for individual surgeons to achieve best practice but also for the system to quickly adjust.

Churchill noted that poor techniques in debridement followed by careless attention to aseptic practice led to delays in wound closure. Our experience with injuries from Iraq and Afghanistan along the entire spectrum of forward deployed to definitive care confirms the value of this imperative for urgent reexploration of all wounds at each new level of care. Indeed, the importance of adequate irrigation and debridement is a central tenet in the JTS clinical practice guideline (CPG) dedicated solely to this topic, updated as recently as 2021. In both the modern JTS CPG and this chapter, the subject of topical antibiotics as an adjunct to treatment of war wounds is covered.

The central topic of this chapter is the use of topical and oral sulfa compounds for the treatment of combat wounds. Although these were successfully implemented in both Dunkirk and Pearl Harbor, outcomes in North Africa proved disappointing. Potential explanations for this discrepancy include longer transport times to definitive surgical therapy and the rapid development of antibiotic resistance. Indeed, multidrug-resistant organisms (MDROs) plagued the most recent conflicts in Iraq and Afghanistan. Routine culturing to monitor for evidence of colonization and judicious use of antibiotics to counteract further development of resistance proved successful in decreasing rates of MDROs within wounds. However, new war wound pathogens also emerged including invasive fungal infections (IFIs), which became common in the Afghanistan theater in patients suffering dismounted complex blast injuries. In congruence with Churchill's observations, the definitive treatment for these infections is most frequently amputation.

The lesson of the inadequacy of antibiotics as a replacement for adequate wound irrigation and surgical debridement remains relevant today, even after the discovery of many new antibiotics thanks in no small part to the record-keeping and advocacy of Dr Churchill. Future generations of military surgeons would be wise to heed, or risk painfully relearning, that antibiotics are "only an adjunct to sound surgery."

SUGGESTED READINGS

Hutchings MI, Truman AW, Wilkinson B. Antibiotics: past, present and future. *Curr Opin Microbiol*. 2019;51:72-80.

Hospenthal DR, Crouch HK, English JF, et al. Multidrug-resistant bacterial colonization of combat-injured personnel at admission to medical centers after evacuation from Afghanistan and Iraq. *J Trauma*. 2011;71(1 suppl):S52-S57.

Joint Trauma System. War Wound and Debridement and Irrigation. Accessed August 2, 2023. https://jts.health.mil/assets/docs/cpgs/War_Wounds_Debridement_and_Irrigation_27_Sep_2021_ID31.pdf

Tribble DR, Ganesan A, Rodriguez CJ. Combat trauma-related invasive fungal wound infections. *Curr Fungal Infect Rep*. 2020;14(2):186-196.

North Africa

6

Arrival in Algiers

On March 10, 1943, Major Kenneth F. Lowry, of the 2nd Auxiliary Surgical Group, made the following entry in his diary, which goes into some of the history of North Africa. He was in southern Tunisia, vicinity of Tebessa, at the time.

March 10, 1943

Capt. Tom Ely of Jonesville, Virginia, is an authority on history and also a diligent student of Latin. Several nights ago after lights had gone out and we had all tucked in, with a bit of priming Tom gave us a thumbnail sketch of the history of North Africa. He began with the founding of Carthage on a bit of ground which Queen Dido, a Phoenician, purchased from the native Numidians about 878 B.C. We were then taken through the rise and fall of Carthagean empire which ended with the defeat of Hannibal and his army and the complete destruction of the city of Carthage by the Romans about 146 B.C. Then followed the growth and ultimate collapse of the vast Roman empire which included all the civilized world of that time.

After the fall of the empire around 300 A.D., the Arabs overran all of North Africa, going as far as Spain and into France where they were defeated at the Battle of Tours around 700 A.D. The Arabs continued their hold in Spain until the time of Ferdinand and Isabella who were able to drive them out. Spain then became an empire. About this time the Turks were growing in power, having brought about the fall of Constantinople in 1453. This brought to an end the Eastern Roman Empire. Following this the Arabians in North Africa sought protection and put themselves under control of the Turks. This marks the beginning of the Barbary States, each governing itself with its Bey or Sultan. A flourishing pirate trade was built up; the governments of which derived great profit from the trade but pretended to know nothing about its source. It was unsafe for any merchant ship to enter the Mediterranean.

(continued)

Finally the United States sent several ships to Tripoli in 1803. These included the Constitution, the Constellation and the Philadelphia. This gave origin to the U.S. Marine phrase: "To the shores of Tripoli." In 1830 the French under General Lyautey began to colonize Morocco and Algeria. Tunisia came in as a protectorate; the French left the Bey as the nominal head of the government.

Tom's discourse on North Africa must have lasted two or more hours. With little side lights and intimate details, he held every one of us entranced. I do not think I shall ever forget the pleasant evening we twelve officers have spent in this ward tent.

At one time after the war I found an excellent history with the title, *North Africa, 7000 Years*. Like all books it was expendable and I have been unable to find another copy. The long history blends with the legends and mythology of the dim past.

LETTER TO THE SURGEON GENERAL

When I had left the United States I carried only a Leica camera and a valpak, with some spare uniforms and shirts. My bedroll was lost on the way over. I never saw it again.

Flying south from Miami over the West Indies to Georgetown, British Guiana, then with a pause at Belem on the Amazon, I reached Natal, a coastal city of Brazil in the state of Rio Grande de Norte. The plane had lost a wing tip somewhere over the jungle, so a delay of some days followed.

Later, I wrote a letter to Fred Rankin in the Surgeon General's Office. Some of the excerpts that follow give a grim picture of the sanitary conditions along the route of the Air Transport Command (A.T.C.).

A LETTER TO FRED RANKIN

"*British Guiana:* Held up here for a few days for plane repairs. The station hospital here is well-equipped and an excellent one. Maj. Church is the C.O. and appears to be a competent young surgeon. They do not have much work to do—a few traumatic cases from the camp. Everything is shipshape, however, and despite the fact that they are in the jungle, sanitation seems excellent. All along this route V.D. is a major problem. The rate ran consistently at 250-300 per 1,000 per annum from Oct. '41 to Sept. '42—all white troops. Then with an informal understanding with two of the houses that brought about medical inspection of the girls and established a pro station in the houses, the rate dropped to 26, 90, 66 and 60 for successive months. Objections by the bishop of the region forced them to take out their pro station, and the rate now appears to have risen to around 200.

"Lt. Kelley is A.T.C. surgeon, and Lt. Carter, Air Base Surgeon. They help out at the station hospital and all seem to be working together with first rate *esprit de corps*. The spirit of this post stands out as a bright spot in contrast to those seen later on.

"*Belem:* Fortunately I spent only one night here, as it seems to be a God-forsaken hole right in the mouth of the Amazon. My information came only at dinner from an Air Force surgeon assigned to A.T.C. He seemed to be a disconsolate and discouraged young gentleman, waiting for his transfer orders. Altho in a heavily infected malarial region, control measures do not appear adequate. The town itself is said to be very bad from a sanitary standpoint. Heavy contamination of water supply, and even of bottled water. Amoebic dysentery very prevalent. Examination of 70 applicants for food handlers showed all but 5 had amoebae in stools. An order of ice cream for mess from best hotel was followed by 80-90 cases of diarrhea in camp. V.D. rate around 125. Chiefly chancroid and G.C. The surgeon finds very little enthusiasm for the acceptance of his suggestions.

"*Natal:* As in Belem there is great difficulty encountered by medical officers in securing command responsibility for carrying through elementary sanitation measures. General Marshall has personally called attention to slovenliness, haphazard work and poor maintenance in this portion of the A.T.C. route. When it is obvious in sanitary measures, it constitutes a real hazard.

"The only bright spot is that Station Hospital No. 194 arrived at Natal about four weeks ago. This is a good group, and they are starting to clean up. Their building is still under construction, and their equipment has not all arrived—but they are busy with camp sanitation. The problem of native help, particularly food handlers, is a tough one. There are no dishwashing machines available and the natives will not put their hands in hot water. From 1,600 to 2,000 meals a day are served in the officers' mess alone. This means a constant reuse of dishes and tableware.

"Diarrhea is frequent. Follicular tonsillitis reaches almost epidemic proportions, particularly a few days after a large group of transients pass through from the north. Trench mouth is very prevalent—in fact I got a touch of it myself.

"The nearby town is in quarantine for typhoid. Three years of drought in the hinterland has brought a migration to the coastal cities. Reduction in coastal shipping has increased poverty. Last Wednesday there were 22 funerals of infants under one year. In January 192 infants, 100 under one year of age, died.

(continued)

"Thousands of native workers come into the camp daily. (4,000 in the engineering work alone.) Many squat on the reservation in hammocks at night. They defecate in the bushes close to the construction jobs. The flies are thick, and fly spray is badly needed to make headway against a bad situation.

"Inspection of passengers embarking at Miami should be more rigid according to the officers at Natal. Five cases of measles have been seen among the passengers in 10 days. One tactical officer had a fever of 103° in hospital in Miami, but embarked the next day—now he is held here with fever, mediastinal and cervical nodes—presumably lymphoma.

"I didn't get to Recifi but from a conversation with a surgeon from there judge things are not much better. 3,000 prostitutes are housed on an island with no inspection after they are given a card to admit them to work there. V.D. rates in the Navy are running over 500. It is interesting to note a high incidence of syphilis here as well as at Georgetown, relative to G.C. Presumably because of the expanding employment of young girls from the bush country.

"I am aware of the fact that all this does not concern me, or you, but valuable Army personnel is passing along this route in increasing number. Conditions are ripe for a spread of disease both to the north and eastward. The medical officers are doing their best—and conditions at Georgetown demonstrate that the situation can be licked. The difficulty appears to lie higher up. I hope you will chuck this in the wastebasket if I am speaking out of turn. Label it Confidential Scrap."

FLIGHT TO ALGIERS

After a replacement part arrived and repairs were made, I left Natal at 8:35 P.M. on March 4, 1943. The take-off was not without its anxious moments, for a plane taking off the night before had fallen and burst into flames as its heavily loaded gasoline tanks exploded. The plane used by the Air Transport Command for the Natal-Dakar crossing was a C-87, a converted B-24. There were no seats in the fuselage, but the four or five of us who were to spend the night aboard made ourselves fairly comfortable on piles of luggage. This was the first trip of the plane's crew on this particular run. Other than an encounter with an electrical storm close to the equator, the flight was a smooth one and Cape Verde Two a welcome sight when it appeared below us.

Dakar: On arrival over Dakar at 7:25 A.M., the plane landed on a chickenwire runway about eighteen miles from the city. The first vision was a classic Senegalese carrying a green silk parasol. Huge trees bare of leaves studded the landscape—just the way Africa should look, I noted. Vultures sat in clusters on the barren twisted limbs or circled in search of carrion.

The Air Transport Command Medical Officer at Dakar was Lieutenant F. C. Dohan, medical resident at the M.G.H. in 1934-35 and thereafter in Philadelphia. In the afternoon Dohan drove me into Dakar. The road was lined with Senegalese natives. A favorite costume appeared to be a white nightshirt version of the Arabian burnoose. Many were in rags. In the city the natives were better dressed with colorful cottons.

A home for the aged—Maison de Repos—had been loaned by the French for conversion into a station hospital. The commanding officer was Major Boyd of Baltimore. Medecin-General J. D. Ricou as Directeur du Service de Sante des Troupes was a genial official who promised the full cooperation of his Bureau in providing information regarding epidemic disease in the Dakar area. The malaria season reached its peak in July and August. The natives had been inoculated against yellow fever on an extensive scale. Sleeping sickness was found only back "dans le bois."

Islamic Senegalese were at prayers or clustered in the markets of the Medina. There were many French in the city—little convent pupils were walking in file under escort of their shepherdess nuns and a group of black boys were under the guidance of a priest.

On return to the airstrip I spent a comfortable night in the barracks, although it was rumored that a black mamba—"the most poisonous snake in Africa"—had been killed in the latrine a week before.

Marrakesh: We landed at Marrakesh at 4:00 P.M. and were driven to the Hotel Mamounian, whose gardens and balconies are familiar to travelers to Morocco. There I shared a room with Colonel Bowman, in charge of A.T.C. communications. After the first hot bath since Miami, I joined my fellow passengers on this safari in a drink of chilled muscatel followed by dinner.

After dinner we strolled to the "perpetual funfair of Marrakesh"—Place Djema'a el-F'naa (Congregation of the Departed). Here the snake charmers, the men with performing apes, the acrobats, the woman who drinks boiling water, and many others were displaying their tricks and skills to clusters of hill-folk. Circles were formed by the smokers of hashish, seated on the ground with long-stemmed, tiny-bowled pipes. Glowing bits of charcoal were passed to keep the pipes alight. Near the center of the circle was some object—a chicken with ruffled feathers or the skull of a gazelle—on which the smoker focused his gaze and beheld it transformed into a djinn or other apparition. Hashish is also known as *kif,* meaning "repose."

Thousands of human heads have been displayed on the walls of the city of Marrakesh even in the present century. Decapitations were still going on in 1909. The heads were salted and fastened to the walls by passing a wire through an ear.

In the market the stalls were filled with native products. The dark and narrow streets were crowded with Moroccans—a term which means having a mixture of Arab, Berber and Ethiopian blood. We were persuaded by the driver to visit a native house, so entered a dark hole in the wall that led down a few steps into a tiny room where a girl had a charcoal fire under a copper kettle. We were then led up a winding stair into a room furnished with a double bed. A rug on the floor provided seating. The madame produced three little girls—the oldest not over fourteen years of age. We gave them cigarettes and departed. The driver failed to collect his commission that evening.

The following morning we left Marrakesh for the three hour flight to Oran, and the next day on to Algiers, my destination.

In view of the direct flights now scheduled by jetliners between the principal cities of the world, the question may well arise why, in 1943, the route between Washington, D. C. and Algiers was so circuitous: Miami-Georgetown-Belem-Natal-Dakar-Marrakesh seems a strange way to go to Algiers. The main reason, of course, is in the difference between jet and propeller power; but there was also the inexperience of the crews being recruited rapidly into the Air Transport Command.

AT ALGIERS

I arrived at Algiers at 11 A.M., March 6, 1943, and was met by Colonel Standlee, the Deputy Surgeon, Allied Force Headquarters, and taken to the adjutant general's Office to register.

The headquarters of the medical department was set up in a building known as Church Villa close to the general staff headquarters in the Hotel St. George. The following letter, written by Perrin Long in 1956, describes Church Villa and my arrival at A.F.H.Q.

LETTER FROM PERRIN LONG

1956

It seems as though it was only yesterday that I was with "Pete" in the bleak little Office in Church Villa in Algiers, on the road with him in North Africa, Sicily, or Italy, or in the areas which were successively occupied by the Medical Section of A.F.H.Q., in or near the great palace in Caserta. The "Consultants," as we were called, were generally in the back room, always within easy call of The Surgeon, but otherwise out of sight. Fortunately, under "Pete's" leadership we were kept "in mind": by the various Surgeons under whom we served.

And speaking of Surgeons, I am reminded of our first name calling, British Director of Medical Services (D.M.S.), A.F.H.Q., Major General Sir Ernest Cowell, who really startled "Pete" the first morning after the latter's arrival. For weeks, General Cowell had been asking, "When will the Consulting Surgeon, American, arrive?" We had been saying that we expected "Pete" Churchill to come in February. Each morning, at what General Cowell called "8 o'clock Signal Time," it was his practice to hold an Office conference in which the various problems of military medicine which confronted the members of the Medical Section were discussed. The first morning after "Pete's" arrival the D.M.S. went the rounds, and then ended up by saying, "Peter, have you anything to say?" An amused silence ensued, until "Pete" woke up to the fact that for a considerable time thereafter, he was destined to be "Peter" Churchill in the mind of the D.M.S.

On arrival at headquarters I reported to my superior officer, Major General Albert W. Kenner—the senior American medical officer—and through Kenner to Cowell, the British Theater Surgeon, who in this headquarters assumed seniority.

The medical section, A.F.H.Q., was composed of two divisions: British and American. The British Surgeon outranked the senior American medical officer; consequently he assumed the authority of Theater Surgeon. The mixture of British and Americans was complete in the medical field.

When the Western Task Force had landed in North Africa, an Army headquarters was set up in Morocco under General George Patton. By the time I reached North Africa, Patton had been given command of II Corps which was fighting in southern Tunisia along with the British First Army. Major General Lloyd Fredendall had been in command of the armored division but was relieved after the battle of Kasserine Pass. As Patton was moved up to command II Corps in southern Tunisia, Mark Clark moved in to take command of the Fifth Army, at that time no more than a headquarters and a training center at Oudjda near the border between Algeria and Morocco. It was necessary to protect the rear area which extended to the Atlantic coast, for if Vichy France and Spain had been persuaded by Hitler to close the Straits of Gibraltar, the supply line for II Corps and A.F.H.Q. would have been overland through Morocco.

Mark Clark, as soon as his headquarters had been set up, selected Fred Blesse as Fifth Army Surgeon at Oudjda. Al Kenner, who had come in with the Western Task Force, moved up to the Eisenhower headquarters as U.S. Theater Surgeon, presumably as the coequal of, but, as I have pointed out, actually outranked by Cowell, who was responsible to Sir Alexander, the Chief of Ground Forces under Eisenhower.

There was no American Army in action in North Africa; the largest unit was II Corps—a reinforced corps. The Corps Surgeon was Dick Arnest—Colonel Richard P. Arnest. The Corps Surgeon's Office was in constant touch with Kenner's Office in Algiers. Every night a long telephone call came in from "Speedy Rear" through Constantine, giving a report on the number of wounded in the mobile hospitals ready for ambulance evacuation, and the number of lightly wounded ready for evacuation as "sitters" in returning transport of other types.

I can still picture Earle Standlee sitting in Church Villa until this call came in, faint and scarcely audible over the wires strung by the Signal Corps.

INTRICACIES OF ARMY ORGANIZATION

Al Kenner was an able officer, respected greatly by General Marshall, and it was commonly rumored that he was to be the next Surgeon General. He was not a surgeon in the sense that he performed operations. "Surgeon" is an ancient title in its military usage. An internist becomes a Surgeon when he serves as Surgeon General or Corps Surgeon.

Kenner had the problem of Churchill, a full colonel, arriving in his headquarters unfamiliar with anything military, except perhaps a salute. He took me into his Office several times for long helpful talks on the formalities of Army procedure. Kenner also straightened me out on the many intricacies of Army Organization, particularly pertinent to an overseas theater in combat where the lines of command authority and staff function are sharply drawn. He was quiet and patient, and I developed respect for him immediately. He told me that I should remember that I had no authority to give commands or issue orders; that any authority I had was derived through his position and that even this was limited.

One thinks of a colonel or a general in the Army as having a command, but this is not true in the Medical Corps, particularly in a theater which is in combat. Then the distinction between the line of command authority and the position of technical advisers and staff officers becomes sharply drawn. A colonel in the Medical Corps who is commanding officer of a hospital has command authority within his unit—*internal* command. A hospital has a detachment of enlisted men for whom he is the commander. He is not under the Theater Surgeon but under the line officer in command of the tactical force to which his medical unit is assigned. The Surgeon General has command authority over a certain number of general hospitals; but when a hospital is assigned to the "ground forces," it is beyond his control.

My function in relation to a tactical unit such as II Corps or, subsequently, the Fifth Army was purely that of a "visitor." The autonomy of a tactical unit in combat is complete. No one could enter the Fifth Army area without permission from General Mark Clark. The only exception was by a direct order from a higher headquarters, and this was a device used rarely, as it implied that some officer on the staff of the combat unit was derelict in his duty. As a further example, the Surgeon General could not enter the Pacific area because MacArthur would not invite him. Only if the Chief of Staff in Washington *ordered* MacArthur to let him in could the Surgeon General inspect the hospitals in Japan.

In North Africa, a hospital assigned to II Corps to support the combat operations came under the command of General Patton. The Theater Surgeon was on the staff of General Eisenhower. If I thought a medical officer in an evacuation hospital was not doing a proper job and should be replaced, I had no authority whatsoever to replace him. I could report the situation to Kenner and talk it over with him. Kenner, depending upon his relations with II Corps Chief of Staff, might persuade him, through the hospital commander, to transfer the incompetent surgeon to other duties. The only way the Theater Surgeon could remove an officer by command authority would be to go to Eisenhower's Chief of Staff, have him issue an order to General Patton, who, in turn, would order the hospital commander to do so. Such a roundabout channel was too complicated for practical purposes. This was the Army system in 1943 as Kenner explained it to me; it had not been explained to me in Washington.

Kenner returned to the United States on March 26, 1943, and was succeeded by General Blesse who came from the Fifth Army to become Theater Surgeon, U.S.A. Fred Blesse was indoctrinated thoroughly with the ostrich technique of keeping one's head under cover and one's neck from getting extended. He told me immediately that I was not to write personal letters to friends of mine in the Surgeon General's Office; in other words, all personal channels of communication were cut off. Actually this was not as bad as it sounds. Even if I had communicated with Washington, it would have been impossible for the Surgeon General to do anything about it. Later in the war the Surgeon General set up "Essential Technical Medical Data," a monthly report, directly from the Surgeon of a theater to the Surgeon General. Then we could describe our technical problems directly to those officers in the Surgeon General's Office who, we knew, wanted to hear about them. I could then write an account of what was going on surgically with the knowledge that it would get into the hands of Fred Rankin's staff. For a long time the Surgeon General merely received the incoming reports and filed them; he did not let his staff see them. Finally, Michael DeBakey, then in the lower levels of the Surgeon General's Office, found this out and got hold of the reports so that I knew that I was communicating with DeBakey and Nick Carter, the two righthand men of Rankin. Rankin was busy trying to get things done in accord with what he learned through this channel, but it was a devious route of communication.

Communication between an overseas theater and the Zone of the Interior (Z.I.) presented an ingenious paradox of Army organization. I have described the restrictions placed on communication with individuals in Washington. There were reasons for this regulation. An indiscreet letter going to my friends in the Surgeon General's Office might have jeopardized Fred Blesse's position. He did not know me and he did not have a voice in choosing me for the assignment. Some remark of mine might have traveled from the Surgeon General to General Marshall and back to General Eisenhower. The Army guards against so-called "end runs." Blesse also worried because Perrin Long was looking out for the personal health of some of the members of Eisenhower's staff, particularly General Hughes, the Chief of Staff. An indiscreet word from Perry to Hughes might undermine Blesse's position.

Soon after I had arrived in Algiers, it had become apparent to me that no one at headquarters had any real idea of what was going on surgically. Kenner talked at length about taking care of burns on the beaches in Morocco, but neither he nor anyone else seemed to have rational notions about what to do for them. Perrin Long had been sent down from the European Theater of Operations (E.T.O.) where he had been on Hawley's Professional Services Staff, and was at A.F.H.Q. in Church Villa as Medical Consultant. Perry had been trying to formulate some policies about the use of sulfonamides, a subject on which he was one of the best-informed men in the United States, but otherwise there had been no attempt to examine, much less to formulate, policies for the management of the wounded. Surgical policies were at loose ends. This was early March, the landing had been in November. My first job was to find out what was going on, a task made doubly complex by the fact that A.F.H.Q. was supporting the British First Army in the north as well as II Corps in southern Tunisia. So there were two complex military situations to find out about: one predominantly British and the other American.

In this learning phase, Brigadier John Weddell was my mentor. He was a regular officer of the Royal Army Medical Corps with experience in World War I and also at Dunkirk. Weddell served as Surgical Consultant to Cowell, so we worked closely together. He made available to me all of his sources of information about the management of casualties and took me on several visits to the British hospitals in the vicinity of Algiers. The Americans had no hospitals in the Algiers area except a small station hospital for headquarters. This contained few, if any, battle casualties; so, my baptism to war casualties came on trips with Weddell to the British hospitals near Algiers.

At that time there was an intermingling of British and American wounded. In theory there were separate streams of evacuation, but we were working as an integrated force in the battle of Tunisia and there were American units under British command in the First Army area and there were British outfits under American command in II Corps. I saw many American wounded in the British hospitals. The British were old hands at the business; we were learning. They had a different system and were short of personnel and equipment. The group of British surgeons with the First Army lacked the experience that the western desert surgeons had been through. They had, however, profited from a freer exchange of information than our surgeons had enjoyed. In the early Ethiopian and western desert campaign, Heneage

Ogilvie had been Chief Surgical Consultant and had written sound directives and established wise policies concerning the management of battle injuries. This knowledge had been transmitted by their War Office to the new command under Alexander and the First Army so that they were well indoctrinated.

SOUTHERN TUNISIA

I worked at A.F.H.Q. in Algiers until March 16; then Weddell and I set forth on our first field trip together for a week's tour of southern Tunisia. (See Chapter 12, The Tunisian Campaign) There were many documents to review. Before going to North Africa nothing about the tactical setup had been divulged to me. I had no knowledge of what units were there or what was the magnitude of the undertaking or of the tactical and strategic aims. These matters seeped slowly through my skin. At headquarters Standlee, Kenner's chief executive, had a large map on his wall with the placement of American hospitals in southern Tunisia, Algeria and Morocco, so I became acquainted gradually with their constantly shifting positions. It was a dynamic pattern, changing every day.

In Tunisia I met Dick Arnest for the first time. The Surgeon of II Corps was a fine, wise man who saw to it that Perrin Long and I could visit the Corps' hospitals whenever we wanted to. We were fortunate he was the type of man he was. Someone who was insecure would not have let us move freely where and when we wished. We could not have learned what we did learn and thus prepare ourselves for what was coming.

A corps is ordinarily a subdivision of an army; but in North Africa, instead of an army, II Corps was the tactical unit in combat: two or three divisions and other troops. A term that came into usage later, fits it—a task force. The combat function of II Corps was that of an army but without the equipment and table of organization that build up the large structure of a field army. The 1st Division, the 9th Division, part of an armored division, the Rangers—all functioned as an integrated tactical unit. II Corps' purpose was to keep the Germans (who were retreating from the western desert toward Cape Bon in Tunisia) in a corridor along the coast instead of letting them strike inland and cut off the lines of communication of the British First Army. The latter was moving along the northern shore of North Africa.

The attempted German breakthrough at Kasserine Pass demonstrated that II Corps did not, at that time, have enough equipment and manpower to establish adequate defense in depth against German tanks. Our medical organization was equally sketchy. The only small hospital that could be placed forward to receive the seriously wounded was the 48th Surgical Hospital. This was a mobile hospital designed for urgent surgery; it had been conceived on paper following World War I. Only one such unit was made, and this had been sent down from the E.T.O. It was too large and too heavy to be really mobile. It had three functional components: one so-called *operating* unit and two *holding* units which were equipped with cots. Nurses were assigned to the holding units. The operating unit functioned in conjunction with one holding unit; then the operating unit was designed to move forward with the second holding unit, leaving the first to care for its nontransportable wounded until they were ready to be evacuated. When empty of patients, it was ready to leapfrog the other holding unit and move forward with the operating unit. The hospital was not only too heavy for mobility but was not well equipped.

The small (400-bed) evacuation hospital had not yet been designed, so that the only available hospitals were the 750-bed evacuation hospitals, which were too heavy for mobile warfare, and the 48th Surgical Hospital. Air evacuation in C-47's was available back into the Oran area and to Morocco. Here general hospitals were established.

The armored division of II Corps was equipped with a "treatment station"—a mobile half-track truck which could be converted into a shelter for surgery. It had no holding unit. The idea was prevalent that a surgeon could operate on the tailboard of a truck, but who was to take care of the patient after the operation was a question no one had faced.

The fantastic vision of the heroic surgeon following the dust of battle just behind the tanks and doing operations was still in vogue. Experience with German tank warfare and the resulting mobility of enemy forces was ignored and I doubt that it would have been helpful if it had been known.

Dick Arnest had requested a "medical regiment," which then was composed of clearing companies, ambulances and collecting companies. In addition, a division takes with it battalion surgeons and their aid stations. A division had only one clearing company, and some divisions were poorly-equipped with collecting companies. The medical support of a division was a matter of heated debate at that time. In addition to the hospital units then, II Corps had at least a part of a medical regiment which provided ambulance and clearing companies.

Arnest and his executive officer—Lieutenant Colonel William Anspacher—faced with long distances and the transport of the seriously wounded, had taken the clearing companies from the medical regiment, set them up forward of the 48th Surgical Hospital, and staffed them with surgeons from the 2nd Auxiliary Surgical Group who had come in as free-lance surgeons at the time of the landing. Clearing companies with surgical teams, not attached to a division but working directly under the Corps Surgeon, provided first-priority surgical care for the seriously wounded. They had inadequate equipment, were understaffed and could improvise only a small holding unit in some crude shelter. These young surgeons were doing a superb job, but they had no guidance except what Bill Anspacher, who had had very little surgical training, and Arnest, who had had none, could give them. They were relying on the advice they could get from the evacuation hospitals behind.

At the time I arrived, Howard Snyder had been taken from the 77th Evacuation Hospital on temporary duty to help solve the surgical problems. If I had failed to use as excellent a surgeon as Snyder, who was already in the good graces of Arnest and Anspacher, and had tried to insert someone of my own choosing, I would have run into friction immediately. One necessity in the Army is to make the best of what is available if it's working, and build on it when opportunity presents. Otherwise there is the risk of upsetting a machine that is in action. The best I could do was to apply a few drops of oil and then try to identify the problems and prepare for the next undertaking.

UNDERSTANDING THE ARMY

A military operation under any circumstances is a succession of calculated risks. Military *training*, so-called, may be looked upon as a conditioning of the individual to value the effective action of the group above the convenience or safety of the individual. The concerted or integrated effort rests on an intuitive base, but it can be developed on a purely intellectual level, which is the way I had to acquire it. In consequence, I sometimes think I understand the Army and am more articulate about its essential nature than some men who have been in it all their lives and who respond intuitively but are totally inarticulate about why they do so. A brief talk I gave at the Army Medical School a few years ago has been printed and reprinted—and I recently had another request from Germany that it be reprinted again in the bulletin issued to U. S. Army hospitals there.

An army in combat is extremely sensitive to any remarks that can be interpreted as criticism. Mike DeBakey came over to Italy from the Surgeon General's Office and I took him through the Fifth Army combat area. From there he went to Europe and visited the Army areas there. One chance remark about blood transfusion with a reference to what he had seen in Italy was interpreted as a criticism of what they were doing. He was asked to leave the Army area and the recommendation came to Hawley in Paris that he be sent back to Washington or court-martialed. I happened to be in Paris in Hawley's Office when Mike came in, not knowing what it was all about. I explained to Hawley what a wonderful fellow Mike was. It was the Army Surgeon who thought that someone was criticizing the quality of care he was providing.

FINDING HELP

Because the American undertaking in North Africa at this time was on an austere basis, pared down to minimum staff organizations, Long and I had to find help wherever we could. We turned directly to our colleagues in the hospitals and learned from them rather than importing more inexperienced surgeons and physicians, and thus running the risk of inexperienced men trying to tell the hospital staff what to do. I traveled the length and breadth of the theater and talked with many surgeons before I made up my mind how to tackle the problems of the care of the wounded. Long and I were in a far more flexible position than existed in the E.T.O. where, during a long period of waiting, they built up for the cross channel invasion. The E.T.O. had an enormous professional services division.

As I have said earlier, the laboratory for the testing of ideas in World War II was the North African-Mediterranean Theater, not only in medicine and in the care of the wounded, but also in many of the tactical operations. That North Africa was a *learning* theater was something I welcomed, realizing very early in the game that what was needed were facts on which to develop the teachings of experience rather than the enforcement of preconceived ideas. As a result—when I was able to add the services of a consultant— instead of sending back immediately for a consultant in neurosurgery or orthopedics and so on, I turned to the hospitals and selected men who had actual experience with wounded soldiers.

We were constantly working under a rigid policy to keep the headquarters staff small. A major problem of a commander in the field is to avoid the building up of an enormous staff that busies itself with paperwork. Our number of assigned officers was kept at a minimum. It was soon apparent that the original concept which I had discussed with Admiral Stevenson was going to be the one that I wanted to develop: namely, a few trained observers to find facts and to identify and outline problems so that they might be solved. I was at the top level as far as formulating surgical policies, although I needed authority to implement them. I was not going to get authority for the elaboration of surgery in North Africa because the theater was on too austere a basis. Later on in Italy, more became possible.

Linda C. Benavides, Jennifer M. Gurney, and Brian J. Eastridge

This chapter highlights the importance of effective advising and communicating to both prevent disease and nonbattle injuries (DNBI) and improve care for battle injuries (BI). Churchill first discusses his circuitous travel from the United States to Algiers and the issues with DNBI that erode the fighting force. He then focuses on his task of improving surgical care in a mobile theater and how best to employ surgeons and medical assets.

As Churchill traveled the Air Transport Command route (Miami-Georgetown-Belem-Natal-Dakar-Marrakesh-Oran), he visited multiple station hospitals along the way. He learned of rampant DNBI ranging from diarrhea to venereal diseases and how surgeons successfully convinced line leaders to embrace preventative medicine practices, thus decreasing DNBI rates and thereby boosting medical morale. These improved outcomes illustrate the impact of communicating in a manner that commanders understand to ensure mission success while optimizing preventative health and care of patients.

Upon arriving in Algiers, Churchill realized that he and his medical colleagues had extremely limited authority and command visibility since medical assets in the combat theater functioned under the operational command of the line officer. Churchill noted that "the consultants . . . were generally in the back room, always within easy call of The Surgeon, but otherwise out of sight. . .. My function in relation to a tactical unit such as II Corps or, subsequently, the Fifth Army was purely that of a 'visitor.'" To exert influence without command authority, Churchill leaned heavily on seasoned Army staff and British medical personnel to mentor him in effectively navigating various challenges. As one example, Churchill identified a gap in casualty outcomes data collection leading to a lack of policies guiding the management of the combat wounded. British medical personnel, specifically Brigadier Weddell and indirectly Dr Ogilvie, mentored Churchill in casualty management and policy development.

Upon taking a "field trip" to southern Tunisia, he realized the US military medical organization was ill-prepared for mobile warfare with surgeons at far forward locations lacking equipment, holding capability, and guidance. Like many in Army and civilian leadership, Churchill viewed North Africa as a "learning theater" to "develop the teachings of experience rather than the enforcement of preconceived ideas." Throughout these early months, he was "formulating surgical policies" to improve mobility, equipment, holding capability, and practice guidelines for his surgeons that he sought to fully implement in Italy.

Medical leaders on the modern battlefield face many similar challenges including "ownership" of battlefield medicine and right-sizing the deployed medical footprint. As Ogilvie famously stated, "Good surgery must be done as far forward as possible. If it is too good, in the sense of too elaborately equipped, it will not be far enough forward, and if it is too far forward it will not be good enough." In the same spirit of Churchill's vision of North Africa serving as a "learning theater," the Joint Trauma System (JTS) should serve as a continuous learning health care system. The JTS and DoD Trauma Registry (DoDTR) have evolved to provide data on combat casualty care and outcomes. This capability has enabled "real-time" performance improvement and the production of relevant evidence-based clinical practice guidelines that will enable us to preserve the lessons of World War II and the more recent conflicts in Iraq and Afghanistan and even improve care for the benefit of future warfighters.

SUGGESTED READINGS

Joint Trauma System. History. Accessed September 11, 2023. https://jts.health.mil/index.cfm/about/origins.

National Academies of Sciences, Engineering, and Medicine. *A National Trauma Care System: Integrating Military and Civilian Trauma Systems to Achieve Zero Preventable Deaths After Injury*. The National Academies Press; 2016.

Ogilvie WH. *Forward Surgery in Modern War*. Butterworth & Co. Ltd; 1944.

7

The Army Learns About War

Almost Thirty years have passed since the United States entered World War II. It is still disturbing to recall how unprepared our nation was for war and the lack of knowledge that was displayed by the officers of the regular Army Medical Corps about the conduct of other wars. Perhaps this is one of the reasons I have postponed writing about World War II, hesitating lest I offend some of the officers whose friendship I valued. Also, there is a deep-lying conflict of interests that defies solution.

This conflict of interest centers on the responsibility of a commander to win a battle although to do so means the sacrifice of soldiers. "The Charge of the Light Brigade" motif has made the compelling nature of a decision of command immortal. The medical officer wields no comparable command authority—his function is to rescue and repair the damage sustained in the "valley of death."

The reaction of a medical officer to this difference in purpose is recorded vividly in the diary of Major L—, M.C. Under the date of January 6, 1943, in Casablanca: "Early this evening, General George Patton came out and talked to us. . . . As medical men we could not entirely agree with some of the principles which he dictated. In substance he said, 'If you have two wounded soldiers, one with a gunshot wound of the lung, and the other with an arm or leg blown off, you save the s.o.b. with the lung wound and let the g.d.s.o.b. with an amputated arm or leg go to hell. He is no g.d use to us any more.' Perhaps it takes this hard boiled attitude to win battles, but. . . ."

The daily demonstration of the function to save life in close support of combat troops is in itself no insignificant contribution to the military effectiveness of an army recruited from the population of a democracy. The preservation of the personal dignity and integrity of the individual constantly adds untold complexity to the organization of the services that must accompany the citizen-in-arms to the battlefield—but without this consideration, a sustained military effort may well be impossible to achieve. The logistic burden imposed on the Army by its Medical Corps is enormous.

The Army assumes many other "logistic burdens" to maintain the human dignity of its citizens-at-arms. There is the Army Post Office, for instance, which provides a young man on the frontlines with letters and transports his letters back to his family and friends. The Red Cross, the Canteen, and so forth provide him with doughnuts, literature, comic books, toothbrushes and toothpaste. He has clergy to hold religious services and, if he dies, the Graves Registration Service moves in to supply a mattress cover and place him in an overseas cemetery. Even this may not be his final resting place, for later his remains may be exhumed and taken back to his native land.

In contrast, in World War II when a Russian was killed it was customary to poke him back into his foxhole, cover him with a few shovelfuls of dirt and leave him in an unmarked grave. The long months of toil of the Graves Registration Service after World War II received little publicity. The Russians could not understand our concern and thought we had some ulterior motive. They couldn't understand why the United States had any emotional concern about where some particular citizen had died in battle.

To the combat commander the logistic problems imposed by the Medical Corps give rise to conflicts and misunderstandings. It is important that the medical officer of a combat unit maintain a close contact and understanding with his commander. It may be necessary for him to say to the unit commander: "If you bivouac your troops on this island or on the shores of this shallow lake, you can expect an incidence of malaria which will deprive you of one man out of every ten." The commander may decide to do it, but it is important that the medical information be received and taken into account in every tactical operation. All that is necessary is that the commander be made aware of the fact that he is going to lose one man in every ten and adjust his tactical plans correspondingly.

In peace or in war, a man studies medicine in order to take care of sick and injured people. He may do this for years in a peacetime army to the exclusion of all other interests. Suddenly a war confronts the nation and the regular Army doctor must emerge from the fluoroscopic dark room and become the surgeon responsible for the total care of patients in dozens of military hospitals.

Efforts have been made to solve this dilemma by the creation of a Medical Administrative Corps. But again, as in civilian life, it has been found that a hospital is best administered by a man who has had medical education and experience in caring for sick patients.

It came as a surprise to me to encounter gross ignorance among my A.F.H.Q. colleagues about the experience of the A.E.F. in World War I, the Spanish War of 1936 to 1939, and even of the experience of the desert warfare in Libya in which Rommel and Montgomery were engaged.

There was a comparable ignorance of the medical officer coming from civilian life into the framework of an Army in combat. General Patton was basically correct in voicing his admonition because the civilian doctor invariably turns first to the seriously wounded or dying man. If he can be transported further, he is immediately evacuated to a hospital where lifesaving measures are available.

The French term "triage," meaning "sorting," came into use in World War I. This was used to determine the placement of forward hospitals in the war in Spain. Both the sorting of casualties according to the nature of the wound and forward placement of an improvised "first priority" hospital were introduced in North Africa.

JOLLY'S THREE POINT FORWARD SYSTEM

One of the few books I had tucked into my luggage to take to North Africa was *Field Surgery in Total War* by Douglas W. Jolly. This described the "three-point forward system" developed in Spain and influenced my thinking greatly. Jolly's book was unknown to our A.F.H.Q. group of medical officers. Even the word "triage" required explanation.

In Spain the system of forward hospitals was reorganized and the "three-point forward system" introduced to separate the functional elements of the British casualty clearing station of World War I. These functional elements were:

1. Classification Center (triage) in advance of the farthest forward hospital.
2. No. 1 Hospital for the most urgent cases.
3. No 2 Hospital for the less urgent cases.

This principle of *triage based on the urgency of the wound*, with separate hospitalization for the two categories of cases, subsequently became the basic principle followed by the U.S. Medical Corps in World War II. To a great extent it resolved the dilemma between the mutually contradictory "military" view and the "surgical" view and established clearly that the function of the Army medical service is to save life irrespective of the future military potential of the individual battle casualty.

In Spain the use of the Red Cross as protection for hospitals and ambulances was abandoned in the earliest days, for they attracted rather than prevented attack (Jolly). As a consequence, the development of the No. 1 Hospital was kept at the level of a mobile surgical unit. A Renault truck adapted from the French "autochirurgicale" and known as the "auto-chir" was used for the transport of surgical material including operation theater furnishings. An ambulance provided transport of personnel and their personal baggage. The auto-chir was poorly suited to serve as an operating theater, and for this purpose as well as for the housing of patients, use was made of tents, wine cellars, underground shelters and caves, or railway tunnels.

BRITISH EXPERIENCE IN MIDDLE EAST DESERT WARFARE

In the second Libyan campaign, which had opened on November 18, 1941, the Royal Army Medical Corps attained mobility for their forward surgical teams that made the relatively cumbersome and static British C.C.S. which served so well in the last war as a forward surgical station appear obsolete. Two three-ton desert-worthy four-wheel-drive trucks comprised the transport but neither lorry was designed as an operating room. A large penthouse tent, specially made to be erected round the unfitted lorry, and to enclose it completely provided shelter for operating. This unit was not self accounting and relied on a parent installation for supply replenishment. During combat it was attached either to a forward C.C.S. or a field ambulance.

Triage was limited to the selection of cases from the ambulances of a convoy and the passing of the remainder farther to the rear. The basis of selection varied from day to day, or hour to hour and took into consideration the number of casualties; the capacity of the surgical team; the holding capacity of the whole unit; the ease or difficulty of evacuation, and the means available; the distance and time to the next point to the rear where surgical aid may be had; and the tactical situation.

The unit (C.C.S. or field ambulance) to which the mobile field surgical team (F.S.U.), was attached was held responsible for the matter of how to hold and how long to hold patients after operation, and there was general agreement that it was usually best to operate early, no matter how soon the patient must be evacuated. It was considered desirable that the mobile surgical unit itself be relieved of all responsibilities not directly concerned with operating. It was recognized that evacuation by air was ideal because the alternative, inevitable in five-sixths of the casualties, was by ambulance or even ordinary truck, over 100 miles of open desert, where the speed of an ambulance did not exceed ten miles per hour.

Nursing facilities in the desert were inevitably crude. It was necessary to evacuate patients after operation within twenty-four hours when possible, but they were sometimes able to hold the worst cases two or three days. Casualties were heaviest during the first month of the campaign and during the whole of this period the only available accommodation was tents. The wounded men lay on stretchers on the bare ground, and most of them were evacuated on the stretchers on which they were brought in, for it was seldom necessary or wise to lift a man off his stretcher for operation. Each man, unwashed and unshaved, wore his fighting clothes, dust-covered and blood-soaked, torn by flying metals and ripped and cut to expose the wounded part. The "wards" were not a pretty sight.

Great emphasis was placed on the ability of a mobile surgical unit to get to work or to pack and move off in a matter of minutes; and the one-table vehicles, designed as an operating room on wheels, were considered eminently suitable for the "guerilla surgery" that was being undertaken—but in practice remained attached to the C.C.S.'s.

These specially-built vehicles, which were gifts from America, were appraised critically in the Middle East and the judgment rendered remained valid throughout the war. Ogilvie commented as follows:

"On paper the idea is irresistible. The planning intrigues the surgeon, the detailed designing is a welcome diversion to the engineer, and the presentation of the finished product appeals to the charitable society or the wealthy donor."

After presenting the advantages and the drawbacks he confesses that "in practice the vans in M.E. have been attached to C.C.S.'s" where their special merits have not been called into action.

This extreme swing of the pendulum toward mobility that started with the blitzkrieg not only was a reaction away from the static C.C.S. of World War I but also was shaped by both terrain and tactics of desert warfare. The urge for mobility is understandable when the first warning of the approach of an enemy column may be a shell from approaching tanks. Regarding the terrain:

"We have fought the war along a strip of coast, practically in a straight line, and hospital sites exist wherever you choose to unload your tents. The straight line lengthens, but as it does so the advanced base moves forward, and the final base is linked by the smooth travel of air on sea." (Ogilvie to Weddell, April 5, 1943.)

Ogilvie, in his report entitled *War Surgery in Two Commands*, further describes the western desert as

"a vast country with long distances . . . undulating desert that is sandy in places only, usually firm enough for the passage of every kind of vehicle. Over these the units of two large armies move like ships on the sea, navigating by compass or previously placed marks, rather than by geographical features. As at sea, the only obstacles to movement are rocky ridges and mine fields, and air observation dominates all tactics, so that dispersal and concealment are the key to protection. Here, where the line of battle may move 40 or 50 miles a day in either direction, the surgical services must be equally mobile. The surgeon can get anywhere, but his outfit must be self-contained and reduced to bed rock simplicity."

Viewed in retrospect and as other than an evolutionary adaptation to a specialized environment, forward surgery in the western desert may be criticized for the emphasis placed on mobility and early operation without sufficient regard to the care of the patient. The vision was sound, however.

"Nothing but the best is good enough for the surgical treatment of patients in the forward areas. It is here, rather than at the base, that the fate of the wounded man is so often decided; whether he lives or dies; whether his limb is saved or lost; whether his wound remains clean and healthy or becomes infected and keeps him in the hospital for months. By the time the patient reaches the base, the subsequent course of the injury is largely determined. The logical conclusion is that there is no room for makeshift surgery in the forward areas. Within the limits imposed by local conditions every effort should be made to operate with the same care as is exercised under normal circumstances."

About New Year's, 1941, an Australian division had taken up positions around the perimeter defense of Bardia. An Australian surgical team was attached to the main dressing station of a field ambulance near Fort Capuzzo, and all casualties were directed through this station. The critically wounded were retained for treatment by the surgical team, while other casualties were passed on to a "light" C.C.S. working below the escarpment a few miles from Sollin. From this unit, wounded were evacuated over the unbelievably rough road to a C.C.S. at Mersa Matruh and from there by rail to a base hospital at Alexandria.

In discussing frankly the merits or even the necessity of operating on the wounded in forward areas under the conditions that then existed, Lieutenant Colonel Julian Smith, A.A.M.C. (*Australian and New Zealand Journal of Surgery 11*:153, January, 1942) comments as follows:

"One believes that a primary function of the medical service is to assist in the evacuation of the wounded to a place of comparative quietude and safety, where they can receive surgical treatment and thereafter be held until fit to travel to base hospital. That the wounded man should receive treatment as soon as possible is beyond all argument. If tactical considerations have prevented a casualty clearing station from being reasonably accessible, then the critically and severely wounded must be dealt with at the main dressing station level. The surgical service should here be provided by a team sent forward, and not by the personnel of the field ambulance. Operations should be strictly limited to those who are severely wounded, the less severely wounded being passed back to casualty clearing station, distant though it may be. After a severely wounded man has been operated on, he must on no account be evacuated forthwith, but must be held until fit to travel without risk. This is no question of military tactics—it is a cold surgical fact. Therefore, in all forward operating centers provision must be made for holding wounded for some days after operation. The practice of treating all wounded in forward areas, without discrimination as to severity, will lead to confusion. The greater the number operated on, the greater the number which must be held. Field ambulances are not equipped to handle large numbers of patients who have been operated on, and the addition of a surgical team does not adjust this deficiency. A field ambulance should never attempt to abrogate the functions of a casualty clearing station."

In further reaction to excessive enthusiasm for mobility, Smith quotes the following incident that occurred during the campaign in Syria: "There is the true story of the surgeon well trained in the niceties of civil thoracic surgery, in charge of an operating team, who had apparently seen little of the ravages of war. In the course of the conversation with a member of the writer's unit, he stated his intention to operate on chests as far forward as possible, moving quickly from place to place; such excursions, he anticipated, the mobility of his unit would allow him to make. He was asked with whom during the course of his thoracic barnstorming he would leave the patients on whom he had operated. He answered that they would be billeted in farmhouses and the like, and left to the tender mercies of the occupants. By what happy chance had a knowledge of surgery been widely disseminated through the peasants of Syria? What strange nomadic taint prompted such an outrageous proposal?"

Ogilvie, in *War Surgery in Two Commands*, also expressed his reservations:

"Whether with a mobile theater or a standard field surgical unit, the forward surgeon in Middle East is now on wheels and equipped for tailboard operating. The idea that he will save lives by going up to the outskirts of the fighting is, however, illusory. When the ebb and flow of a modern battle between mechanized forces over country that offers no natural obstacle is remembered it will be realized that the further forward a surgeon is, the more local will be his scope, and the greater the number of wounded who fail to contact him but go further back. He can do his best work only if his site is accessible and known to a group of forward collecting units, that is at the converging point of well known tracks."

The Middle East consultant also repeatedly stressed the futility of operating on, and evacuating rapidly, casualties with abdominal wounds.

"After operation they must be kept till they have established equilibrium—for four days at least, often for ten. In early battles many patients were evacuated by air after a relatively simple abdominal operation, and died in consequence. It is now (end of 1942) the practice to send a certain number of beds to each forward centre for the nursing of abdominal cases."

Again, with reference to abdominal wounds:

"These differ from all others in that without skilled operation and specialized after-treatment at an early date the majority will die. Patients should not be evacuated till they have 'got over' the operation and are clearly improving."

There was seen, therefore, in the Middle East a strong departure from the static C.C.S. as well as movement of the surgeon forward, but the placement of the F.S.U. in the straight line of evacuation of all casualties in a field ambulance station or a forward C.C.S. without the forward triage point which was an integral component of the Spanish "three-point" system. The lack of this triage is illustrated by Major Peter Ascroft's statistics that show in an analysis of 239 operations (other than minor) only 8 procedures for penetrating wounds of the abdomen and 15 closed fractures and dislocations. The surgeon was placed forward, but spent a great deal of his time in operations that were urgent not because of the nature of the wound, but because of the difficulties of evacuation imposed by the terrain and the tactical situation.

That progress had been made from the catastrophic days of the blitzkrieg is apparent in comparison with the following statement by Major Jeffrey, R,A.M.C.:

"In a base hospital of 2,000 beds (La Baule near St. Nazaire) functioning until the final day of evacuation of the B.E.F. from France (18 June 1940) several thousand wounded passed through in the last six weeks. In this 2,000 bed hospital there would not be more than three or four intra-abdominal wounds and a dozen intrathoracic wounds. The principal explanation must be that the men so wounded did not survive; at any rate long enough to get them to hospital."

At this point it must be admitted frankly that no system for providing adequate surgical care for the wounded has held up in the face of an onrushing enemy offensive movement. The blitzkrieg of 1940 repeated the pattern of August 1914 when, after the subjugation of Belgium, the right wing of the German forces under von Kluck swept over northwestern France against sporadic French and English resistance. During this time the Allied surgical field work was an extremely arduous, not to say impossible, undertaking. The lines were constantly falling back, which allowed for practically no organization for field hospital work or even the assembling of the wounded, much less caring for the dead. Scarcely would a regimental stand be made and allow the surgeons to form a hasty plan to group and succor the wounded, when the order would come to fall back. There was nothing to do but apply as many first-aid dressings as practicable to the wounded in the immediate neighborhood of a surgical unit, and then leave them on the field to care for themselves, where those who survived necessarily became prisoners.

It is against the background sketched above that the course taken by the U.S. Army Medical Corps in the development of forward surgery can best be interpreted. The same elements repeat themselves; the lack of planning at the outset, the need to bring surgery forward and the necessity for mobility weighed against the cold surgical fact that proper resuscitation and postoperative care are of importance equal to the operation itself in determining whether a wounded man will survive.

LANDING IN NORTH AFRICA

Records of the management of the wounded in the early phase of landing in North Africa are fragmentary and may even be contradictory. My own diary records the story of the landing in Morocco as related by General Kenner early in March, 1943, four months after the events occurred.

Kenner, as Surgeon of the Western Task Force, landed in the vicinity of Casablanca "with very inadequate help but everyone did a superb job." Approximately 400-burn casualties were treated at a provisional hospital clearing station established on the beach. Ample supplies of plasma were available and only four or five cases were lost. Shore to ship evacuation was feasible at first but within a day or two became impossible because of a twelve-foot surf. Many of our casualties were treated in French military hospitals by French surgeons.

On the night the Armistice was announced, Kenner learned that some U.S. Army casualties were in the Casablanca military hospital. Loading a truck with medical supplies, and driving a jeep, he entered the city and was received cordially by the commandant. Machine gun fire and sniping were still going on that night.

At Oran, the 77th Evacuation Hospital entered in two sections: the first at 1700 hours, November 11, and the second at 0500 hours, November 12. Two hundred and sixteen casualties wounded in action under treatment in two French hospitals were turned over to the surgical personnel for care. One hundred and sixteen of the wounded were at Bauden's Hospital and 100 at the Civile Hospital.

E.D.C. Comment: "Treatment at both hospitals had been done almost exclusively by the French," I recorded in my diary. "The sanitary conditions were very poor and many patients had had no food for three days. Since the French had no plaster of Paris, the many simple and compound fractures as well as extremities with extensive tissue loss were not in casts. Some had been splinted (inadequately) and some not at all. Two patients were still in Army leg traction splints; both were uncomfortable and had developed pressure necrosis. The French had practiced wide excision of wounds, very liberal implantation of sulfanilamide and a tight gauze packing. This last procedure caused marked discomfort as well as other deleterious effects, and the packs were loosened or removed as quickly as possible. Records consisted of scraps and bits of paper in, to us, unreadable French. There was, naturally, no clothing, except that which the patients had on entrance, and bathing of patients had been almost nil. Soap was practically nonexistent.

"Equipment available to care for the wounded consisted of two sets of emergency instruments and two boxes of sterile dressings, plaster of Paris and drugs (picked up here and there), all carried in our luggage. This was augmented by instruments owned and carried by individual officers. We had no instruments or supplies from our own equipment which was unloaded several days after the acute need.

"For practical purposes, nearly all open wounds were infected, about 40 per cent of these enough so as to require hot packs or drainage. In most cases treatment of these wounds had been delayed and improperly done and their condition further aggravated by dressing with none too sterile dressings and inadequate equipment."

In the landing at Algiers, affairs were little better. An extract from a report by Major Paul L. Dent, M.C., provides a vivid picture of the lack of organization of the medical service from the point of view of the commanding officer of a detachment of surgical teams.

"On November 8, 1942, the 39th Task Force, part of the 9th Division, anchored off Charley Red Beach near Surkouf, thirteen miles east of Algiers about 1:00 A.M. The Navy medical personnel set up an aid station on the beach after the beachhead was secured. The plan was to evacuate casualties to the ships until it was thought safe to land a clearing station. This plan was never carried through because the sea was too rough to land equipment. At 1:00 P.M., November 8, 1942, the ship received a radio call to send medical personnel ashore. Captain Dent and Captain Mansfield were asked to go ashore and determine what medical equipment was needed. We landed about 4:00 P.M., but were never able to contact the ship again, due to roughness of the water. No more landing barges were dispatched. Captain Mansfield and myself assisted the Naval personnel in the Aid Station, Sunday evening and night, November 8, 1942. The only supplies available were dressings and morphine. We could not evacuate casualties to the ship and had no instructions from the Task Force Surgeon as to the disposition of them on land by the morning of November 9, 1942. We evacuated some twenty odd patients to the dispensary at the Air Field, Maison Blanche fifteen miles southeast of Algiers, by truck and French ambulances. We were no better off here in the way of equipment, but did have a building and Captain Mansfield and myself had to do the cooking, feeding and complete care of the patients. Not having received any instructions from the Force Surgeon, we loaded the casualties in French ambulances and Captain Dent rode with them through the lines to the French Army Hospital in Algiers. After explaining our situation, the French Commandant was very sympathetic and promised to care for our casualties until our own medical installations could be landed and set up.

"We evacuated to the French until Wednesday night, November 11, averaging about twenty to thirty casualties a day, mostly from the heavy bombings of the air field where we were located.

"Captain Roller, who was in charge of the collecting station with the Task Force, landed on Sunday, November 8, but had no equipment.

He loaned four of his enlisted men to us Tuesday, November 10, to help care for the patients.

"Our ships docked at Algiers on the evening of November 11, and we set up in a school building in Maison Carrée, with Captain Yancy's Clearing Station. Our two general surgical, one orthopedic and one shock team did our first surgery here, on November 12, 1942.

"At 4:00 A.M. November 13, I received orders to report to the Task Force Surgeon's office immediately. We received orders to move with Captain Yancy's Clearing Station and Captain Roller's Collecting Station, to the vicinity of the Fort de l'Eau. We all set up together in a school building in the town of Fort de l'Eau.

"Moving for my group was very difficult. We had no transportation. All the other units were short on transportation, and we had to wait until they were moved so that we could borrow their trucks.

"During the following week, casualties were evacuated to us from the Air Field at Maison Blanche. Most of them were due to bomb fragments, antipersonnel mines and booby traps. They all had multiple wounds including extremities, abdomen, chest and heads; in all, twenty-two casualties required major operating procedures. We evacuated casualties to the 94th General Hospital (British) as soon as possible: six to twelve hours. We had no facilities for postoperative care and no trained personnel to care for the patients.

"On November 22, at 3:30 P.M. orders were received to move to a winery at Les Quatres Chemins, about ten miles North of Algiers. (Clearing, Collecting and Surgical Group.) Moving was complicated again by lack of transportation.

"The winery was small, filthy, cold and damp and did not have space for work at all, so our equipment was not unpacked. We were bothered frequently by air raids and the raining of shrapnel on the roof.

"On November 23 at 10:30 P.M. we received orders to move, but this was cancelled shortly after. November 23 and 24 were spent in trying to find a fit location to move to. Captain Roller and Captain Dent roamed the country in the mire and mud looking for adequate quarters with no assistance or direction from headquarters. Finally on November 25, we moved to another winery near Bafa Hassen, the men sleeping on top of the wine vats and the officers under the vats. The buildings were very damp and cold and there was no available way to heat them. There was no tentage available to set up here, so we only treated a few minor injuries.

(continued)

"On November 28, 1942, we received orders detaching us (1st and 2nd Surgical Teams, 1 Orthopedic and 1 Shock Team) from the 39th Task Force and attaching us to Special Troops EAF. The same day at 1:30 P.M. the surgical group received orders to the British Cottage Hospital in Algiers. Again we wasted a lot of time and energy trying to procure transportation. Headquarters issued orders but furnished no means of executing them. Surgical Team #2 and Shock Team #1 were ordered to the Petit Lycee Headquarters of Special Troops in Algiers on November 29, 1942. The Petit Lycee is situated near the docks and the two teams were to set up an Aid Station there to take care of the bomb casualties. Jerry stopped his raids, so there was no work.

"Surgical Team #1 and Orthopedic Team #1, at the British Cottage Hospital, with a nice place with sufficient equipment, received very few casualties.

"December 7, 1942, orders were received transferring the Shock Team to British Cottage Hospital and the Orthopedic Team to the Petit Lycee. We were alerted and asked by Major Creighton, acting Surgeon to A.F.H.Q., what equipment we needed for a ten day period of action. We furnished a list which included one hundred vials of plasma. We had only four vials and could not obtain more. The British installations had sufficient amounts but would not divide with us. We also needed heating units for sterilization, autoclave and drums, transportation, orthopedic instruments and gauze. None of these supplies was available."

II CORPS IN TUNISIA

The following extracts from the report of the Surgeon, II Corps, provides the necessary background for an understanding of the problems of forward surgery in the southern Tunisian campaign. The conduct of forward surgery was obviously the starting point for the Surgical Consultant of the theater.

"On 1, January 1943, II Corps was designated to proceed from Oran to Tunisia and participate in operations. The period 6 January to 21 January was occupied in planning and in concentration of troops in the Constantine-Tebessa area. For the operation there was set up one armored division, one infantry battalion and various corps troops consisting of anti-aircraft, anti-tank, tank destroyer battalion, etc., as well as various service elements. A French force of approximately 5,000 was attached to the Corps on the left.

"The concentration of supplies in the Tebessa area was begun immediately. The base of supply was in Oran and difficulty was experienced in obtaining the necessary special items of medical supplies and equipment. During the second phase of the operation an advance depot was set up in Constantine.

"The medical units concentrated in the Tebessa area consisted of the following:

"9th Evacuation Hospital, 750 bed;
77th Evacuation Hospital, 750 bed;
48th Surgical Hospital, 400 bed;
51st Medical Battalion;
2nd Battalion, 16th Medical Regiment;
1st Advance Section, 2nd Medical Supply Depot.

"Upon arrival in the Tebessa area, the 9th Evacuation Hospital was established 12 miles south of Tebessa. The 48th Surgical Hospital established one hospitalization section at Feriana, the other section moving to vicinity of Thala. The 77th Evacuation Hospital was held in reserve until 14 February, when it established lightly 12 miles south of Tebessa. The advance section of the Supply Depot was established 10 miles south of Tebessa.

"At the time of the Kasserine Pass breakthrough (16 to 20 February) all medical installations were withdrawn to vicinity of Aine Beida. Seven hundred patients were moved with the hospitals because of lack of facilities for evacuation to the rear.

"Immediately following 21 February the defense line was reformed and additional units concentrated in the area with a view toward taking the offensive tactically. The major units brought into the Corps at this time were the 9th Infantry Division, 34th Infantry Division and the remainder of the 1st Infantry Division. This gave the Corps a total of three infantry divisions and one armored division, together with additional Corps and service troops. The total troops under Corps control numbered about 90,000. A request for additional medical facilities, one field hospital, one 400-bed evacuation hospital and additional ambulances was made. None of these was secured until the end of the second phase after the peak load of casualties had passed.

(*continued*)

"The Corps line during this period extended from the vicinity of Maktar through a point east of Sbeitla to east of Gafsa. With the limited troops available a number of small separate forces were organized. In order to cover these various forces, it was necessary to utilize Clearing Platoons of the two Corps medical battalions, reinforced by surgical and shock teams, as small forward hospitals. These units were located as follows: one west at Maktar, one at Sbeitla, one at Gafsa and, for a short period, one at Sened Station, east of Gafsa. These units were mobile and could be moved quickly. Additional surgical and shock teams were attached to Corps, giving in all six surgical teams, four shock teams, and one orthopedic team.

"Initial medical supplies were adequate and there was no difficulty in maintaining an adequate supply of items contained in medical maintenance units. The greatest difficulty in supply was encountered in replacing items of organizational equipment for hospitals and field units. It was necessary to augment the T/BA equipment of hospitals materially in order that they might function efficiently at near full capacity.

"Evacuation from forward units was accomplished by the 51st Medical Battalion and the 16th Medical Regiment (2nd Bn.). This latter unit was placed entirely in support of the 1st U.S. Armored Division. Evacuation to the base was entirely by air until 16 February when it was stopped by unfavorable flying conditions. A section of the 6th Motor Ambulance Corps of the British First Army then supplied evacuation by road to the 61st Station Hospital at El Guerrah.

"The first major operation by the II Corps in Tunisia covered the period 17 March to 9 April, inclusive, and is known as the Second Phase of the Tunisian Campaign. The front covered a line Gafsa—Maknassy—Faid—Fondouk. The 1st U.S. Armored Division took the offensive initially, operating toward Maknassy. The 1st U.S. Infantry Division moved south toward Gafsa. The 34th Infantry Division was in a defense position in the vicinity of Feriana later taking the offensive against Fondouk and Faid, while the 9th Infantry Division was committed to action in the El Guettar area.

"In support of this four division attack was the 9th Evacuation Hospital, the 77th Evacuation Hospital and the 48th Surgical Hospital. The first section of the 48th Surgical Hospital was moved into Feriana and received the early flow of casualties from Gafsa—El Guettar area. On April 22, the second section was moved to Gafsa and handled casualties from both Maknassy and El Guettar. The 9th Evacuation Hospital located at Youks-les-Bains received transfers from the 48th Surgical and many initial casualties from the forward areas. The 77th Evacuation Hospital established first at La Meskiana moved to Tebessa. These two 750-bed Evacuation Hospitals were hard pushed to handle the peak load of casualties.

"A platoon of the 51st Medical Battalion was set up in the French Hospital at Gafsa with two surgical and two shock teams. The clearing platoon of 'D' company, 2nd Battalion, 16th Medical Regiment was located at Sbeitla and covered the reception of casualties from the 34th Division until the 15th Evacuation Hospital was set up on 10 April at the end of the operation. The 2nd Clearing Platoon, 2nd Battalion, 16th Medical Regiment was located 15 miles west of Maknassy in support of the 1st Armored Division.

"Evacuation to the Base was by air from the field at Youks-les-Bains, by rail from Tebessa to Constantine, and by road to El Guerrah."

AN EXPEDIENT

It is to be noted that the use of clearing platoons, reinforced by surgical and shock teams, as small forward hospitals was an expedient to provide medical service to small separate mobile combat forces on a wide front, otherwise covered only by two 750-bed evacuation hospitals and one surgical hospital. In this sense it was an effort to bring surgical aid forward, but without planned triage or adequate facilities for the management of a concentration of the most seriously wounded. The result was that the reinforced clearing platoons functioned as miniature evacuation hospitals, performing initial surgery on as many casualties as they could handle and, under stress, passing the patients who could travel farther to the rear (**Figure 7.1**).

In addition to these provisional hospitals, there were also the treatment stations of the 47th (Armored) Medical Battalion of the 1st Armored Division equipped with operating trucks to perform emergency surgery.

It is not surprising, in view of these many independent units staffed by personnel inexperienced in wound management, to find confusion of function and procedure. It is perhaps more surprising to note the high quality of surgery that was performed, and that from this brief experience the concept of a pattern of forward surgery emerged that required little subsequent modification.

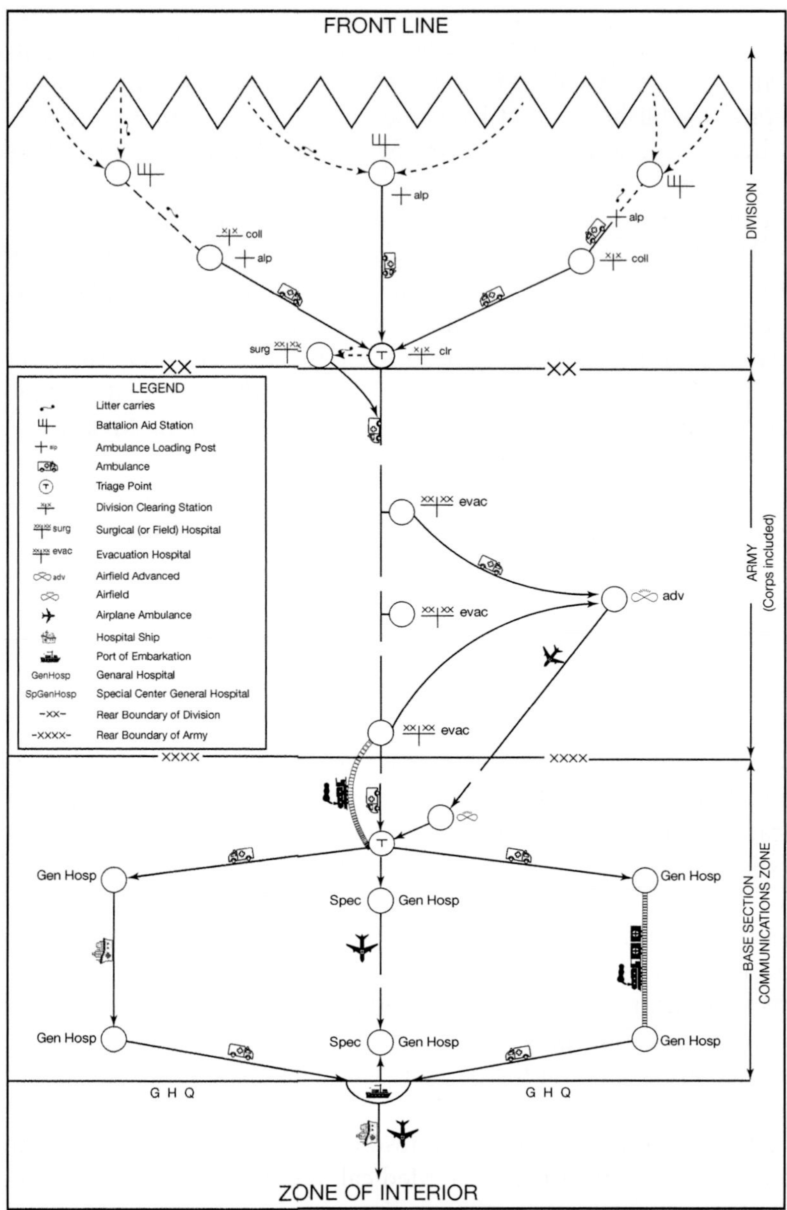

Figure 7.1 Diagram of medical facilities in a theater of operations.

The status of forward surgery at this time was presented in the "1943 Annual Report of the Surgical Consultant to the Surgeon, NATOUSA" as follows:

NORTH AFRICA THEATER OF OPERATIONS,
UNITED STATES OF AMERICA

"Most of the work was done under quite adverse circumstances, without the essentials, to say nothing of the niceties and decorum of a well-regulated operating room. Clearing Stations, corps or division, are not adequately equipped for the performance of major surgery. The personnel of the surgical teams attached to Clearing Platoons during the recent campaign devoted at least 50 per cent of their time and energy making preparation for the care of the wounded. An adequate supply of pre-sterilized linen was not available. Hours were spent laundering and sterilizing our used linen in a miniature autoclave, which proved entirely inadequate. The lack of any suction apparatus, particularly in abdominal surgery, was keenly felt. Lighting facilities were, for the most part, inadequate and uncertain. One abdominal operation, with multiple small and large bowel perforations, was performed with the only source of illumination being furnished by flashlights. Imperative evacuation of patients soon after major surgery is not conducive to their recovery. The need for immediate evacuation of our patients was secondary to our proximity to the front, a poorly defended front line with sporadic fluctuations, and our lack of hospital facilities and trained nurses for postoperative care.

"That surgery can be done in a Clearing Platoon is admitted but in so doing its function is seriously impaired and maximum efficiency of the Surgical Teams is not obtained. We, who were elected to fill in the gap between the front line and the Evacuation Hospitals 100 to 150 miles to the rear, during the Tunisian Campaign, in an installation not designed for major surgery, will welcome the opportunity of doing our work in the future under circumstances more conducive to the recovery of our patients."

Jamison S. Nielsen, Martin A. Schreiber, and Kenneth L. Mattox

A caution and a challenge appear in the opening paragraph of this chapter. "It is still disturbing to recall how unprepared our nation was for war and the lack of knowledge that was displayed by the officers of the regular Army Medical Corps about the conduct of other wars." Sacrifice is often necessary to meet military objectives. That does not mean human suffering and life lost remain a foregone conclusion—preparation saves lives. Actions to mitigate casualty numbers speak both to a nation's values and to its combat effectiveness. Unfortunately, the unpredictable timing and frequency of war present significant impediments to preparation and skill maintenance. As is the case of wars before and since, difficult lessons in the care of combat casualties were relearned in World War II.

It is well established that during interwar periods, focus, funding, and training all shift away from battlefield medicine. Allocation of finite resources contributes significantly to this cycle. As Churchill notes, "The logistical burden imposed on the Army by its Medical Corps is enormous." Without funding or attention, lessons learned were lost. Fortunately, the past was able to speak through the book *Field Surgery in Total War* carried in Churchill's luggage. Aspects of the "three-point forward system" can be seen in Figure 7.1 (p. 98) that bears a striking resemblance to the current Roles of Care structure.

Colonel Churchill makes the case that human dignity justifies, if not demands, the primacy of medical care. Other services such as the Post Office, Red Cross, the Canteen, chaplains, and the Graves Registration Service are given as examples whose primary function is soldier dignity. The dignity discussion factors into treatment priorities in limited resource settings: treat those with the most severe injuries or those with greatest continuing utility in the fight? General Patton's sentiment (in more colorful language) that a soldier with a traumatic amputation should be allowed to die reflects a utilitarian "military" approach. The institution of "triage based on the urgency of the wound" to "save life irrespective of the future military potential" reconciled the opposing "military" and "surgical" views.

After settling the triage debate, the issue of *where* and *when* surgical care occurred remained an open question. Larger hospitals had more personnel, a greater array of specialists, and more supplies, but they were far removed from the point of injury and were much less mobile. Forward, smaller, mobile hospitals were more nimble and closer to the fight but had fewer capabilities. The ultimate solution learned through trial and error favored forward resuscitation and surgery. "Nothing but the best is good enough for the surgical treatment of patients in the forward areas. It is here, rather than at the base, that the fate of the wounded man is so often decided." The forward mobile surgical team structure remains, but discussions regarding scope and scale to match need continue to the present day.

Roughly three generations following World War II, the conversations and practice decisions surrounding combat casualty care bear a striking resemblance to those described in this text. Those entrusted with command authority must strike a balance between providing guidance based upon sound doctrine and agility to respond to a complex and dynamic operational reality. Just as in Colonel Churchill's era, today's military surgeons should advise line leaders, inform doctrine, and assume appropriate risk to minimize death and suffering during war.

SUGGESTED READINGS

Cubano MA, Senior Editor. *Emergency War Surgery*. 5th ed. Office of the Surgeon General, Borden Institute; 2018.

Jolly D. *Field Surgery in Total War*. Hamish Hamilton Medical Books; 1940.

Mabry RL, DeLorenzo R, Challenges to improving combat casualty survival on the battlefield. *Mil Med*. 2014;179(5):477-482.

Remondelli MH, Remick KN, Shackelford SA, et al. Casualty care implications of large-scale combat operations. *J Trauma Acute Care Surg*. 2023 Aug 1;95(2S Suppl 1):S180-S184.

8

Diary and Letters of a Forward Surgeon

MAJOR KENNETH LOWRY was leader of a surgical team of the 2nd Auxiliary Surgical Group. His brother "Frosty" was his assistant. Ken Lowry was older than many of the surgeons in the Group and in civilian life had conducted a general surgical practice in Ohio. The Lowry brothers were painstaking and reliable surgeons, especially conscientious in following the course of their patients after they had been evacuated to the rear.

The Lowry team landed in the vicinity of Algiers. They then moved to Gafsa in southern Tunisia. Here they supported the Rangers and the Kasserine Pass threatened breakthrough. I first saw Lowry in the French barracks at Feriana on March 19, 1943. We remained good friends.

The following are some excerpts from his diary and letters. (See Chapter 12, The Tunisian Campaign under "First Trip with Weddell," for other entries in his diary.)

MAJOR KENNETH LOWRY DIARY AND LETTERS

January 24, 1943—Sunday P.M. *(Letter)*

Our operating room and hospital is located close by in one of the French hospital buildings. This is of modern construction with tile floors. The walls are of stone and cement, or stucco. As there is no heat we have put up a G.I. stove in our O.R. and another in our postoperative ward. There was no equipment, whatever, in this building but Capt. Poupart, the C.O. of the French hospital, has been very kind in loaning us some equipment which they are not using. Of course there is much to be desired as we have no x-ray, no suction or anesthesia machine, and our methods for sterilizing and autoclaving are most inadequate. Our sterilizer, for example, is only slightly larger than the one in my office and is heated over an old kerosene stove. Our gowns, gloves, and linens are autoclaved in a small pressure cooker which is also heated over the kerosene stove.

January 25, 1943—(Diary)

What a night we just had! Through yesterday and last night we have thirty-four casualties. Frosty and I ran both operating tables almost constantly, not finishing up until 4:00 A.M. They were bringing in the wounded so fast we could take care of only the more seriously injured. I am sure I can say that the care and attention some of these German patients are receiving is equal to what we give our own. We have hatred, of course, for the race, the government and all it stands for, but not for the individual.

Our first casualty was a Lieutenant from Jersey City with a ragged gunshot wound through the inner aspect of right upper arm, and another through the right wrist. One of the Germans had (1) severe shock, (2) severe hematoma of anterior abdominal wall with no penetrating wound, but clinical evidence of intra-abdominal injury. On exploration, he was found to have a large tear in his anterior stomach, liver, mesentery and omentum, and a large extra-peritoneal hematoma in the left flank. I am at a loss to explain his injuries unless due to blast. Another, an old Arab, had a penetrating sucking wound of his anterior chest wall and a mangled right hand. We débrided and closed his chest wound and amputated his forearm. Although he nearly died on the table, he picked up and was in good shape when we evacuated him this A.M. Another had a compound, badly comminuted fracture dislocation of the left elbow, multiple fractured ribs, and a severe hemothorax. I was up at 7:30 A.M., saw all the operatives and evacuated them back to the 9th Evac. by ambulance. We dislike evacuating so early but we are not equipped for any extensive postoperative care and, anyway, we have been directed by higher authority to hold our patients no longer than twenty-four hours. Our proximity to a not too strongly defended front line also makes it advisable for us not to get bogged down with postoperatives.

January 29, 1943—(Diary)

This has been a very busy day. Early this A.M. Mme. LeFebvre told me that Capt. Poupart wanted me to see one of his French soldiers who had been injured in a motorcycle accident. The Captain suspected a ruptured liver with intraperitoneal hemorrhage. I rather disagreed with him as there was no outward evidence of shock, pulse was normal, abdomen not rigid, and there was no evidence of fractured ribs. I suggested giving him a hypo for his pain and promised to see him later if they wished

(continued)

me to do so. As I was telling the boys about it, Frosty casually asked about his blood pressure. Outwardly, I tried to appear cool as I said I had not taken it, but inside I was most perturbed and soon found an excuse to leave the circle and although I ambled out slowly, I hurried, when alone, to the operating room, procured a blood pressure manometer and hustled back to the French dispensary. I found his B.P. 80/40, his pulse, now, not so good and his right upper abdomen definitely tender. I talked with Capt. Poupart and told him of the change in his patient and advised immediate surgery. As the French Captain was not a surgeon, and since it was one hundred miles back to the nearest French hospital at Tebessa, he asked if we would operate. When I assured him we would be only too glad to take the best care possible of him, I did not take into consideration Army red tape about which I know little. I was briefly but definitely told that we could not operate on him—Army Regulations—Bah! During considerable argument, which I would like to forget, the soldier was rapidly going into severe shock. He could not possibly live to get to Tebessa, so, in spite of Army Regulations we operated. Frosty and the French Captain assisted, while George gave the anesthetic and Dan helped run plasma and glucose into his veins. We felt fortunate to keep him alive until we got through. What he needed, of course, was blood and lots of it, but there was no time to wait until a suitable donor (French) could be obtained, typed, and cross matched. When our incision reached the peritoneum it was blue and bulging. He had the most tremendous intra-abdominal hemorrhage I have ever seen. How we needed suction apparatus! We found multiple deep, crushing lacerations of the liver, some of which seemed to extend almost through. While I compressed the portal vein and hepatic artery, Frosty mopped out. Two large packs were placed around the liver and brought out through a stab wound in the right flank. Exploration also revealed two small lacerations of his spleen which under other less grave circumstances would have called for a removal of that organ. We were forced to risk a delayed secondary hemorrhage from that source, and get out. He has now been given two transfusions of blood and will be given more tomorrow. George tells me that his B.P. had gone down to less than 50/30 while on the table, but it is now 120/80 and his pulse is of good volume. His R.B.C. is only 1,400,000 so he needs plenty of blood yet. I have been asked to get the patient out so that will be done and no record made of his care in our hands. I still insist, however, he will not be moved till it is safe for him. Permission was obtained sometime later from the Corps Surgeon to work with the French and assist on care for any casualties which they were not prepared or equipped to handle.

February 2, 1943—(Letter)

We have been very, very busy. At one time we were in our O.R. for eighteen hours without a let-up. In fact, it was during this particular time that I did not have my clothes off for forty-eight hours. Frosty and I are both feeling fine and thrilled with our work and experiences.

February 2, 1943—(Diary)

Beginning at 4:00 P.M. on the 31st, casualties began pouring in. We started operating at once and kept at it through the night, not stopping till 10:30 next A.M. Just now, 8:00 P.M., two more ambulance loads have come in. Frosty reports that casualties are on litters all over the floor of the dispensary. Surely we are taking an awful lacing between here and Maknessey. From one company of over two hundred men, thirty-two are now living.

I certainly have a real operating crew. They are all willing to work until they drop and with never a word of complaint. We have had all types of surgery; sucking chest wounds, abdominal wounds, compound fractures, and amputations of arms, legs, feet, and thighs. Some have had an arm or leg either partially or entirely blown off, so we have no choice. To date we have lost only one case here, a lower one-third thigh amputation with multiple wounds of the left leg and thigh. He was in profound shock in spite of 1,500 cc. of plasma, 500 cc. of blood and lots of glucose. The operation did not increase his shock, but neither did he improve. More blood might have helped. *Blood is so precious! So urgently needed!* What we do give is being obtained from our own personnel who are most willing, but they really need it themselves after putting in long hours without rest or sleep.

We could not find a donor for a splendid chap from Maine last night. He was in severe shock and needed something in addition to plasma and glucose, so Frosty gave his blood, took a short rest and went back to operating again. We had to amputate his right lower thigh, do a débridement and open reduction on a compound fracture of his left tibia and fibula and then remove a shell fragment from the left temporal region. He was evacuated back in good condition this evening.

They are strafing the road between here and Tebessa every day, killing and wounding our men, burning our supply and ration trucks. Rommel is reported in Gabes, eighty-five miles from here. Our rations are only C and even those are very skimpy. We are often hungry.

(continued)

February 3, 1943—(Letter)

I cannot help but add one remark which I have observed in our work. Dried human plasma is saving hundreds of lives that would surely otherwise be lost. Of course whole blood is better but is more difficult to obtain.

February 4, 1943—(Diary)

I went out to the cemetery with "Chappie" for a burial service for several of our boys. There are now sixty-seven (American) graves in our little cemetery. Only two of these, including our Corporal, died in our care. The others have been brought in dead.

February 11, 1943—(Diary)

We just had two thoracic cases that were quite interesting. One, an English soldier, had a sucking wound which we had to close without locating the bullet because of his poor condition. He had some cord symptoms and I fear the bullet may have lodged in his spinal canal. How George does need an anesthetic machine. These patients could be operated so much more easily and with much less risk under endotracheal anesthesia. We have had one or two very close calls trying to do them under pentothal, so we are doing nearly all of them under local and are doing just as little as we can to get them in condition for transportation back to the 9th Evac. where Colonel Berry can take care of them.

Lt. Col. Wiley, Lt. Col. Anspacher from Second Corps Headquarters and Major Howard Snyder, Chest Surgeon of the 77th Evac. were here overnight and left this morning. One of them had brought a bottle of real honest-to-goodness aged in the wood whiskey. It must have been strong for I surely got to feeling good before the evening was over. We had some very interesting discussions on operative treatment, value of plasma in shock, blast, and concussion injuries, etc. We learned we had used close to one hundred units of plasma since we have been in Gafsa and that is probably more than any other group in No. Africa.

February 13, 1943—(Diary)

Gee, but we have been busy. Ranger casualties began pouring in at 8:30 A.M. yesterday. We operated straight through till 1:00 A.M. today. We had many interesting cases; one, a sucking chest wound with a bullet hole through his right external ear, entering the right mastoid region, going down into the neck; many extremity cases. There was one gunshot wound entering the right popliteal, coming out of the calf of the right leg, apparently severing the popliteal artery. A large hematoma was found. When he was evacuated his leg was warm but there was no anterior or posterior tibial pulsation. It might be saved, but I don't know. Frosty had an Italian prisoner with a compound fracture of the neck of the right humerus. In fact, that part of the bone along with considerable muscle was shot away. Blood and nerve supply, by some miracle, was O.K. He did a nice débridement and reduction.

These Rangers are certainly a swell lot. They are made up entirely of hand-picked, commando-trained volunteers. They are not the least hard-boiled and tough like we expected they'd be, but we find them mild-mannered, well-behaved and all anxious to get back to duty. They took their injuries without a complaint.

February 14, 1943—(Diary)

Yesterday we had an officer with a subdural hemorrhage due to his walking into a mine he had set himself. He had three head wounds and multiple wounds of extremities. At the beginning of the operation his pulse was 58 and his B.P. 240/90. We débrided and explored his head wounds then found and ligated the source of bleeding. At the end of the operation his B.P. was 110/70 and pulse 120. He was evacuated immediately.

We just learned that the Arab with the sucking chest wound and right forearm amputation had done very nicely—in fact, well enough to be led before a firing squad (French) and shot as a spy. The French soldier with the liver injury has been evacuated further back than Tebessa hospital so is apparently doing O.K.

February 16, 1943—(Diary)

It is now 8:00 P.M. We are in a wall tent out in the middle of a sandy plain between two mountains (Kasserine Pass). The wind is blowing a gale and we wonder if our tent will stay up. It is bitter cold, too, and as I try to write I find it necessary to stop and warm my hands occasionally over one of our coal-oil heaters. Thank God for those even though the heat they give is slight.

While we were eating supper Sunday, Capt. Huber who had come down to Gafsa in the afternoon and Capt. Lichtenstein returned from a meeting and informed us that we were to pack and leave immediately.

(continued)

It seemed most apparent that we were not going to put up a fight for Gafsa. The Germans had, that morning, started a drive north of us and we were taking a lacing. Within two hours we were loaded on trucks and on our way. When we hit the main road from Gafsa to Feriana we found ourselves in the largest wholesale evacuation we had ever seen. The road was clogged with a steady stream of trucks loaded with men and equipment. The French and the Arabs were on the move also, on foot and using every conceivable conveyance imaginable. Everything about the retreat or withdrawal was quite orderly. It was a beautiful moonlight night and we travelled in a strict blackout and kept a sharp lookout for Jerry planes.

Midway to Feriana we were met by Major Wilkinson (Exec. Officer of 51st) who told me our team would stop off at Feriana and work with the 1st platoon, taking over buildings which were then being evacuated by the 48th Surgical Hospital. We stopped, as ordered, but had to wait until midnight to begin moving in as the 48th had not completely evacuated. They left several patients too sick to transport, among them the brain case we had operated the 13th. At about 1:00 A.M., Capt. Mansfield and Lt. Berlin of Major Dent's team (2nd Aux.) came in with orders to take over and told us to report back to 51st Headquarters near Tebessa. We decided to remain there for the night, however. Next morning I met Major Dent and, through him, learned that I might pick up one or two pyramidal tents from the 2nd Corps bakery. As we went on our way again we saw hundreds of troops going through the hospital area on foot, and on the road many troops, French and Arab civilians with what personal belongings they could load in a cart or on the back of a jackass.

We arrived at the 51st just before noon and found them out in pup tents. I borrowed a vehicle and went to Corps Headquarters on several errands. They were so well concealed in thick wooded mountains that I had a heck of a time finding them. I then went to the Corps Surgeon's Hdq. to enlist his aid for the pyramidal tents held by the bakery. The Corps Surgeon was out but there was Lt. Col. _________, later known as "Beartracks" (because of his big feet), asking the Asst. Corps Surgeon for our team to go with one of his platoons to a nice, choice spot in the open. Well, here we are, the worst place I can imagine in which to do any surgery. The air is full of dust and sand; everything is covered with dirt thirty seconds after it is exposed. Might as well state that the Asst. C.S. did not think it would be at all patriotic to ask for tents for ourselves; for patients, that would be different.

When I arrived back at the 51st, Frosty, Dan, George and our E.M. were already dug in and comfortably fixed up in their pup tents. Golly, how I hated to tell them. We left at 6:00 P.M. and travelled over about the roughest roads we have found yet, arriving here at midnight. It was so cold our hands and feet were numb. The entire hospital set-up of tents was spread from one hundred to one hundred and fifty feet apart. Any patients admitted for shock, operated, and then taken to a ward tent would have been carried one-fourth to one-half mile. We were again informed that that was "Army Regulations."

February 19, 1943—(Diary)

On the move again. We were just above Kasserine Pass when my last note was written. About 6:00 A.M. next day, we were awakened with the news to move out in a hurry; Rommel's forces were within six miles of us and still coming. During the night I had awakened several times and had heard trucks and tanks on the go so I was more or less expecting something, although I kept hoping they were moving up. Not being particularly anxious to work for Rommel, we tore down in a hurry, really glad to leave that dust bowl. As we were just ready to leave, some Jerry planes came over making us all scurry for the ditches. We truly believe that a red cross painted on a large tent fly not taken up yet, was all that saved us from a strafing. We could not return by the road we had come as it had been mined. About three o'clock we pulled into a forest on a mountain top and had our chow. It was very cold but we built a fire and did manage to get our feet warm. Major Barker, Exec. Officer of the 16th, arrived and he and the Lieutenant had a brief conference over maps. None of the rest of us were allowed a "sit-in." We received our orders only from the Sergeant, and they were always the same—"Let's go! Let's go! Come on! Get the lead out—!"

Our destination for this move proved to be another woods about six miles south and west of Thala. It was after dark and quite cold. Frosty and I put our pup tents together end for end, and did manage to shut out some of the cold. We got tucked in and were really pounding an ear when about 12:30 A.M. we again heard that Sergeant's infernal "Let's go!" This time he added that we had just one-half hour before shoving off, so he got no argument as we realized the seriousness of the situation. Again we travelled in the moonlight, passing Roman ruins at Haidra, and about 4:00 A.M. came to Tebessa where we caught glimpses of more ruins.

We drove on through Tebessa to Youks les Bains. Here we ran into the 48th Surgical and part of the 9th Evac. Hospital officers. The 48th was just setting up, taking all the 9th Evac. patients as the latter are being

(continued)

forced to move back from their location on the other side of Tebessa. One cannot help but wonder *when* we are going to win this war. The 48th have just received my brain case from the 9th and tell us he is somewhat better. I wonder how he can stand all this moving around. (Note—Regret to say this patient died three or four days later.)

We drove on through Youks les Bains a mile or so, into a field then out, and after a wait of a half hour or more, back in the field again and there we sat until daylight. We tried to get a little sleep sitting up but at daybreak we were on our way again, but not far. On a barren hill we stopped, unloaded the trucks which moved out immediately. I had tried to contact Major Barker or the Lieutenant but was unsuccessful. Again we were feeling stranded, cold and miserable. All we needed was to be put with an outfit for action. To my dismay I learned that Corps Headquarters was in the process of moving back some fifty miles, also that 9th and 77th Evac. had started a fifty mile move to the rear. Rumors were filtering in with casualties that we were taking one awful lacing. Many of our troops had been surrounded and captured. We had lost one entire tank battalion along with countless supplies, gasoline, guns, ammunition, etc. Retreat? Yes, we were retreating, are retreating. It is rumored that preparations are being made for a final stand in the heights or mountains of Tebessa. Had we held them at Kasserine? Had we been ordered? Well, no one seemed to be sure of anything. Retreat is a ghastly word. Only one who has been a part of or involved in a retreat can realize the full significance and horror which the word implies.

The E.M. have pitched their pup tents together in a deep wadi (ditch) that gives them good protection from the wind. They also helped us pitch the wall tent the 16th had loaned us and we carried our belongings and surgical chests inside for protection against prowling Arabs. This A.M. we made preparation for another move and awaited the promised truck to move us, belongings and equipment. When the truck came it was two-thirds full already, so it would not have been possible to accommodate all of us. After a short delay, we were on the road with the other vehicles going back toward Constantine.

We are now camped on the top of a wooded mountain about two miles off the main highway. I think we are near Ain Bete. Across the valley we can see the tents of the 9th Evac. Hosp. We have a GI stove and for the first time in five days we are warm and comfortable.

Our enlisted men are out in pup tents but our tent is open house for all our men. They come in here to eat, shave and bathe. It is raining so they are all in here now. We certainly have a swell group of men and we consider them just as good as we are. I only wish I could get them in a wall tent. I had to put up a fight to get this one for ourselves.

February 22, 1943—(Letter)

We are on the move again, but this time it is forward. At the present time I am sitting with the driver of a truck in a picturesque little valley off the main road between Tebessa and Haidra. It is pouring down rain. The poor cook and his crew had to prepare our dinner of C rations and coffee out in the rain. Of course we had to stand in the rain to eat and we all felt the coffee was diluted one-fourth before we finished with it. The rain is like ice on our hands. I understand we are headed for Thala but must wait on Major Wilkinson who is looking the situation over first. We are now at least one hundred and twenty-five miles from where many ruins of ancient Roman cities remain.

We have our set-up in tents and have replaced an English casualty clearing station. We could put everything in buildings, but they are pretty dirty and we are somewhat afraid of lice. Last night we slept out in the open. In my sleeping bag I was quite cozy, but it was so cold that my hand got numb while I was finishing my final cigarette. The sun came out today and it surely did feel good.

February 24, 1943—(Diary)

Apparently the situation in Thala was considered too precarious. A terrific battle was said to be in progress there between German tanks and our artillery, yesterday. This finds us at Slata. The last thirty or forty miles of our trip was somewhat eventful. Had we not been delayed in that peaceful valley yesterday waiting for Major W. we would have been caught in the middle of one of the most devastating strafing and bombing incidents I have yet heard of.

As we came along later, there were any number of bomb holes in the roads with burning trucks and vehicles of all kinds. This made necessary many wide detours through the fields. The Jerries certainly had raised hell. There were four English ambulances among the forty or more burning vehicles which had been deliberately strafed.

February 25, 1943—(Letter)

We did have a grand set-up at our last stand (Slata). We had our surgery tent up in wonderful shape and were looking forward to action. Yesterday

(continued)

we cleaned out the building where the British officers had stayed so that we might move in. Then the bad news came, through Major Wilkinson, that we were to move back immediately. That meant that we did not get to even lie down in our gorgeous quarters.

Our convoy of trucks took a supposed short cut over the roughest road I have ever been on. It really was a terrific ride. We left at 7:30 P.M. and arrived in this bivouac area at 3:30 A.M. It was cold, but a clear night, so I put my bedding roll on the ground, blew up my mattress, and crawled in. It took me quite a while to get my feet warm, as they were like chunks of ice. As I looked up into the sky the great dipper seemed directly over me and the stars were so beautiful, but I was too exhausted to enjoy even this beauty very long.

I am now sitting in my pup tent. It is raining and my mind is pretty much on my tent for the night. I have it fairly well ditched but I feel inclined to go out and dig some more if this rain keeps up.

This moving from place to place is really very tiresome. One officer rides with the driver of each truck or ambulance. Absolute blackout must prevail at all times, that is, no lights except very dim, red tail lights. We do not understand all these moves—some of course we do—others seem foolish to us.

March 14, 1943—(Diary)

According to plan, Lt. Col. Batch, Maj. Dent and I went into a meeting at Corps Surgeons today, starting about 8:30 P.M. It was a long miserable drive of about fifty miles as they are now some place near Haidra. Here, to my happy surprise, I found Maj. Bob Garlinghouse. He was certainly a sight for sore eyes and I thanked him profusely for lugging that big sack of mail all the way from Casa. for us. Norris Frank was also there and the three of us had a grand visit after the meeting was over. Lt. Col. Palmer and several of his henchmen of the 16th were also on hand. The entire meeting was devoted to the handling and use of surgical teams in Clearing Stations. Col. Arnest, the Corps Surgeon, and Lt. Col. Anspacher seemed to be quite sold on us and the work we had done but it seems that some pressure is being brought to bear from or through the Surgeon of A.F. Hq. to try in a nice way to string halter us to some extent. In fact, according to higher headquarters we may not even do bellies and chests in Clearing Stations. Our protest to that was loud and long. If we were to do only first aid work, they certainly did not need any surgical teams up in Clearing Stations. We were requested to do no more plating of fractures, not that any trouble had resulted but if it did we would not have a leg to stand on. I think that criticism is entirely justified. Also we were asked to use no tannic acid or coagulants on burns—only sulfathiazole or sulfadiazine ointment. This is a good suggestion, but they better take the tannic acid away from the Battalion Aid Stations for that is where it is being used. They have been smeared before we see them, so we give them a little plasma if they need it and send them on.

March 24, 1943—(Diary)

We moved out of Gafsa about 10 P.M. The road wound around the oasis and in the subdued light of a full moon, the tall date palms, pools of water, and small winding streams were most picturesque. We travelled over a very rough mud road through the ruins of Senid, finally pulling up in a muddy field next to the 47th Medical Battalion and had supper. It was 1 A.M. Frosty and I had eaten with the 51st officers at Gafsa, but we were ready to eat again. I decided to spend the remainder of the night on a stretcher in an ambulance but Frosty, George, and the E.M. laboriously unloaded and put up their cots. Poor Frosty had just finished blowing his air mattress up and getting his sleeping bag warmed when the Sergeant let loose his informal "Let's go." I decided to stay put on the litter in the ambulance. It was impossible to sleep. The road was so rough it almost threw me to the floor several times. This gave me a good idea of the torture a wounded patient suffers in being evacuated over these roads. Maybe as Dent was advocating, it would be more humane to evacuate a postoperative patient back immediately following his surgery while still under partial anesthesia. I have since asked a couple ambulance drivers how long it takes to get a patient back to Gafsa and they said about ten hours (in other words, about five miles an hour).

We arrived at our present location near MaKnassy at daybreak. Almost everyone just stretched out on the ground and went to sleep. About 11 A.M. I was called to the 47th Medical Battalion to see some casualties. They had moved up with us and are set up in the next field. I was quite interested in seeing their surgical operating truck set up and in operation. The truck has a built-in fixed operating table with built-in cabinets and lights. A tent is put up which surrounds the truck on both sides and to the rear providing ample space for two operating litters on each side of the truck. These units have certain advantages, the chief of which is the rapidity with which it can be set up and put into operation and, likewise, torn down again. Frosty and I did a sucking chest wound in the truck and found that we were rather cramped for room. There

(continued)

was an abdominal which we decided to do in our own tent. He was in severe shock and had quite extensive injury to his descending colon as well as multiple perforations of his small intestine. The colon was exteriorized.

March 27, 1943—(Letter)

First of all, let me assure you that we are now quite comfortable and contented in our pyramidal tent. I will admit we are rather close to the front, but we are not in the least uneasy. Wounded soldiers do not stand transportation well and I personally would not complain if we were even a bit closer.

The temperature here is much nicer than any we have had. Often the days are so warm that we can sit with our shirts off, soaking up the sunshine. However, the nights are quite cool, necessitating the bit of heat we can coax out of our coal oil stove.

Our set-up is, of course, now in tents, and these are quite satisfactory. My only objection is the minimum seventy-five yards between the tents, which this platoon commander insists upon. I will admit in the event we were ever bombed, our chances of escaping injury would be much better this way.

I believe we are beginning to know and understand the officers of this platoon better than when we were with them before. Being busy professionally is, I am sure, bringing about a feeling of comradeship. These officers are all young and are eager to learn more about surgery. Frosty and I have made up two teams by using two of them as assistants and George is giving another some training in anesthesia. With this arrangement Frosty takes first call for twenty-four hours in seeing cases which the admitting officer thinks might need our attention, then I see them the next twenty-four hours. While he is on first call, I am on second call and vice versa. Usually we operate only the severely wounded, nontransportable cases and evacuate the others to the rear.

We have been quite busy in spurts. One night Frosty and I were both operating all night. On another night while Frosty was doing an abdominal with a belly full of blood and several holes in the bowel, the lights went out. He did almost all of it with one of the men holding a flashlight. There are lots of adversities, but one can't have everything, so we do the best we can under the circumstances.

From our set-up, the thunder of artillery fire is clearly audible. In fact, now we are almost used to it. On our first two nights, it looked like a fireworks display. However, for the past two days, a fog-like haze has settled over the entire countryside. This, in my opinion, is due to the terribly thick dust which is constantly being thrown into the air by the never ending traffic of trucks, half tracks and tanks, and, of course, heavy artillery and anti-tank guns. No doubt some of the haze is due to artillery fire and bombing, also.

The other day we had an errand up front, so we had a good look at "No Man's Land," if there is such a thing now. All at once we noticed that ours was the only vehicle on the road. An almost death-like quiet prevailed with no sign of life anywhere. We stopped and were just considering turning around when our artillery a mile or so back of us opened up and began exploding shells on a rather high hill in front of us. Our heavy guns were so well concealed we had passed right close to some of them without seeing them. We learned that the Germans were so well entrenched and dug in on this hill that we had thus far been unable to dislodge them. We visited with the artillery boys for a while and enjoyed watching them in action. Nearby we saw the remains of a Messerschmitt (ME 109) that had been brought down the day before. We had previously seen the remains of the pilot. Upon returning to our Clearing Station, we found that the boys had had a little scare. Some Jerries had been over and had bombed and strafed all around our set-up but had absolutely left us alone. That shows they are definitely respecting the Red Cross. The boys say they had ample opportunity to destroy every one of our tents and trucks. Nevertheless, the men started deepening their foxholes after that. We have ours right in one corner, inside our tent. As yet, however, I have not used it. I should not forget those famous "last words," such as "They are ours," referring to planes overhead.

For the most part, our boys do not take any chances. Really at times it is comical, when some enemy planes come over, to look around, you don't see a soul. After they pass, helmet covered heads start popping out of the ground all over the area. Presently, here comes the rest of them out of the foxholes.

No, I have not heard anything to the effect that they will only keep us over here for a year. I surely hope it is true though. We have heard the rumor that we might go back as soon as this African campaign is over, but that really sounds ridiculous, for the war certainly will not be over then. There is only one answer, Germany must be beaten to her knees, and made to answer for her wholesale hostage killings and atrocities.

There has been a small herd of camels grazing nearby, about three hundred yards from our tent, so this afternoon Frosty and I walked over and took several pictures of them. Two young baby camels were quite cute.

(continued)

March 29, 1943—(Diary)

Gee, but it is black out tonight. They have hot coffee over in the Admission tent but I'll swear I could never find it. I did well just now to find my way to our tent without falling into a foxhole.

We have been quite busy. We had several sucking chest wounds with numerous soft tissue wounds. Frosty had a descending colon injury last night that was quite difficult. This afternoon I had a penetrating wound of the right lower posterior chest. He had no chest signs but did have some very definite abdominal signs, i.e. pain, tenderness, and rigidity. Without x-ray one must depend almost entirely upon what he sees, hears, and feels. At operation the bullet was found to have gone through the diaphragm and liver and could be palpated on the under surface to the left of the cystic duct. Just now I had a bad compound fracture of the left knee joint due to gunshot wound.

I am now keeping a record of each case. This is not required but sometime I hope to follow them up.

Yesterday I saw the most pitiful case I have ever seen—a traumatic amputation of the right leg with multiple shell fragment wounds up to and including the lower half of the thigh. The right tibia was protruding three inches. The tissue was gangrenous, smelly, and teeming with maggots. This man had lain out in the field for four days. He was brought in to the 47th and given up to die, but he did not die. They gave him fluids and plasma and kept him for three days. We gave him more glucose and plasma. He had no pulse or blood pressure, yet seemed to be conscious. His lips and face were blistered. All he could say was "Water, water" in a far-away indistinct whisper. We felt that surgery was out of the question, so we evacuated him eight hours after admission to the next hospital installation. (We learned later in a follow-up study that he died six hours after admission to this hospital.) Certainly the long ride of fifty miles over unbelievably rough roads contributed to this man's death. In retrospect it is regretted that he was not held at the Clearing Station for further shock treatment and definitive surgery if and when his general condition warranted. However, I feel the end would have been the same. In our business, with each casualty we have only one chance and we honestly try to use our best judgment.

The Germans have attacked us twice today with heavy casualties on both sides. The local situation is still snafu. There is much traffic on the road tonight.

March 30, 1943—(Diary)

I am all in tonight with good reason. I was called out of bed at 1 A.M. to take care of a bad sucking wound of the left chest through the left scapula. Also a compound fractured skull due to penetrating G.S.W. (gunshot wound). While operating, the Jerries came over, dropped flares all around us. After finishing I watched the spectacular fireworks display for a while until I became so cold I had to turn in. However, there was no sleep from then on. We do not know who they were after for there are no other military installations in our immediate vicinity. We would hear them coming, then the explosions on all sides of us shook the ground and our tent. It is a sensation which cannot be adequately described. We wait and wait, outside it is pitch blackness except for the light of the flares. We hear our boys scampering for their foxholes. The off-beat drone of the planes gets closer and closer then suddenly those terrific explosions are too close. We think the concussions will cause our tent to fall in. The ground fairly trembles. It is a relief to be called to surgery again. At least our minds will be occupied. We almost pray for dawn so we can at least see the planes and they can see our Red Cross. Sometimes I feel it would be safer if we could illuminate our Red Cross at night but that would not be fair to other installations as it would give the Jerries a landmark to go by.

I took a picture today of an unexploded 500-pound bomb which the Jerries had dropped about two hundred yards from our tent. This A.M. I did an interesting abdominal with perforations of his ascending colon.

April 1, 1943—(Diary)

By 10 A.M. we began getting casualties that kept Frosty and me running two tables until supper time. Then four of us tore in on a poor chap with at least fifty shell fragment wounds, one of which had completely destroyed his left eye, another had penetrated the left frontal region fracturing his skull, while still another had torn out his right cheek.

I guess we will have to send Corporal P________ back. He is one of the 16th E.M. who works in surgery and is a good boy there, too. He is frightened stiff, cries frequently and just can't keep from running and jumping into his foxhole every time he hears a plane. He was out four times during the night and virtually lives in his foxhole during the day. This fear must be terrible.

(continued)

April 8, 1943—(Diary)

Frosty had a most interesting case on the 5th. This man had a G.S.W. of his right upper arm which had resulted in a compound fracture of his humerus and severed his axillary artery and vein. Obviously amputation would be needed but he had lost a tremendous amount of blood and had no pulse or blood pressure. We put both of our coal heaters under his litter, with blankets down on both sides and over him. Frosty then nursed him along all night, and, with great difficulty, because of his collapsed veins gave him plasma, glucose, and blood. However, when I saw him with Frosty during the morning of the 6th, he had not reacted and still had no pulse or blood pressure. Rigor mortis had developed in his right arm. Finally near noon, Frosty did a rapid disarticulation at the shoulder joint and during the operation the patient developed a faint pulse and a perceptible blood pressure for the first time. He rapidly improved during the afternoon and night and had a good pulse and B.P. when we evacuated him yesterday morning.

(In early June we just missed seeing this patient before he was evacuated to the United States from Casablanca. According to available hospital records and talks with his ward officers, he was ambulatory and in good general condition. There are surgeons who will say the above case is not possible. I will admit that it is most unusual for a patient to remain without a perceptible pulse and blood pressure for thirty-six hours and live.)

I was on first call on the 6th and we had a regular field day of interesting cases. Four were severe compound fractures, one of which involved not only his tibia and fibula, but also his femur on the same side; one, a sucking wound; and another, a torn spleen. We also had several less severe cases. We finished about 1:00 A.M. feeling that we had really earned our salt that day.

On the 7th came Col. Forsee and with him Maj. Howard Snyder, Maj. Dent and Lt. Jergeson. The Colonel and I had quite a long talk. It seems that he wants me to follow up our 2nd Aux. operative cases. I am not too sure whether to be pleased or disappointed with this assignment.

We have been moderately busy today. The Jerries have been shelling our infantry.

May 5, 1943—(Diary)

Yesterday we drove back through La Calle taking a short cut along the coast to Tabarka. It was a beautiful, picturesque drive and gave us an excellent view of the Fort, city, and coast line of Tabarka from a mountain top, just before we descended into the city. To our keen disappointment we learned that the 51st Medical Battalion, with our 2nd Aux. teams, had moved ahead some place near Beja, that morning, and that the 10th Field Hospital had moved in. Although we were almost too late for dinner, Major Plylor had their kitchen fix us a good lunch. This is the first Field Hospital we have seen, although I had heard some rumor at Corps Surgeons Headquarters that some were coming over and that we 2nd Aux. teams might work with them. I discussed this, briefly, with Lt. Col. Ross, the C.O. of the 10th F. H. but he maintained that they were organized only to service the Air Corps.

After he left, we had a surgical conference in our tent with Col. Weaver, Col. Hashinger, Major Dillon (urologist), Capt. Lalich, and other members of the surgical staff. While this meeting was most informal, it was chock full of meat and did not break up until 1:00 A.M. I could not get to sleep, however, for new ideas, new techniques and methods of treatment, kept running wild through my mind.

9

The Algerian Highlands[1]

ONE COLD, gray afternoon in January 1943, I met Colonel Richard T. Arnest, the Surgeon of II Corps, as he was visiting our hospital area (9th Evacuation Hospital) in the highlands of Algeria. He asked me if I knew a Dr. Churchill. I told him I surely did but the one I knew was in Boston. Then he informed me that he had just received word from General Rankin, Surgical Consultant to the Surgeon General, that Dr. Churchill was on his way to North Africa to become the Theater Surgical Consultant. Thereupon I told Dr. Arnest how extremely fortunate he and the whole Corps were that Dr. Churchill was to be our consultant. It was not long after that, that the famous man himself appeared with a large notebook partly filled with fine, perfect handwriting of notes that he had made in the course of preparing himself for his work. These included all sorts of items: conversations with Sir Heneage Ogilvie, meetings with the British Penicillin Team, interviews with the British consultants, and of course all kinds of notes on United States policies and the military medical establishment. More than that, he had made a detailed study into the workings and duties of consultants of all sorts in World Wars I and II and their relationships with the command. The Theater Surgeon was Brigadier General Fred Blesse with headquarters in Algiers. He was succeeded later by Major General Morrison C. Stayer, who was of great assistance in his wholehearted support of Colonel Churchill.

When Dr. Churchill was making his first tour of the front, away from Algiers, with the comforts and chills of that lush city in winter, the Surgeon's offices were in a humble establishment known as the Church Villa overlooking the city and almost next door to the St. George Hotel, which was the home of the mighty, high on a hill overlooking the French Governor General's palace and French headquarters. Further down the slope was the Cercle Inter-Allies and then the city below with the newer Aletti Hotel, that sanctuary of the American officers who passed through or who remained in Algiers temporarily, that group of doughty Aletti Fusiliers.

---

[1]Written by Frank Berry in 1956 and previously published in Surgeon to Soldiers: Diaries and Records of the Surgical Consultant, Allied Force Headquarters, World Ward II, 1972.

Near the medical headquarters was the 29th Station Hospital, especially designed and equipped for the duties, responsibilities and cares of a headquarters hospital. We looked upon our Consultant as advisor, friend and teacher. Howard Patterson and I were almost the only people at first who had known him over the past years, but in almost no time his friendliness, guidance and help were known and available to all. From his own unit, the 6th General at Casablanca, all the way across North Africa to Tunis, as troops and medical units poured in, he roamed constantly, conducting a huge postgraduate course in surgical education.

It was my privilege to visit him two or three times in Algiers, to work with him in the office and through his arrangements I had the opportunity to visit some of the British hospitals where I first made my acquaintance with penicillin. At that time the hangover from World War I treatment with Carrel-Dakin Technic, and the numerous tubes, was still evident and it was quite evident that the program was halting and experimental. Suppurating knee joints were seen with a little tube running in at the top and pus oozing out. Penicillin was injected at frequent intervals and a waxy mixture was often forced in through the tube. The joints were huge and the patients unhappy. Such were the initial days of Dr. Churchill and our own fledgling period, feeling our way with treatments, watching the experiences of others and finally learning under his guidance that adequate, clean surgery, carefully performed, was the primary need in war, that the sulfonamides and penicillin and antimicrobials were adjuncts but never substitutes.

Dr. Churchill was also extremely interested in our thoughts as to the use of whole blood and plasma and his work in establishing blood collecting units and a transfusion service by utilizing the service troops in the area as donors is too well known to repeat here. Suffice it to say that due to his insistence on the utilization of fresh blood and the precautions taken, no instances of difficulties from the use of outdated, contaminated or improperly typed blood ever arose.

Our own unit had proceeded to the east by several stages so that at the end of the North African campaign we were at Mateur, just behind Bizerte. We had commodious quarters and Colonel Churchill became a frequent visitor, as we helped wind up the affairs of the German Army and while he in turn was preparing the medical aspects of the Sicilian invasion.

In the fall of 1943 we crossed over to Sicily and then Italy, where we were established adjacent to the large hospital center in Naples which Pete had helped organize. Here a course in postgraduate surgery was in full blossom, with weekly surgical meetings and frequent visits from the Colonel. We were assigned to take care of the French and their African troops; therefore, we had much material that was of great interest because we had no evacuation policy and could hold our patients until they were well or transferred them back to the French hospitals in Algeria, as we desired.

Late in the spring of 1944, Pete asked if I wished to be considered as the Surgical Consultant for the Seventh Army and of course I jumped at the chance. Whereupon I went back to Algiers and put in another session at the Theater Headquarters which itself was preparing to move to Caserta, a short distance from Naples. The planning for the Seventh Army invasion of southern France, which had been begun in Algiers, was completed in Naples and there were frequent visits between Naples and Caserta to seek help and advice.

In addition to his manifold duties in the field and with planning, through circular letters from the Theater Headquarters, in TB Med 147 written while on a mission to the United States, and in many articles in our medical journals, Colonel Churchill further enriched our knowledge and understanding of military surgery. These were always all accomplished with painstaking care and high literary value, and were based upon his own experience and his thorough grasp both of surgical principles, and the distinction between, and cooperation of, the administrative and professional groups.

Our penetration into eastern France proceeded very rapidly after our landings in August, and in October when the weather had become cold and rainy, the Colonel and his driver with jeep appeared in Vesoul, in eastern France for a short visit and tour of the front. Here our problems of the rapid advance, the bad weather and the holdup of evacuation by air and the availability of blood were discussed. We were due to transfer early in November to the European Command with another old friend, Elliott Cutler, as our Surgical Consultant and advisor, and so this was the last time that we saw Pete in that formal capacity. He and Oscar Hampton visited us again later in the spring after the war was over and at this time we called upon Dr. Sauerbruch in Berlin and Dr. Lebsche in Munich. In Berlin, Sauerbruch was amazed when Pete told him about resecting pulmonary tuberculous lesions, and said, "You know medicine and surgery in Germany have been at a standstill ever since 1930 when Hitler came into power; we have been shut off from the outside world." In Munich we were intrigued as we watched Lebsche do one of his cineplastic maneuvers for a prosthesis of the arm, and were interested in the contrast between the two men, Sauerbruch, big, bluff and blustering, and Lebsche his first "oberarzt" in Munich, shy, delicate and retiring. Although never confirmed, it had been rumored that Lebsche had worked with the underground throughout the war.

The last time I saw Pete overseas was when I returned overland from Augsburg, Bavaria, to Naples and Caserta for a final visit at the old headquarters and to bring the loose ends together of the transfer of the Seventh Army from the Mediterranean to the European Command. I was to have stayed with Pete at his quarters in Caserta but unfortunately at that time he had just been taken to the hospital with a virus pneumonia. Nevertheless, I visited with him frequently and thoroughly enjoyed the group with whom he had surrounded himself in his office as informal consultants. They were finishing their reports, and among them were Oscar Hampton in orthopedics, Eldridge Campbell in neurosurgery, Harvey Allen in surgery of the hand and plastic and maxillofacial work, Fiorindo Simeone in surgical physiology, Henry Beecher in anesthesiology, and Howard Snyder, the surgical consultant of the Fifth Army. This was the end of June and the first of July in 1945, and Naples wore almost a fiesta appearance at that time with the war ending and the officers club at Mondragone Beach not too far distant—a charming and delightful spot.

During our early days in North Africa we were disappointed and yet happy that we were able to contribute to his professional manpower problems by first sending Pelham Glasier as Chief of Surgery to the 29th Station Hospital in Algiers, and later Howard Patterson as Chief of Surgery to the 95th Evacuation Hospital with the Fifth Army. Both more than justified the confidence placed in them by Pete. Howard was with the 95th when it was bombed at Anzio and had done such fine work with them that he was promptly transferred to the 93rd Evacuation Hospital which was sent to Anzio to replace the 95th. We had the good fortune in the Seventh Army to have both of these hospitals with us as we went into southern France and all through our campaign. And so, even though later separated from the Mediterranean Theater, we continued the policies and teachings that had been practiced by Pete and spread abroad to his increasing host of friends.

As to the postwar years the particular experience that I recall with considerable amusement was when he was ill and I called upon him in Phillips House. They announced Dr. Berry but forgot to say Dr. Frank Berry, as momentarily I had forgotten that my namesake was Dean of the Medical School at the time. As I walked in, Pete and Mary were obviously relieved to see a friendly visitor arriving to chat merely on inconsequential matters, rather than one who had come to talk about serious matters connected with relationships between school and hospital. Our closest postwar relationship has really consisted in the meetings of the Excelsior Club, born from the war years largely at the suggestion of Eldridge Campbell, and each year we look forward to meeting with him and Mary and catching up with what has happened over the past years.

10

Retreat of Africa Corps From El Alamein

AFTER THE TUNISIAN campaign the route up the coast of Tunisia was littered with discarded equipment, clothing and personal possessions of the soldiers of Rommel's Afrika Corps. In this rubbish Major J. Lawrence Pool found fragments of the diary of a German private. Major Pool, neurosurgeon of the 9th Evacuation Hospital, translated it and I am indebted to him for permission to reproduce it. The diary was dated March 1, 1943.

A retreat is a humiliating and disastrous experience for a military force that has been victorious. It is also commonly attended by a sharp rise in neuropsychiatric disorders and infections from delay or neglect in the care of wounds.

GERMAN SOLDIER'S DIARY

The Command for the Retreat

We could scarcely believe it at first when we heard our Commander in Chief utter the word *Retreat*. Had we not halted all attempts of the English to break through? Had not the enemy suffered heavy losses since the beginning of his offensive? Had he not lost 300 tanks? For eight days he had pounded our positions with unprecedented weight of munitions. And yet he had only broken through our northern lines. But we held just the same! We were still not licked. And now, "To the Rear?" The whole front? We couldn't grasp it. But it must be the best solution from the broad point of view. We, like every soldier, understood only our own little bit. We knew nothing of the situation as a whole. But now, with the crumbling of our long distance campaign, we learned afresh of the enemy's enormous advantage in material. Firing of a great weight and mass hammered our positions so that we all wondered that so little had been damaged. The enemy had everything in overabundance, while we had to be sparing with everything. That was the answer to the riddle.

Thoughts of the Retreat

With something of a sentiment of disaster we began the retreat. Our personal psychology had to be completely changed from *Forwards* to *Backwards*. That wasn't easy. For we had not been prepared for it. We went since everyone went, and had to; alone, we were helpless. And as often as we met our fellows on the march to the rear, we greeted this one and that one with a queer dumb look—as if each wanted to inquire, "Just why are *you* going back? Is the forward zone too hot for you? *We* are going to stay. Why not *you*? Aren't things really going well any more? Who's to blame? *You* or *who?*" But no one alone had run away. No one gave voice to these thoughts. The command had been given *Back!* and so to hell with it! Each one simply must have heard the general order to fall back. And actually, we could only be thankful to our leaders that they didn't let us be mowed down all together, but were trying to arrange a more favorable position.

General Field Marshal Rommel

Every day at least twice we saw our General Field Marshal Rommel. Either in the company of his colonels or looking eastwards from a hill near the Via Balbia. Each time we asked ourselves when will he finally give the order "Halt everything! Here is our new front!" Each time we saw him we were all struck anew by the questions: "*When, How* and *Why?*" and:—What will he do? Surely he has a plan. A goal. Surely at this very moment. But his undisturbed calm gave us the answer without words: He would do it soon; right now he knew why.

Retreating Infantry

A picture I'll never forget. On the first day of our withdrawal, we overtook with our trucks the retreating infantry. Whole companies in goosestep were marching to the rear like caravans. There weren't enough trucks for everybody. They had to carry out the retreat on foot. Round them everything else was motorized. We would soon be overtaken and attacked by enemy tanks. And very soon we even spotted enemy tanks in the distance, now coming up at us, now at a tangent to us, cutting across country. We could hinder them, but the infantry must march

(continued)

until the very last minute, when the tanks came up and opened up in unequal attack. We badly wanted to help these troops. They had been the first ones to fight, the last to retreat. Had they not held the very forward lines during all the preceding months? But where could we get so many trucks to carry them all? Hence many of them had to resign themselves to the very tough solution of being taken prisoners of war.

We Were Bombarded

Another picture that has unforgettably forced itself upon me. It was just after noon. A clear blue sky. We had picked up one of our 21 cm. mortar batteries. Their gigantic guns, mounted on colossal trailers, rattled along like monsters of prehistoric times. In their wake they left a thick cloud of dust. Suddenly, over us, overtaking us came 18 heavy British bombers, already quite well known to us. "Everybody under their trucks! Scatter! Lie down!" We even saw our jeeps scatter helter-skelter. Already the first bombs were falling and the first splinters flying. We jumped up—hid in the next hole in the ground! And now ensued the grandiose spectacle that I'd seen so often in magazine pictures—but here, for the first time in reality:—an air attack on a column of transport vehicles. With blow after blow bombs crashed to earth, bursting and exploding. But they all fell to one side. Our cannon, still covered, lay chained to the trucks pulling them. Nothing happened. Everyone stood up and went on. That's surely only the beginning, I thought. Now they'd pound our columns in a steady rolling bombardment. But this was their only attack. Up to Halfaya Pass the British planes didn't bother us any more. Their radius of action certainly reached that far. But we didn't experience the annihilating pursuit tactics that brought us Germans the speedy end of the war in Poland and France. Couldn't the British do it; or didn't they want to? Was he too foresighted or too unprepared? Or did he rate our ME too hot for him? It might be all these together. Only once did it seem as if he wanted to carry out a systematic liquidating action from the air. We lay in our positions on the Via Balbia near Sidi El Barani. During the whole night we had free lighting. A British air squadron was trying to light up the ground below them with countless flares. Stick for stick, with almost pedantic precision, he bombed every target that seemed worthwhile. But our bunch of vehicles was scattered over the countryside. He couldn't inflict much damage. I lay in the shadows of our trucks. Over me a flare was wandering in the breeze. With it the truck's shadows wavered, and in the shimmering truck shadows I too, lest I be spotted from above.

It's a horrible feeling to lie unprotected in the open fields, at night, hunted by your enemy, with flares. It's as if someone with a lantern went down in the cellar looking for a mouse hiding in a corner from which there was no escape.

We Have Nothing and Help Ourselves

We come to Marsa Matruk. No more gas, no water, no food. All used up. Who's taking care of us? The staff is no longer present. Just as ourselves, it too is on the march. So we must all help ourselves. We will no longer be taken care of, so we must grab what we can. There's a fuel dump. At it! In fevered haste we cram our trucks full. With gasoline cans and tins. As much as possible. Quickly, for every second may bring an air attack, and catastrophe. Finally, we're ready. Over there stands a ration truck. It must be blown up so Tommy won't get it. First quickly fetch out everything we can possibly take along. And so it went during the whole retreat. There a filling station. Is anything in it? Look! Yes, gasoline. Load it aboard. We spent the night at Tobruk. Fireworks were exploding to our right. Had Tommy landed? No. A rations truck was burning up. O.K.! Into it, for its 80 sacks. We must live, we must eat. From the roaring furnace we pulled out the boxes. With canned meat on to Bengasi. A ration depot. Door jammed. No entrance. Our Ober-Lieutenant was not dismayed. He took care of the situation, got in, and it lasted us for another couple of days.

Retreat or Flight?

In the first few days of the withdrawal our trucks sped along the Via Balbia at top speed, westwards. Could hardly go fast enough. One overhauled the other. Finally because of "overtaking fever" the road at Marsa Matruk was completely jammed. Motor columns stood side by side 12 rows deep, thicker and thicker. Suddenly: Panic! Tommy planes over us! Get away! In the getaway there'd be great confusion. The first captured Tommies used this chaos to escape. We watched them go. Bombs fell. A truck caught fire. Luckily there were only four planes. What if the whole R.A.F. bombed us! Don't think of it! If that sort of thing went on, how would it all end, I thought to myself. But no others came. From now on, dug-in positions would be manned, by us, by our batteries. We were protecting the east, now here, now there. The enemy never knew: Is this a new front, or a rear guard action, or scouting troops? In any case he had to find out, and that cost time, which was exactly what we needed to withdraw the army in orderly fashion. Along the Via Balbia infantry with loaded rifles

(continued)

ensured food discipline, which was stern. Rations had to travel. Thanks to these rearguard troops and infantry, the retreat was orderly, and could be carried out in complete calm. Thus the dangerous massing of vehicles and the road block that occurred at Marsa Matruk didn't happen again.

Capuzzo

Slowly and carefully Tommy pursued us. Only once during the time we were protected by our rearguard, did he launch a brilliant thrust, a regular Hussar's charge. That was so contrary to all custom that we did not reckon on it, and therefore were surprised, plenty. That was at Capuzzo. Overnight we lay in our positions. In the gray of morning we started to change our position. We were going back to the Via Balbia. But there Tommy was ready for us with countless tanks that showered us with a hail of shells and machine gun bullets. That cost us a heavy toll in dead, wounded and prisoners. Even today it is not clear to me how so very many enemy tanks could have stolen upon us in our position that night. I myself as observer clearly heard the ever louder clanking of one Tommy tank in my area. But I heard only ONE, and in the gray of morning many Tommy tanks were swarming upon the horizon. I guess at least 30. Peppered by machine gun bullets, we tried to collect ourselves for retreat. But where? Tommy pressed on. No time could be lost. Our captain was captured. So the remaining officers held the batteries together, what was left, and led them to the highway back of Agaila. Each of us who lived through the intermezzo of Capuzzo will forever vividly remember it, and the question of whether, as well as how, the misfortune could have been prevented, will keep us busy as long as we'll live. We will never find an answer. For Mars, the God of war, is capricious. On even the most careful soldier he sometimes turns his back.

Cyrenaika

So we went on, starving men without strength, through the fruitful region around Cyrenaika. It was like the Garden of Eden. So strong was the contrast. Before, standing at the front, was the enemy. Not now. Before, wasteland; and now sober suburbs with neat little white houses, gardens and orchards. And mountains, like our Alps, with high pale-green vegetation and great gnarled trees. We breathed deep. That's the way it was at home. And when we went on again, past Bengazi to our accustomed element, the wasteland, the picture of Cyrenaika, a bit of home, remained fixed in our minds like a refreshing drink.

The Arabs

During the whole retreat the Arabs accompanied us the entire length of the Via Balbia, often in whole gangs. They picked up biscuits fallen from the men's pockets. Why did they tag along with us? Why didn't they stay back? Had they had such a tough time with Rommy? Were the Arabs better off with us? Or did they follow us only because we betrayed the scorched earth policy?

Our Journey

What the journey and, above all, the travelers must suffer and still suffer during these weeks is beyond description. The traveler not only by day but even at night had to sit at the wheel, often with no hope—alone a test of nerve of the first water. Steady repairs, towing on and off the road, favors to others, took most of our time. How often it all seemed hopeless, yet it all went well. "Have you an extra can of gas?" was the great question. And the second most frequent question was "Can you tow me—just six feet?" One half to the other. It was thus we all reached our goal.

From Marsa Matruk to Tunisia

Our batteries were ready and newly set up by the highway. Again as rear guard. But now for the first time we awaited the enemy from an established position. The forereaching English Army should be halted for a long time with a small force. It worked. For several weeks. We knew we were in a situation where the tempo of our retreat slowed down. The Tommy's advance would be stopped more and more. Until he came to a standstill in Tunisia. Here in Tunisia we had the advantage which the British had at Alamein: easy contact with our bases. By this advantage we balanced the ever mounting force of our enemy. Our strength again held sway. And we were winning time to start new operations as soon as possible.

11

A Look at an Evacuation Hospital

ATTEMPTS TO BASE a novel or story on the happenings within a single hospital during a war are rarely successful. They tend to focus on the romances and intrigues of a small circle of friends banded together in the formation of the outfit, its shipment overseas, a holiday in Paris and, in World War I, a brief period of receiving wounded soldiers at a situation far in the rear. The commanding officer is either the villain or butt of the carryings-on of the staff of officers, nurses and enlisted men.

Nevertheless, the true picture of a war can be seen only by a glimpse into the daily life of an individual hospital unit. Each had its own personality, its own trials, its own sweat and its own tears. Circumstances brought me into closer contact with the Roosevelt Hospital-affiliated 9th Evacuation Hospital than with any other mobile or general hospital, including the M.G.H. 6th General Hospital. The 9th Evacuation Hospital was a "heavy" (750-bed) mobile hospital often expanded to house over 1,000 patients under canvas. They usually had a small wall tent which was at my disposal for days or weeks at a time. Its staff contained many surgeons and physicians whom I came to know intimately and with whom I have maintained warm friendships long after the war.

In Operation Torch, the 9th Evacuation Hospital came in convoy from Southampton under escort of the *Pennsylvania*—the same battleship that had escorted the convoy in which Frank Berry had traveled to Liverpool in World War I. Coming into the Mediterranean, the unit was put ashore in North Africa at Mers el Kébir near Oran. They had told a few friends in England that they were going to North Africa but were regarded as completely confused—such an absurd idea was ridiculous. A large part of the equipment was loaded in a second ship with the supply officer, Harrop, in charge. This ship was sunk in the Mediterranean.

The Commanding Officer was Colonel William Stone, a National Guard officer from Missouri. He was a kindly and friendly gentleman who liked his pipe and a game of bridge and was content to let his staff run the hospital. This explains the hospitable reception of consultants and other visitors to the hospital. Rigid-spined commanding officers do not welcome visitors—they undermine military discipline.

On arrival at Mers el Kébir, the staff marched to a staging area at La Senia and then moved to Tlemcen where the tents were set up and patients were received from the local area. It was at Tlemcen that Harrop, who had been given up as lost, reappeared unexpectedly. His arrival was greeted by "Harrop is here! Harrop is here!" The dental officer, hearing the shouts, mistook "Harrop" for "Arabs" and ran "on the double" to headquarters to spread the alarm that the Arabs were attacking. Tlemcen is deep in Algeria and far more Arabian in atmosphere than French.

From Tlemcen the 9th Evacuation Hospital moved to the head of the Kasserine Pass in support of II Corps' combat in southern Tunisia. When the threat of the breakthrough by the African Corps was recognized, the Corps Surgeon's Office, at 5:00 A.M., ordered the hospital to move back sixty to seventy miles. Berry and two men, one of whom was the quartermaster, drove back under a full moon to the site selected by Arnest's staff. The selected site was on shale rock and tent stakes could not be driven into the ground. The quartermaster was a tent expert formerly with the Ringling Circus, so he knew his craft. An alternative site was chosen in the vicinity of Ain Beda. The hospital itself took off at midnight and by morning the weather had turned stormy and windy.

After the Kasserine Pass threat had passed, orders were received to move forward again to Youks les Bains. Their 500 patients were transferred to the 77th Evacuation Hospital and to British hospitals.

Coming from New York City, the hospital quite naturally had in its detachment many men of Jewish faith. When first set up at Tlemcen, what became known as the "Jewish revolt" took place. This "revolt" was based on the belief that no Jewish religious services were provided in the hospital. Ordinarily this matter would have been handled by the commanding officer, but it was solved by Frank Berry who invited the spokesmen of the group to a discussion of their grievances. The official table of organization of a 750-bed evacuation hospital provided *one* Chaplain, the Reverend Bob Woodruff, an Episcopalian. He had been authorized and schooled by Jewish, Catholic and Protestant faiths to conduct services for each faith. Only the larger general hospitals had three chaplains.

Notices of the services of the three faiths had been posted on the bulletin board at the staging area and at Tlemcen. When confronted with this, the "revolters" admitted that they had not looked at the bulletin board and consequently had not informed themselves of the Jewish service. The whole thing subsided. Anxieties and gripes rose like the proverbial tempests in a teapot and called for the same wisdom and patience that a doctor learns in his relationships with patients and their families.

At Tebessa, the 9th Evacuation Hospital received a present of a large keg of rum, courtesy of the Air Force. Whenever the 9th moved, there was always a careful check to be certain which truck had the rum. Pel Glazier, later transferred to be chief of surgery at the 29th Station Hospital in Algiers and now a leading surgeon in Albany, New York, thought it wise to check more thoroughly on the *contents* of the keg. He held a lighted match to the bung hole, so he could see how much rum was left. It was good rum for the explosion singed Pel's eyebrows.

After the invasion of southern France up the Rhone Valley, the Seventh Army and its hospitals were transferred to the European Theater. Mather Cleveland, Consultant in Orthopedic Surgery, E.T.O., notified the 9th Evacuation Hospital of a proposed visit and asked them to assemble all their orthopedic surgeons so he could hold a conference with them. We had never been that formal in our theater. Berry told him there was only *one* orthopedic surgeon and that was the Chief of Surgery. Battle fractures were all cared for by Jim Thompson and Casselbaum. They supervised the plaster bandages and spicas.

12

The Tunisian Campaign

AFTER THE landings in Morocco and Algeria had been made secure, the Tunis-Bizerte area had become the primary objective of Anglo-American-French forces. Allied forces moving eastward from Algiers were stopped by the Axis approximately forty-five miles from Bizerte on November 17, 1942. The French army and naval units in North Africa were presumably under Marshal Henri Petain in Vichy, and a stream of orders was received from him to repel the American and British invaders and cooperate with Nazi forces in Africa.

TUNISIA REACTS TO NORTH AFRICAN LANDINGS

In Tunisia, General George Barré commanded the army and Admiral Louis Derrien commanded the naval force. Coastal defense batteries were immediately put on combat alert by Admiral Derrien and naval units were ordered to repel invaders. General Barré, after confirmation from Petain, issued an order to enemy troops "to defend the empire against no matter who will try to gain a foothold." As German planes began to land at Tunis airfield, guards were placed around the field by Barré to prevent any hostile acts by civilians. An attempt was made to remain neutral, then learning that Axis ships were about to appear at the port of Bizerte, they decided to open fire on them. This definition of the Germans as their enemy aroused great enthusiasm among the soldiers and sailors of the Bizerte area, and when Derrien—before an hour had passed—annulled the order favoring neutrality, widespread consternation ensued.

German planes brought antiaircraft batteries, and air transports landed troops and material at Bizerte. Ships were admitted to the port by order from Vichy. Barré moved army troops to establish his headquarters on the road to Constantine. On his way to confer with Barré on the thirteenth, Derrien received orders from Admiral Jean L. Darlan to throw the Germans into the sea, bottle up the harbor and withdraw his naval forces to an area near Tebessa. The following day a message from Marshal Petain commanded him to "defend North Africa against American aggression . . . I order the army of Africa to exercise no action and in no circumstances against the Axis forces."

Barré, in the meantime, had established a defensive position about forty-five miles west of Tunis and his troops were under orders to oppose any Axis units approaching from the east. Derrien, in contrast, demanded opposition to American attack and forbad hostile action against Axis forces; he then capitulated to the Nazis. Despite further pressure, Barré held firm and active combat ensued.

This kind of confusion, indecision and rapid change in attitude had been the first reaction to the landings in all North Africa, not only among the military but among civilians as well. A buildup of German strength in Tunisia followed immediately. Hitler gave Kesselring authority to attack Allied shipping in Algiers and to send troops to Tunisia. Men and equipment poured into the Tunisian bridgehead, building Axis strength to 17,000 German and 11,000 Italian troops by the end of November. Italian troops were sent from Libya to the Gabes region to close the gap between the Tunisian bridgehead and Rommel's forces.

The first German senior officer placed in command of forces in the bridgehead was General der Panzertruppen Walter Nehring, who had been with Rommel in the Afrika Corps. He had been wounded in the arm on August 31, 1942, and, although he had been sent back to Berlin for treatment, the wound was still suppurating. Nehring reached the bridgehead on November 14 and soon became pessimistic in his view of the situation. His unhealed wound began causing severe pain. Early in December Nehring was recalled and replaced by Generaloberst Juergen von Arnim on December 9—"a surly, sullen officer who walked with a slight limp." Arnim continued the buildup of men and material in Tunisia, extending the Tunis-Bizerte bridgehead south to Gabes. By early February his strength mounted to 75,000 German and 25,000 Italian troops. But with the buildup of Arnim, reinforcement for Rommel received low priority because the battle of Stalingrad was absorbing Nazi strength. It has been said that the reinforcement given Arnim at this time showed how important the Tunisian action was regarded by Hitler and Mussolini.

Before considering the pattern of the Allied offensive in Tunisia, the geography of the country requires review. And, as in so many campaigns in history, the weather played an important part—rain, cold and mud. By the end of 1942, it was apparent at A.F.H.Q. that the Allies had lost the race for northern Tunisia. The long distances, lack of transport, shortage of spare parts, lack of airfields and shortage of reserve units brought the Americans face to face with the realities of a winter campaign even in a Mediterranean land. Also, there was still the danger that Rommel could turn west and cut the lines of communication stretching from Algiers toward Tunis. For these and perhaps other reasons, attention was turned to southern Tunisia.

The Tunisian theater of operations for American combat, as defined by Martin Blumenson, was triangular in shape, the northern boundary extending from Constantine to Bizerte—250 miles. From Bizerte south along the coast road through Sousse and Sfax to Gabes is the eastern side of the triangle, again 250 miles. From Gabes to Constantine across the arid highlands of Tunisia and Algeria is roughly 300 miles and this line forms the third side of the triangle. The road from Constantine to Gabes, through Tabessa, Feriana and Gafsa to the coast of Gabes offered the opportunity to drive a wedge between Arnim in the north and Rommel approaching Tunisia from Libya. Rommel was at Marsa el Brega with 70,000 troops but Gabes offered a more strategic site for him to stabilize a stronger defensive position against Montgomery's Eighth Army. Rommel did not share Hitler's and Mussolini's vision of holding Libya or even Tunisia. He was too able and experienced in warfare. In Rommel's mind the task before him was to salvage as many men and materials as possible by getting out of Africa.

Extending south from Tunis behind a narrow coastal plain is the Eastern Dorsale mountain chain that ends at Gafsa. The Petite or Western Dorsale branches off the Grande or Eastern Dorsale and terminates in the Atlas Mountains near Tebessa. Passes in these two mountain ridges were to form the battle sites in southern Tunisia. Leading to Sfax were the Maknassy Gap or Faid Pass; to Sousse were Fondouk or Pichon; in the Petite Dorsale are the passes of Kasserine and Sbiba. Faid Pass in the Western Dorsale is joined to the Kasserine Pass by a road crossing the fifty mile plain of Sbeitla (**Figure 12.1**).

From earliest times, these passes, particularly the Kasserine, had been the sites of furious battles between the native Berbers and the invaders of the region—the Carthaginians and the Romans. More than a place of combat, the Kasserine region was a place of encounter, a frontier where the uncouth jostled the cultured, where a vortex of agitation and brutality attracted soldiers, traders, and adventurers in search of excitement and fortune.

This was the Kasserine Pass where Rommel, leading the Afrika Corps up the narrow coastal corridor, threatened a breakthrough.

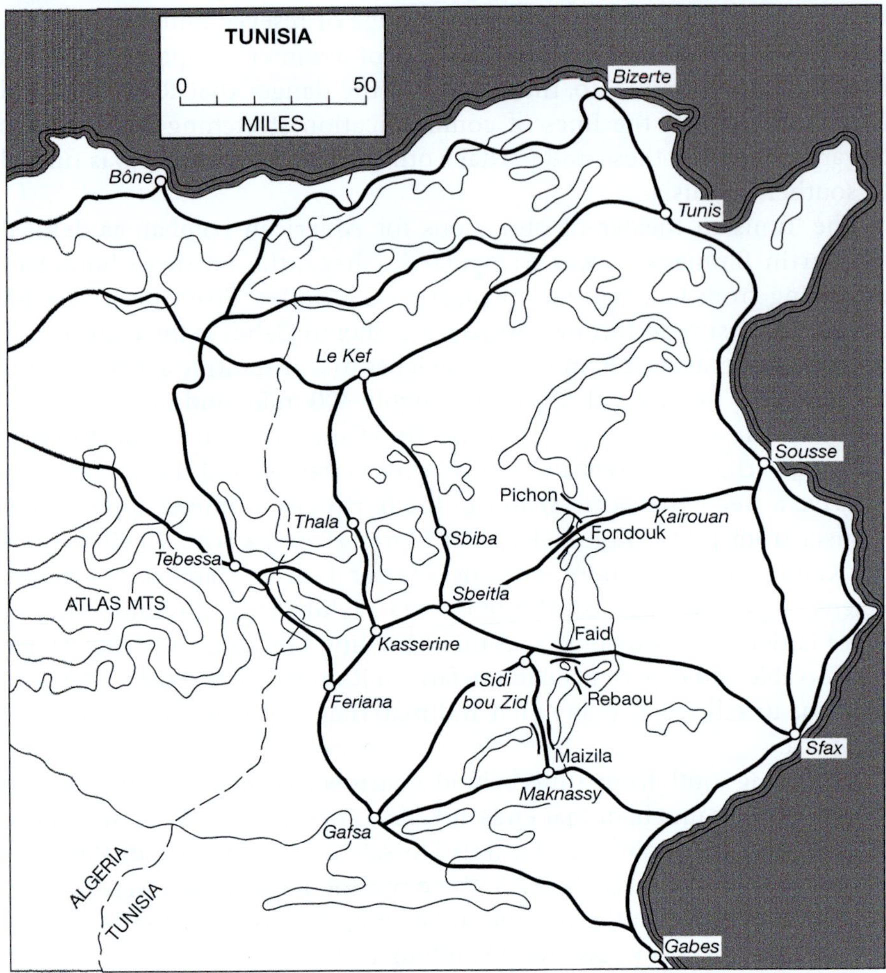

Figure 12.1 Battle sites of the Tunisian campaign (November, 1942, to May, 1943).

FIRST TRIP WITH WEDDELL

My first travel orders in the theater were issued on March 15, 1943, and read as follows:

E.D.C. Comments: Brigadier J. Weddell and Colonel Edward Churchill 0199980, MC will proceed from this station on or about March 16, 1943, to El Guerrah, Ain Beidia, Souk ei Arba, Setif, and such other places in the North African area as may be necessary on temporary duty in order to carry out the instructions of the C in C and upon completion, to return to proper station. By command of General Eisenhower, signed by the Adjutant General.

This trip with Weddell was my introduction to the medical support of a front in active combat in contact with the enemy. Our tour was centered on medical installations behind the British First Army and it gave me a close view of the British system of management of the wounded that had evolved from the experience in the western desert and the efforts of Heneage Ogilvie as Consulting Surgeon.

It was commonly said in southern Tunisia that there were twenty-eight acres of C-rations that had to be eaten before B-rations would be issued. The dump of C-ration crates did not have to be guarded because "even the Arabs will not eat them." The impact of a diet of C-rations on me is evidenced by my detailed notes of lunch at the Hotel de la Colonie in Bouria on March 16. An omelet whipped up from fresh eggs with vin de pays made a not-to-be-forgotten impression. Our stop for the night was "laid on" at the British 31st General Hospital in Oued Athmenia with the "Surgical Specialist" Heatley, of Dublin. A general surgical team of the 2nd Auxiliary Surgical Group, headed by Jim Sullivan, was on loan to this hospital.

Weddell and I were given beds in a recovery room alongside the operating theater. In the morning we were awakened by the clumping boots of a British orderly and further roused by a cup of scalding coffee placed on the bedside table. As the orderly clumped off he carried with him our boots to be cleaned and polished. The tender loving care of leather is deeply ingrained in the English. A story told by Mrs. Charles Mayo of her husband, one of the Mayo brothers, illustrates the point. They were entertaining a group of English surgeons as house guests and Charles got out of bed in the middle of the night to close a window. He didn't come back, and finally Mrs. Mayo went downstairs and found him polishing their guests' boots in the kitchen! They had placed their boots outside their doors as is the British custom.

At Constantine we turned south through El Guerrah, Ain Mela and Ain Beida, fascinated by the magic of the Arabic names, and stopped at the 77th Evacuation Hospital at Meskiana. This 750-bed hospital was the University of Kansas affiliated unit, commanded by Colonel Burnett, with Lieutenant Colonel James B. Weaver serving as Chief of Surgery. After a night at the 9th Evacuation Hospital at Youks les Bains, and a visit to the 48th Surgical Hospital then at Bou Chebka, we stopped at the old French barracks in Feriana to see Ken Lowry who had recently been visited by Perrin Long and Ned Boland. Their visit was described in Lowry's diary as follows:

"It rained and blew all day and was quite cold. In the barracks fixed up for surgery we had one stove going. The enlisted men run a shuttle system on the cans used for seats around the stove, and we officers stand back and look at the stove. Even that helps a little, just knowing there is a stove with a fire in it."

(continued)

"During the day the Corps Surgeon dropped in with two big-wigs, another full Colonel and a Brig. General. Finally I was asked by the Corps Surgeon if I wished to voice any complaints. We both laughed, then I said: 'Do you really want me to open up?' He nodded in the affirmative, and as Frosty said later: 'I let him have both barrels.' Briefly, I took up the lack of numerous needed instruments and equipment, lack of transportation facilities, and the status of our living as field soldiers. As we say in the Army, I really 'blew my top,' but it may do some good."

The stop Weddell and I made at Feriana was recorded by Ken Lowry in a more cheerful mode. The date of the entry in his diary was March 19, 1943.

"The wind has died down so it is not so cold. We feel quite honored by a visit from Col. Edward Churchill of Mass. General Hospital fame. He is Consulting Surgeon of A.F. Hdq. He was accompanied by a British Brig. General and Col. Arnest, our Corps Surgeon. We appreciated their apparent sympathetic understanding of our problems and I have every hope that some benefit to all Auxiliary Surgical Teams may result from our discussion. As an illustration, certainly not overdrawn, I asked if they could visualize themselves crawling out of a pup tent at 2 A.M. and attempting to dress in mud and a downpour. Then going to a cold surgery tent to do a decent laparotomy. We do not complain about hardships and discomforts that are secondary to the hazards of war, but surely many discomforts are unnecessary. They agreed that we had been getting a pretty raw deal and had been pushed around too much. Our not having the 2nd Aux. Commanding Officer over here certainly had contributed to this treatment. Col. Churchill then told me that Col. Forsee, our C.O. with the remainder of the 2nd Aux. Surgical Group, had landed in Casablanca and he hoped that Col. Forsee might be up to see us in the near future."

On March 19, Weddell and I turned north to Souk Ahras, stopping at several British hospitals, C.C.S.'s and F.S.U.'s. The following night No. 1 Casualty Clearing Station billeted us in a villa that was part of the lead mine at Jebel Malouf. The next morning we were joined by Brigadier Cantley, the administrative officer of this British First Army sector. Cantley had encountered family tragedy during the Air Battle of Britain and insisted on finding active service against the Nazis at the earliest opportunity. Either Canley or Weddell took turns as observer in the open roof port of our car. It took experience to distinguish between a stork and an approaching Messerschmitt.

The next day Weddell, Brigadier Cantley and I stopped at No. 18 Casualty Clearing Station. The 25th Field Surgical Unit was attached and both were sited near the famous Thibar Monastery, which produces "Fine Tibarine," a liqueur distilled with herbs in a combination that remains a closely guarded secret. There I met for the first time A. L. d'Abreu, then a dashing young British surgical officer who became a lifelong friend with interchange of visits between Boston and Birmingham, England.

Major Guy Blackburn was with the 52nd Field Surgical Unit attached to the main dressing station near Teboursouk. He had seen 4 cases of gas gangrene in the last 20 casualties, and a total of 9 in 250 wounds. Four patients died. Blackburn saw little need for the use of x-ray, in fact estimated a real need for x-ray examination in only 2 of the 250 casualties. In these, I noted, "he thinks an expert roentgenologist would have been required. Pentothal is used universally but only for operations of approximately 20 minutes' duration. When a major procedure, such as for a battle fracture of the femur or a wound of the abdomen, is required, ether is essential. Ethyl chloride or chloroform is used only for induction."

"Cyclonal sodium," another entry in my diary reads, "is being supplied to certain British units instead of pentothal. It is said to be entirely unsatisfactory because of tremors, lack of relaxation and slow recovery."

During a discussion of gas gangrene, many of the surgeons we spoke to said they had seen it only in wounds of the lower leg and attributed it to interference of the blood supply by swelling and subfascial hemorrhage. Casualties brought to the F.S.U. showed gas-forming infection at the time of arrival. Cantley advised the administration of anti-gas serum in all wounded with compound fractures of the tibia. The possibility of benefit from block of the sympathetic ganglia was advanced by Larry Pool.

On March 23, we returned to Algiers, stopping at Setif to discuss the treatment of burns with Major Raven. He showed us many "petrol burns"—the type, mentioned earlier, caused by heating ration cans on open gasoline fires.

In a letter dated March 24, I made the following comments about this trip with Weddell:

> *E.D.C. Comments:* "I have just returned to my Hdqrs. from a 1,200 mile auto trip through forward areas. Not too close to the lines, but in one place in the British sector there was fighting going on 6 miles down the road. The signs reading a few kilometers to Tunis were disquieting. Germans respect hospitals, all of which are marked with the red cross. German aviators when taken to a hospital always ask whether it is marked or not. Saw a good many wounded prisoners—far from being the "Herrenvolk" they are supposed to be. The 8 day trip took us through some very beautiful country. Parts were like New Mexico—desert with bare hills and mesas—and part like

(continued)

the Adirondacks, some of the mountains with snow-covered tops. Groves of olive trees—cork trees, but in general no real forests.

"The North African 'Arab' is everywhere. You can't pause on the road for five minutes without drawing a small crowd. They resemble the natives of Mexico or the poorer groups of American Indians. They live in little adobe houses—or in many places just hovels made of an adobe wall—roof poles and the whole thing covered with straw. Many of these thatched hovels are hardly 4-5 feet high. Smoke from fires within seems to seep through the straw. Their clothes are rags—and I should guess were rags before the war, and will be long afterwards. The roads are lined with the Arab men in small groups going somewhere. Where they are going or where they came from is hard to say. Sometimes they ride on the backs of very diminutive burros—very occasionally on a horse or a camel. They till the land, shepherd their sheep or drive a herd of dejected looking beeves.

"In the towns the natives cluster on the streets or in their market areas. Their stores are single small rooms with a few boxes of dirty dates, figs, dried herbs or some strange looking fragment of flesh hanging among the flies."

"French influence is widely spread but down at the heels. Exploring the kitchens of a French restaurant I found a flat top range in the middle of the floor and a fine array of copper utensils on the wall. The Germans must have overlooked them, for despite the tin wearing thin, they were serviceable. In good shape this was a first-class place."

TRIP WITH FORSEE

Jim Forsee, the commanding officer of the 2nd Auxiliary Surgical group, came to Algiers on March 28, 1943. This was his first trip into Algeria and Tunisia to locate the members of his group who came in at the time of the invasion and were widely scattered in medical units, both American and British. Several of the teams were working in the British hospitals in and around Algiers. As we visited these hospitals, we made ward rounds and discussed surgical problems.

One burning issue at that time was whether internal fixation of battle fractures should be performed in the forward area. This topic never failed to provide a heated argument. It was one of the controversial subjects concerning, which we sought information.

On April 1, 1943, Forsee and I left Algeria in a "command car" at 10:00 A.M. A World War II command car was a heavy, ponderous but powerful piece of Army transport with high clearance. It was particularly useful in detours around demolished bridges where fording a stream was required.

Following a long trip through convoys of trucks and over the mountains, we put in at the 35th Station Hospital, which was being set up in St. Arnaud by the Commanding Officer, Lieutenant Colonel Foss and the Chief of Surgery, Captain Harold M. Smith. British engineers were fixing the building. A small opera house was in an adjoining building and was to be used for patients. A French troupe gave a concert under Red Cross auspices in the evening. The little opera house had not been used for some time but soon was filled with service men, American and British. A scattering of officers and nurses sat in the boxes that formed the horseshoe. We sat in the loge municipale, top tier, center. The program was semiclassical—piano, accordion, violin and a soprano singer. Then a trained dog act and finally a "pop" singer who got the audience singing with her—"Roll out the Barrel" and "Alouette."

On the following day we stopped at the British 31st General Hospital to see a neurosurgical team of the 3rd Auxiliary Group (Haynes and Gaynor). "Heatley, the Chief of Surgery," my notes read, "agrees with Shawstone's policy of not encouraging surgeons in forward areas to 'mess about' with head wounds. They start in to do what appears to be a simple job, but find themselves deeply entangled with a prolonged and difficult procedure that requires suction, diathermy and the judgment of an experienced neurosurgeon. Heatley is all for bone plating and believed if the War Office would give them plates they would use them correctly."

Forsee and I visited Eastern Base Section (E.B.S.) Headquarters and several of our station hospitals in the region.

April 3 was spent at the 48th Surgical Hospital where I explored more thoroughly some of the methods being utilized in the treatment of the seriously wounded.

On April 4 we went into the ancient oasis city of Gafsa to photograph a clearing platoon in a French barracks infirmary. Here we saw the surgical team of Major Dent. Snyder, Anspacher and I drove about the city while Forsee stayed with Dent. One corner of the old fort has been reduced to a pile of rubble. Nearby were two deep Roman swimming baths fed by warm water. Looking down forty feet to the surface of the water, the bath was seen to be filled with soldiers in the nude. Ancient Roman inscriptions, arches and nearby palm trees completed the picture. Beyond the city was a sign famous in North Africa: "The British First Army welcomes the Eighth Army" (**Figure 12.2**).

Along the track to El Guettar, Forsee and I stopped at the surgical unit of the armored division. From there we went forward to see a heavily fortified German position in the mountains on the right side of the valley being pounded by our artillery. This point was blocking advance down the valley.

In the open desert floor beyond the Schott El Guettar was the collecting station of Company B, 9th Medical Battalion. H. P. Limbacker and George Cummens were the medical officers on duty.

E.D.C. Comments: "These battalion medical officers lead one hell of a life but are doing superb work," I noted. "Their tent was surrounded

(continued)

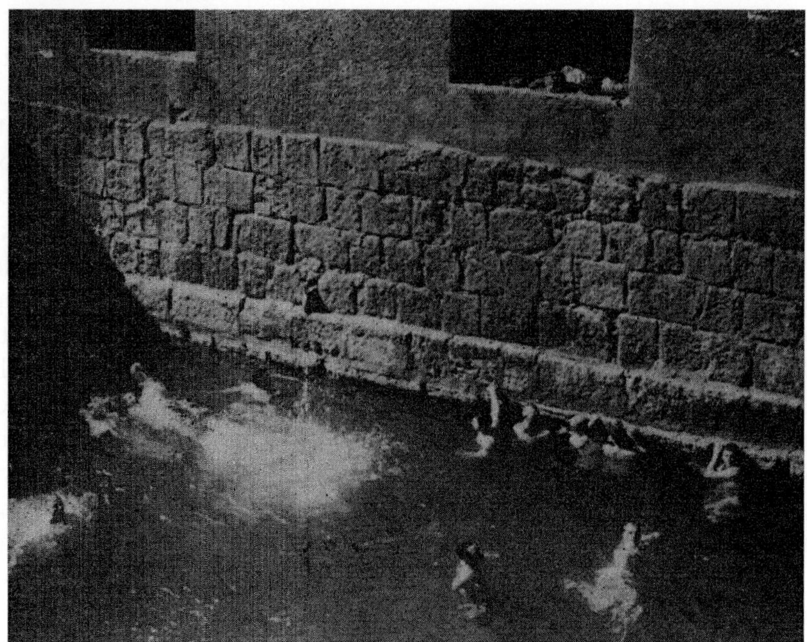

Figure 12.2 U.S. soldiers in a Roman swimming pool in Gafsa, Tunisia.

by foxholes, many obviously arranged for a prolonged stay. Army equipment, tanks and gun placements were widely dispersed on the surrounding desert as air attack is frequent. At present it is impossible to reach an advanced aid station during the day. It is located in a wadi and any vehicle draws German fire. Ambulances collect the wounded under cover of darkness" (**Figure 12.3**).

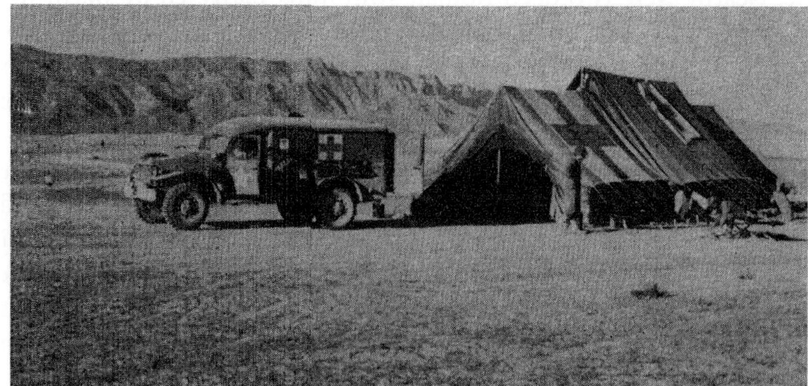

Figure 12.3 The collecting station of Company B, 9th Medical Battalion, on the desert beyond Schott El Guettar.

"The front is a wild but beautiful scene. The sky was cloudless and the jagged mountains stood out in sharp relief. In late afternoon the shadows of the red cliffs were brilliant blue. The desert was flat, with dust from moving transport here and there. No convoys, however, as in this area they must move at night. Small groups or pairs of soldiers were with every stationary vehicle or gun emplacement—all widely separated from each other. Foxholes were the only shelters. All were facing down the valley and alert for a plane that might come over at any moment. Here identification of planes is no matter of casual interest as strafing is a constant danger. There were many British Spitfires in the air—fortunately they were the genuine articles—not Boojums!"

We turned back, through Gafsa, to spend the night at the 48th Surgical Hospital. According to a letter I wrote a few days later: "I shared a tent with a chaplain. In the morning he was on his knees with his mirror perched on the bed—shaving. Whether he said his prayers at the same time I couldn't quite make out. A real example of Army efficiency!"

Later I was asked to award the Purple Heart to a captain who had received a chest wound. A short comment seemed appropriate to indicate that it was the first one he had received and also the first one I had conferred, so the occasion was notable. Giving Purple Hearts to all wounded is a good custom if it is not made too perfunctory.

I spent an entire day nosing about the 48th Surgical Hospital and found many surgical problems. A wounded soldier was having a chill following the intravenous administration of plasma. This type of reaction, the medical officers said, was frequent with British plasma but not with American. I soon found that the tubing provided with U.S. plasma was not discarded, as it was meant to be, but saved to use for saline and British plasma administration. Water was being brought to the hospital in a truck from the "water point" below Gafsa, presumably chlorinated according to Army regulations. It was pumped into a metal drum outside the operating tent, then drawn from the drum into a gasoline tin. It was then used to wash the tubing which was then rinsed in water from the same source that had been boiled for one hour. The tubing was then autoclaved. *Pyrogens gafsaensis!*

A junior officer on duty in the resuscitation tent, I recorded, told me that

E.D.C. Comments: "when a surgeon orders 'resuscitation' but the casualty shows no evidence of shock, 250 cc. of plasma is given 'to avoid a rumpus.' When signs of shock are present, 500 cc. is given in approximately one hour. Then glucose and saline infusion is given until whole blood is available. There is nothing to be gained by giving plasma more rapidly because

(continued)

whole blood will not be available sooner than one or two hours. When it is thought necessary to give plasma more rapidly, the filter is removed. There may be delay between the completion of resuscitation and surgery. The junior officer told me that a patient was ready for operation at 5:00 A.M. that morning, but operation did not start until 11:00 A.M., despite there being empty tables and 'no rush was on.' The delay is sometimes so long that the casualty requires "resuscitation" a second time. The shock squad feels very bitter about this."

I was obtaining all the information I could about the need for whole blood. I recorded in my diary that: "Snyder has in his notes the following comments: 'A few more lives might be saved if a more convenient method of blood transfusion were available. A source of blood for transfusion other than from clearing station personnel should be provided.'"

Several detailed records were studied to determine the time consumed in evacuation, resuscitation and surgical delay. One of these is given as an example:

E.D.C. Comments: G.F., A.S.N.—Howitzer backfired at the breech on April 4 at 1740 hrs. Field Tag and first aid 1750 hrs. Collecting Station 1840 hrs. Arrived Surg. Hosp. 48/2000 hrs. Gives 400 cc. plasma, 1500 cc. blood, 250 cc. plasma. Ready for surgery April 5 at 0500 hrs. 1000 cc. glucose-saline. Operation: 1100 hrs. Compound comminuted fracture right humerus, right ulna and left humerus. Traumatic amputation left hand, necessitating amputation at upper third left forearm. Débridement multiple wounds face, chest and legs.

Wounding to hospital—2 hrs., 20 min.
Resuscitation—9 hrs.
Delay in surgery—6 hrs.

The problems calling for expert surgical judgment seen at the 48th Surgical Hospital surpassed in difficulty any that I had encountered previously in surgery.

On April 6, we moved on to the 77th Evacuation Hospital near Tebessa. In our discussions of forward surgery at this hospital, certain policies of wound management became crystallized. For example, according to my notes:

E.D.C. Comments: "No perforating wound of the urinary bladder is to be closed without establishing suprapubic drainage—a urethral catheter is not adequate; there is no place for a 'hanging plaster' as a transportation splint for fracture of the humerus; gas gangrene is not an indication for amputation. When performed, amputation is a concession to an infection that is already out of control or which has not been eradicated by more conservative measures. In extensive muscle injury without fracture, a lightly padded plaster cast is sufficient. With widespread use of unpadded (skin) plaster instances of pressure on bony prominences will be certain."

As soon as a consensus was reached on some method of wound management, it could be incorporated in a "circular letter" and reach all medical officers in the theater.

Eight or nine transfusions of whole blood per week were being given at the 77th Evacuation Hospital. Men in their own organization were used as donors. It was difficult, they had found, to obtain the consent of lightly wounded casualties to act as donors. I found this attitude understandable because a powerful stimulus to act as donor is the thought that: "I may need it when I am wounded." When someone is already wounded, this stimulus is lacking. Another reason for unwillingness to give blood is the unexpressed worry about one's own wound—"it may be worse than the doctors think." Or—"giving blood may weaken me so that complications will set in." Even the most minor injury results in some degree of apprehension. Also, it should be recalled that the time was early in 1943 and being a blood donor was not the common thing it is today.

Howard Snyder had come overseas with the 77th Evacuation Hospital and had been designated their thoracic surgeon. Grosjean, who was substituting for him in chest work at this time, told me that he was forced to operate with the old set of instruments and not those selected by the National Research Council Committee on Thoracic Surgery some two years ago.

The neurosurgeon at the 77th Evacuation Hospital was Major Carmichael and we had many spirited discussions about craniocerebral wounds with the neurosurgeon at the 77th Evacuation Hospital. Like other overseas neurosurgeons, he was itching to repair bony defects in the skull with vitallium plates. This issue was to come up time after time in the theater but I held fast to a decision made earlier—"the place to repair bony defects of the skull is in the Z.I."

INTERNAL FIXATION

On April 9, I dropped in at the 9th Evacuation Hospital and stimulated a discussion of internal fixation of battle fractures by referring to two patients I had seen at the 99th General Hospital in Algiers on March 30. Jim Thomson brought out the preoperative x-ray films on the second patient, G.V., whose case history follows:

> Penetrating and lacerated wound left knee with compound fracture lower end femur. W.I.A. March 26. Given 750 cc. plasma in 1st Clearing Platoon, 51st Med. Bn. Operated March 26 by Major Thomson at 9th Evac. Open reduction and fixation by two wood type screws. Plaster spica. Arrived 99 G.H. in great pain and very ill. Spica cut away from impingement on costal margin. RBC 1,700,000. Hgb. 35%.
>
> This boy I saw again after my return to Algiers on April 12. He went through a bout of infection and the wound suppurated. At a dressing, one screw could be seen partially covered by granulation tissue.

As Thomson demonstrated the preoperative x-ray films, it was obvious that the shaft of the femur was impacted between spread condyles. In his opinion the only solution to obtaining a functional joint was an open reduction and fixation by screws. Certainly his judgment was correct, and, as I noted in my diary, if infection does not result in serious complications, the trial was justified.

The critics of the use of internal fixation, and at a later date Surgeon General Norman Kirk was among them, had little idea of the complex nature of battle fractures. Also it is to be noted that this casualty was facing the need to heal his wound despite having a profound secondary anemia.

Before returning to Algiers, we spent a night at the 38th Evacuation Hospital, an affiliated unit from Charlotte, North Carolina. The Commanding Officer at this time was Colonel Bauchspies. George T. Wood, Jr., was Chief of Medicine, Paul W. Sanger, Chief of Surgery, and William H. Pennington, Executive Officer. William R. Pitts was the neurosurgeon, and Pat R. Imes a general surgeon. Discussions with this group brought out many interesting comments about forward surgery, as the 38th Evacuation Hospital was on the receiving end of many ambulance shuttles.

Andrew T. Schlussel, Daniel J. Grabo, and Matthew J. Martin

The Tunisian campaign holds historical significance for both Allied forces and Colonel Edward Churchill alike. It was a pivotal part of the broader mission to secure North Africa and the Mediterranean paving the way for the invasion of Italy. The campaign underscored the advantages of shared medical assets between the United States and British forces. In his initial battlefield rotation, Colonel Churchill showed a strong passion for adopting promising medical practices rather than maintaining the status quo.

Northern Africa was a dynamic wartime environment that presented many geographic challenges. Faced with delays in transporting injured soldiers from the front lines to medical facilities, Churchill presented the concept of split medical operations, a paradigm that has since become standard on today's contemporary battlefield. The austere environment also uncovered many challenges and controversies in the management of combat casualties. Obtaining and maintaining a sufficient blood supply was not convenient. The main source of blood donation, albeit limited, came from clearing station personnel. Attempts were made, often met with resistance, to obtain consent from minimally injured patients, as they feared their wounds would not heal and complications would ensue. Finally, long delays between resuscitation and surgery, due to a lack of surgical urgency—a factor known today to decrease survival—brought to light the need for all elements of the system working in harmony to optimize outcomes in these austere settings.

As Churchill continued his battlefield rotation, he encountered additional surgical challenges that remain subjects of discussion today. There was considerable debate on the management of head wounds and the responsibility for their treatment. As many deployed surgeons feel today, the theater neurosurgeon at the time recommended against surgeons in forward areas 'messing about' with head wounds. What may appear as straightforward procedures is often fraught with challenges and complications, necessitating the judgment of an experienced neurosurgeon. Interestingly, despite the caution advised for life-saving interventions by non-neurosurgeons, the request to repair bony defects of the skull with metal plates was desired. Churchill deemed that these injuries required specialized medical attention in facilities with a more secure and well-equipped environment.

While plating cranial injuries was discouraged, internal fixation for orthopedic injuries was deemed justified. This topic was notably criticized by Surgeon General Norman Kirk, an orthopedic surgeon, who Churchill reports had a limited understanding of the complex nature of battlefield extremity fractures. Despite the heightened risk of wound complications, this intervention offered the most promising functional outcomes for open comminuted fracture patterns. Additionally, fixation presented an alternative to unpadded plaster casts, which were known for complications such as pressure ulcers and delayed recognition of compartment syndrome.

Further discussions encompassed various policies for the treatment of penetrating wounds to the bladder and the handling of necrotizing infections of the extremities. Once a consensus was reached, these policies were consolidated into a "circular letter" for all medical officers in the theater. This laid the foundation for Clinical Practice Guidelines, which are policies that are widely followed by military surgeons today.

Notably, Churchill had the distinct honor of awarding a Purple Heart to a captain with a chest wound, marking both the soldier's first Purple Heart and Churchill's first presentation of such an award. This remarkable event, performed by the theater trauma director, unwitnessed today, underscores Churchill's commitment to enhancing battlefield surgical care. It also reflects his transformation from an ivory tower academic to a fully-fledged expeditionary surgeon.

SUGGESTED READINGS

Atkinson R. *An Army at Dawn: The War in North Africa, 1942-1943*. Henry Holt & Co.; 2002.

Bell RS, McCafferty R, Shackelford S, et al. (2018). Emergency life-saving cranial procedures by non-neurosurgeons in deployed setting. Joint Trauma System Clinical Practice Guidelines. Accessed May 24, 2024. https://jts.health.mil/index.cfm/PI_CPGs/cpgs.

Gurney JM, Staudt AM, Del Junco DJ, et al. Whole blood at the tip of the spear: a retrospective cohort analysis of warm fresh whole blood resuscitation versus component therapy in severely injured combat casualties. *Surgery*. 2022 Feb;171(2):518-525.

Gurney JM, Tadlock MD, Dengler BA, et al. Committee on Surgical Combat Casualty Care position statement: neurosurgical capability for the optimal management of traumatic brain injury during deployed operations. *J Trauma Acute Care Surg*. 2023 Aug 1;95(2S Suppl 1):S7-S12.

Hess JR, Thomas MJ. Blood use in war and disaster: lessons from the past century. *Transfusion*. 2003 Nov;43(11):1622-1633.

Howard JT, Kotwal RS, Santos-Lazada AR, Martin MJ, Stockinger ZT. Reexamination of a battlefield trauma golden hour policy. *J Trauma Acute Care Surg*. 2018 Jan;84(1):11-18.

Kotwal RS, Scott LLF, Janak JC, et al. The effect of prehospital transport time, injury severity, and blood transfusion on survival of US military casualties in Iraq. *J Trauma Acute Care Surg*. 2018 Jul;85(1S Suppl 2):S112-s121.

13

Prisoners of War

We Came into frequent contact with prisoners in our hospitals. When there was a large number of them, they were cared for in separate wards or in hospitals designed for that purpose. For instance, when an entire German or Italian hospital was captured, it was left intact with its doctors and nurses to care for its patients.

Revealing insight was obtained in captured letters and diaries. These were turned over to G-2, who not infrequently extracted valuable information on morale or specific items of military significance, and circulated them in mimeographed collections to headquarters' staffs. One valuable insight was that, with a few exceptions, we were fighting simple people, not stereotyped Nazi criminals.

EXTRACTS FROM CENSORED AND CAPTURED MAIL

The prisoners expressed what seemed to be universal amazement at the good food, accommodations and medical attention they received in captivity. Many found their captors extremely amiable and regretted that their nations should be at war; but there was not even a beginning of any recognition that Germany bore any guilt.

The following extracts from letters of Italian prisoners may be of interest. Their surprise at the good treatment they were receiving, and their insistence that they were writing the truth, is indicative of the Italian propaganda on the subject of Allied atrocities to prisoners of war.

> Mamma, I want to tell you that my imprisonment at present is such as I would not believe; it is truly the life of a gentleman. For the present I am working as a cook, and I hope to continue. Mamma, I am well pleased with the good treatment of the Americans.
>
> • • • •

(continued)

I'm writing this letter to let you know that I am a prisoner of the English, recovering in one of their hospitals. I never would have thought this about the English at this time. They forget everything and take good care of us and they show us every courtesy and treat us very well. They do everything to make us forget our troubles. In general they treat us very well and like true brothers.

My dear Mother, will tell you at this time that I am well. I am a prisoner in the hands of the English, they are a very good people, educated men and they treat me very well. If I had known that they were such good people I would have tried to become a prisoner before this happened. . . . In the meantime don't worry about me because I am better off with the English than with the Italians.

Now I am in an English hospital on the road to recovery, thanks to the careful treatment of the English Red Cross. In every way I have had excellent treatment, so I urge you to rest easy about me. Here everything is fine. I am not lying, life is excellent as is the heart of the English. They are fine gentlemen—I will never be able to thank them for all that they have done for me.

AN ALLIED OFFICER'S REPORT

Colonel E. C. Boehnke, Assistant Adjutant General, A.F. H.Q., visited the northern Tunisian front and one of the hospitals that was receiving freshly wounded soldiers. His report may in part explain the surprise of prisoners with their kind treatment.

She hummed softly, a cheery tune from some popular play, this small blond nurse, as she dropped on her knees to tend to the wounded soldier who lay on the litter. He was groaning, but in a suppressed way, gritting his teeth and clenching his fists. His foot was shattered, and he lay there pale and worn, unshaven, his uniform torn and soiled. He lay there under the long field hospital tent pitched on this Tunisian plain, with twenty or thirty others who had just been brought in from a front line collecting station. His foot had been bandaged, but during the journey by hand, litter, and ambulance the bandages had become loosened, and it was her duty to rebandage his foot because it would be a little while before the others would be cleared from this receiving ward and taken to where they belonged. She smiled at the boy, reassuringly, never saying a word, but continuing her humming while she quickly and efficiently completed the job.

They went to the next litter—an officer who lay on his stomach because a large piece of shrapnel had torn through his shoulder blade. She touched the Captain's head lightly, tenderly, and brought a faint flicker of a smile to his tired, drawn face. She adjusted the bandage, gave him a cigarette, and whistled snatches from "Rosemarie," and he felt better.

Her next case was not so easy. He was a tall, blond young sergeant whose sharp blue eyes had glistened as he had led his platoon up a hill to silence a German machine gun nest; they had done it, but the sergeant's face was pale now, and his eyes were drained of their blue. A grenade had exploded almost in his face, and pieces of the cold steel had cut cruelly into his chest and abdomen. This case needed immediate attention, and the nurse called a doctor attending another case. While the medical officer quickly examined the soldier, the little nurse hummed again, only this time it was hardly audible. But as two corpsmen carried the wounded man away to the operating tent, she hummed louder and turned to the next litter.

He was a German. She looked quickly at his face, but if she experienced any emotion she kept it hidden. Dropping once more to her knees, she deftly adjusted the blood soaked bandage covering the stump of an arm. She was humming cheerily again, and the soldier watched her curiously. It was his first contact with an American woman, and as he watched her a glint of admiration flickered in his eyes. She had made it easier.

I watched her a long time, this tireless little nurse, in her grey coveralls, as she moved quickly and sympathetically from litter to litter, humming gently, whistling softly, cheering them all, alleviating pain of friend and foe alike. And I wondered how she could do this for eight hours—ten hours—fourteen hours—endlessly, so long as they came in the duty ambulances from out yonder where the cannons boomed. But they tell me she did.

14

The Consultants in North Africa

THE CONSULTING system that was developed in the North African Theater for the U.S. Army was influenced strongly by the need for simplicity and economy in manpower. It did not occur to me to ask for as large a group of consultants in the specialties as was assembled in the European Theater of Operations. This comment in no way implies criticism of what took place in the E.T.O. but is offered in explanation of the shape the consulting organization took in the Mediterranean area.

One of the first lessons I had learned was that the authority of a "chicken colonel" or of a professor, was not sufficient. I had to establish myself as competent in the surgical field, and I found the opportunity to do so immediately. It happened during a tour I discussed in Chapter 12, The Tunisian Campaign. I was staying at the 77th Evacuation Hospital (the University of Kansas unit), having arrived there on April 6, 1943, with Jim Forsee. I stayed over an extra day, waiting for General Blesse to come through. This quotation is from my diary:

E.D.C. Comments: They are a good crowd and know just how to handle a visiting consultant. The first evening I was there we were in the surgical tent when two normal appendices were removed under a diagnosis of appendicitis. I didn't even raise an eyebrow as far as I am aware. On the next day, however, they asked me to see every bellyache in the hospital until I finally picked out a soldier I thought should be operated on for appendicitis.

"The appendix was normal. Then, having properly deflated me, I was asked to see a soldier who had been thrown from a car in a road accident. He had a fractured lumbar spine without cord damage and a serious degree of shock with respiratory distress. X-ray photo had shown a fluid level running (in the lateral position) to the second rib. A swallow of barium had shown what looked like a normal position of the stomach with a considerable collection of barium in the cardiac end. Chest aspiration yielded thin turbid fluid with no striking odor which was said to show streptococci and tetrads but no leucocytes. I made a diagnosis of rupture of the diaphragm with thoracic stomach. The shock was partly due to impedance of the venous return as the patient had a paradoxic pulse. The accident had happened the previous day and urgent symptoms increased, with gastric dilatation and pyloric obstruction. Having advised operation, I was invited to do it and so went ahead. The 9th rib was removed, the enormous stomach was opened and its contents of fluid and air removed by suction; the gastrotomy was closed and the evisceration that consisted of large and small bowel, spleen and omentum as well as stomach was easily reduced. The rent in the diaphragm was sutured. The lung was slowly expanded and the chest was closed without drainage."

I saw this patient subsequently back in Morocco as he was being evacuated to the United States. During this operation General Blesse arrived at the hospital and was brought to the operating room; so he had the opportunity of seeing his Surgical Consultant solving an unusual and spectacular result of trauma which had not been recognized by one of the evacuation hospital staffs. This was my test "under fire" which happened, coincidentally, just when Blesse had taken over the post of Theater Surgeon. Indeed, it was his first trip as Theater Surgeon. At least this episode demonstrated that I was competent in the practical field of wound surgery. I don't think I did more than one or two other operations during my whole tour of duty. The consultant's job was not that of an itinerant operating surgeon.

SELECTING CONSULTANTS

Subsequently, during informal discussions with Blesse at headquarters in Algeria, I expressed my desire for a few consultants who could deal with basic problems on a "troubleshooting" basis. Although Fred Rankin, when I had been in Washington, had intimated that I might turn to him for an orthopedic consultant or a neurosurgical consultant, it seemed to me that we would make greater headway by having "troubleshooters" who would approach broad problems with an open mind rather than surgeons who might come into the theater with preconceived ideas and focus on the technical management of injury.

The first man I selected was Champ Lyons, an M.G.H. man who was already in the Army working on wound infections, a subject to which he had given concentrated thought and effort for several years. A cable was sent to Champ during the week of May 15, 1943.

During the week of May 29, cables were sent to the Surgeon General, asking for Henry K. Beecher and John Stewart. I also wrote to Stewart, who had not yet entered the Army, telling him to let me know—by a code Western Union cable—whether he had been able to leave his essential post. The code I suggested was Number 81—"I have left hospital." This had been designed to assure some family about a soldier's health. When I received this code message from John I knew that he was on his way. John was an expert in surgical shock and body fluids.

It was obvious in Tunisia that some of the wounded were dying not from their wounds but from the faulty choice and administration of anesthetic agents. Particularly in the forward area, the medical officers were using intravenous pentothal and accidents were happening. Also, we were having trouble from morphine poisoning. The British had already encountered it and warned against large doses of morphine. Our aid men were equipped with half-grain tablets of morphine and, not infrequently, a soldier brought in by litter bearers would be given two, three, sometimes more doses because his pain had not been relieved. This meant that he did not have enough circulation (because of blood loss) to absorb the injections which were remaining as depot morphine under the skin. Then when the casualty was warmed and perhaps given plasma to improve the circulation, he would pick up these depots of morphine and exhibit serious morphine poisoning.

Anesthesia appliances were in short supply, particularly specialized ones such as are required for an open thoracic operation. This need we thought had been taken care of in the States when I was a member of the advisory group of the N.R.C. on thoracic surgery. Portable apparatus had been developed by Beecher, particularly designed for use in war, but it had not reached North Africa. Many things were not available in this hasty war in Tunisia. I asked for Beecher, with the knowledge that he wanted to come into the Army if he could find a place where he would be useful.

A fourth member of my consulting staff was recruited from the E.T.O. When General Hawley came to Algiers on a visit in May, he suggested that one or two of our surgeons with experience with war wounds in the Auxiliary group teams could be of great use to his staff in London. I found a surgeon who was anxious to be transferred to the other theater and said that I was ready to exchange him for Fiorindo Simeone, who had joined up with the Harvard unit, which was in the E.T.O. This exchange was cleared and I had Simeone to use as a general troubleshooter in the forward area.

Simeone also had been an M.G.H. resident surgeon. I was laying myself open to the charge of nepotism but there were so few surgeons available who could tackle broad problems that I had to pick from a small group that I knew. It is common practice in the Army to select a staff whose qualities are known. I discussed this—as to whether I was showing favoritism—but no one at that time thought of a consultant's job as being desirable. Most young surgeons wanted to operate during their war experience. I knew Simeone was overseas and available and he was the only man that I particularly wanted who was in the E.T.O. Simeone had been brought up at the M.G.H. and I knew the caliber of his mind—that he could be put on any problem. He had only recently finished general surgery residency followed by a specialized residency in genitourinary surgery. I also knew that he might like to come to the Mediterranean area because he was an Italian. His parents came to Providence as Italian immigrants and Simeone was a self-made man. After preparation in Brown University, he attended the Harvard Medical School with a brilliant record. He had been offered an assistant professorship of physiology at Columbia while he was still in surgical training (**Figure 14.1**).

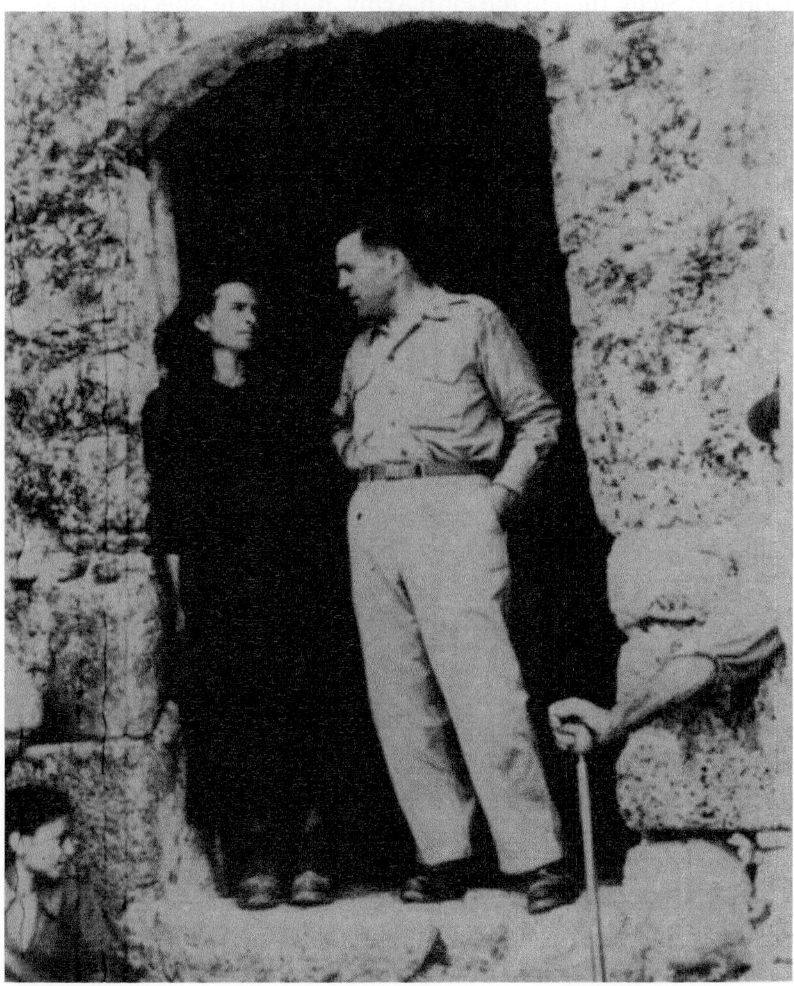

Figure 14.1 Lieutenant Colonel Fiorindo Simeone discovers a sister in the Liri Valley, Italy.

On my first trip to II Corps, I had found that Howard Snyder—who, as I have mentioned earlier, had gone overseas with the 77th Evacuation Hospital—was unhappy being a few miles behind the combat area when there was excitement forward. When I first went to see Arnest, the Corps Surgeon, I found Snyder on detached service already circulating among hospitals and particularly keeping his eye on the isolated surgical teams. He was helping the young surgeons, learning the problems and getting along magnificently with Arnest and his executive officer, Anspacher. It was obvious that Snyder was in the right slot, so I gave my assent to Arnest's inquiries as to whether this was a satisfactory arrangement. Snyder throughout the war became the consultant in the forward area, first to II Corps in Tunisia, then to II Corps in Sicily, then to the Fifth Army in Italy. He "specialized" as a consultant and supervisor in forward surgery. We talked over our problems and worked closely together. I was supporting him and he was feeding problems to me as he encountered them, and we enjoyed a harmonious relationship.

I did not appoint consultants to the rear areas, although from time to time, particularly in the large base section, the Surgeon would use one of his senior hospital surgeons on detached duty to instruct new hospitals when they arrived. My headquarters was always in the rear area and most hospitals were too short of manpower to spare their mature officers for detached service.

Also, I did not want to give over the responsibility for constantly seeing wounded soldiers and their wounds. To see them in the rear enabled me to keep in touch with what was going on forward. Winston Churchill once refused a reorganization which would have made him a "Supreme" Commander. He said he did not care to indulge in "exalted brooding over the work of others." This is what has been called "getting kicked out through the ceiling." To my mind it was important to keep intimate contact with all of the problems presented by wounded men.

A mature surgeon knows that if he is to lead an operating team, a staff of interns and residents or a surgical staff of his peers, he himself must frequent the operating room and wards. To cover the vast distances of the theater, over half of my time was spent in travel—less than half at headquarters. To operate on a patient and then move on, leaving his postoperative care to others, would set a bad example. In consequence, I gave up operating but made every effort to spend my time in the wards and always visit the operating room. It was also important to visit the surgeons in the most forward areas as well as those in the rear.

Although I had no "command" authority as a staff officer, if I were to influence the surgery of the wounded it was advisable to follow a pattern well known to successful commanders. This was well expressed by Rommel: "There are always moments when the commander's place is not back with his staff but up with the troops. It is sheer nonsense to say that maintenance of the men's morale is the job of the battalion commander alone. The higher the rank, the greater the effect of the example. The men tend to feel no kind of contact with a commander who, they know, is sitting somewhere in headquarters. What they want is what might be termed a physical contact with him. In moments of panic, fatigue or disorganization, or when something out of the ordinary has to be demanded of them, the personal example of the commander works wonders, especially if he has had the wit to create some sort of legend around himself." This was the pattern established by General Patton—always flying his flag when going toward the front—and by General Mark Clark.

FURTHER SEARCH FOR CONSULTANTS

One of the gravest injuries was that of compound fractures. A high percentage of war wounds (roughly 72 per cent) were of the extremities. Many of these had fractures of the long bones. This was a field with which I had only a passing familiarity. As I went on tour through the rear echelon hospitals, I found the 21st General Hospital (the Washington University unit) set up in the mountains south of Oran at Bou Hanifia, a French spa. Here I found Oscar P. Hampton, Jr. Oscar impressed me as having had wide experience in the management of war wounds of the extremities. The center of the problems of fracture management was the rear area where methods of traction, splinting and subsequent care of the wounds were concentrated. It was not long before Oscar Hampton was on temporary duty from the 21st General Hospital, working out of headquarters as Orthopedic Consultant.

Later I found Eldridge Campbell, one of the most mature neurosurgeons in the theater, with a general surgical background. He was Chief of Surgery at the 33rd General Hospital (the Albany unit) which first opened in Bizerte during the Sicilian campaign. Eldridge was available for tours of duty as Neurosurgical Consultant.

There were other special needs which as they arose were met by detaching some surgeon, with special knowledge and competence, from his regular hospital post and having him make a tour through the theater. For illustration, the radiologist, Earl Crowder of the 12th General Hospital (the Northwestern unit), made surveys of the radiologic needs and procedures of the theater. The men themselves liked the assignments, but their commanding officers usually resented it bitterly because it left them a little shorthanded.

There were two surgeons in the 12th General Hospital who had national reputations for special skill and competence in caring for injuries of the hand: Michael Mason, a former classmate of mine at Northwestern University, and Harvey Allen. Both were direct descendants of the Kanavel school of hand surgery at Northwestern. Sumner Koch, who carried forward the Kanavel tradition, had a national reputation not only in hand surgery but, of course, the treatment of burns; and Harvey Allen was a disciple of his. I turned to Mike and Harvey for their experience with hand injuries and burns, and later on in Italy we set up a hand center in the 12th General Hospital and tried to concentrate the patients there during the combat in the Apennines.

The surgeons used as consultants can be divided into two broad categories: those like Campbell, who could qualify in the technical field of neurosurgery and head wounds, and those who could troubleshoot in basic areas such as shock, hemorrhage and infection. Most of them had been trained in general surgery before specialization. As I had hoped, the pattern as a whole began to take the form of utilizing knowledge and experience as the need developed and not trying to superimpose preconceived ideas.

The consulting system was not static because consultants were transferred and changed their areas of interest. Subsequently Stewart was transferred to the Air Force when it needed a consultant in Italy. Beecher went on to the broad problems of resuscitation as well as those of anesthesia. Simeone was to shift his interest to trench foot and vascular injury. Champ Lyons had to return to the United States after some time in Italy because he developed hepatitis, but not until he had contributed his share in teaching the principles of wound infection and chemotherapy. The wide range of his interests can be seen in the following letter which he sent to me from Naples during the Italian campaign:

Dear Colonel Churchill,

Thought you might be interested in seeing what I have been doing all this time. I am sure we shall need a stabile penicillin for local application and the wheels are rolling in that direction. I should be unwilling to trust penicillin alone for gas gangrene but would use it with antitoxin and surgery. The clostridia recovered from the African wounds are interesting. Only one Welch bacillus so far. Sporogenes, histolyticum and tetramorphia predominate.

Desert sores seem to be a folliculitis with staph or strept. Some strept. are definitely microaerophilic and little undermining ulcers are present.

Fractured femurs look best when transported in Thomas splints with Pearson attachments and some traction. In plaster casts the thigh atrophies and loss of alignment occurs. Lower legs are holding alignment reasonably well. What are you doing about f. b. in the myocardium. We recently removed one here.

A major problem in chronically septic patients seems to be an excess of extracellular fluid with low hematocrits even after the other values are restored. Penicillin is good but don't expect too much of it in wounds with mixed infection at present dosages. The calculated toxic dosage is 7 million units, so try big dosage if in a jam. Hope they will get enough data here soon.

All my best,
CHAMP

FOLLOWING UP PATIENTS

The placement of medical officers on temporary duty to travel within the theater and report on their findings was an important adjunct to the consulting system. Many surgeons did not have to be sought out, but came to us. For example, during the North African campaign Somers Sturgis asked if he could look around as a plastic surgeon. He did so and made many informal suggestions. This freedom to move about was used as a learning tool in the 2nd Auxiliary Group. These surgeons, during an offensive movement, were busy operating; of course. Many developed such a keen personal interest in their patients that the moment active combat was over and they knew a lull would come, they went back to their headquarters where they were given travel orders by their Commanding Officer, Jim Forsee. He had a thoughtful, almost academic approach to surgery. These surgeons then traveled through the rear hospitals, looked up the patients they had operated on and recorded the results. Forsee and his men began to take over the function of an "end results" study.

The pilot study of this group was that conducted by Ken Lowry. Lowry, after the Tunisian campaign, made an extensive study of the patients he had taken care of and presented a fine report which is one of the basic documents of the theater.

Most important, Lowry's report established the pattern of finding out what happened to a patient—and from that emerged one of the guiding concepts that developed in North Africa: namely, that a wounded man must be thought of in terms of his total care within the theater. He is not like a load of material that is taken to the rear boundary of the division and, by so doing, responsibility is discharged. What is done for a wounded man is determined by what is going to be done at the next hospital. This concept began to place surgical treatment in the fourth dimension of *time* rather than in the usual dimensions of space. A surgeon could say this is the time and place to do the following but not to do something else. From this there emerged the concept which is basic to contemporary military surgery of the *initial* treatment of a wound and then the *revision* and *reparative* surgery. These take place in different echelons from the front to the rear.

WELL-ROUNDED STAFF

Perrin Long was in Algiers before I arrived because he came down from England, not with the Task Force but shortly thereafter. Being Medical Consultant, he had quite a different set of problems to deal with, of course—among them, malaria control and hepatitis. Perry and I worked during the entire war with our desks next to each other, and each respected the other's province. We often made trips together and exchanged information constantly. We also worked together in the field through the Sicilian campaign. We shared a jeep and were with each other most of the time.

Before long, Lieutenant Colonel Fred R. Hanson, a Canadian, joined us as Consultant in Psychiatry. We also had a Venereal Disease Consultant in headquarters, Lieutenant I. A. Dewey. (I discuss the problem of venereal disease in Chapter 17, Prostitution and Venereal Disease.) We had a Preventive Medicine Consultant, Colonel William S. Stone, a regular Army Medical Corps officer—an "Abraham Lincoln" in his integrity and his uncompromising attitude. (The last time I knew Bill Stone's whereabouts he was Vice President in Charge of Medical Affairs at the University of Maryland.)

Lieutenant Colonel Stewart F. Alexander was the expert in chemical warfare, fortunately dealing only with preparedness until the Bari (Italy) disaster, which I discuss in Chapter 26, Mustard Gas in Bari Harbor. Lieutenant Colonel Bernice Wilbur was in charge of nursing until she married Alexander. (According to an item in the *Stars and Stripes*, this was believed to be the first marriage "in U.S. military history in which two lieutenant colonels were united.") She was replaced by Lieutenant Colonel Margaret Aaron. Colonel L. H. Tingay determined the policies in dentistry, an important assignment with direct bearing on the nutrition of the combat soldier.

That constituted the professional consultant structure at A.F.H.Q. in Algeria. In addition there were, in the office of the Theater Surgeon, the usual Plans and Training, Evacuation and Operations Sections—all functions represented at headquarters.

CRITICISM—AND A TRIBUTE

Our relations with the E.T.O. consulting staff were somewhat strained at first because they had envisioned themselves in charge of the invasion of North Africa but had not been permitted to leave England. Shortly after I arrived in Algiers, Rex Diveley, Orthopedic Consultant on General Hawley's staff in London, obtained travel orders and visited North Africa. Rex toured the theater and knew far more than I did about fractures. He had learned in England such novelties as the Tobruk plaster so I invited him to demonstrate it. Our surgeons did not think it gave adequate immobilization and so it was not used.

Meanwhile, criticism had emerged from the E.T.O. about a shipload of casualties sent back to their hospitals. This was immediately after the landing, when everything was chaotic, and they kept spreading the news of the terrible wound surgery going on in North Africa. It takes time to organize and educate civilian doctors in wound surgery, and I have no doubt that their criticisms were valid. After North Africa we knew what had to be done. We had it mapped out, but it took up to the fall of Rome before the theater had the major essentials of wound surgery well in hand.

The close of a chapter on consultants is a fitting place to pay tribute to Brigadier General Elliott C. Cutler, the Surgical Consultant of the European Theater of Operations. Our paths crossed several times during the war. Elliott either called forth an intense loyalty from younger surgeons under him, or a competitive rivalry, similar to that between two athletic teams, on the part of those of equal status. Any remarks of mine that may seem derogatory of the E.T.O. undertaking are to be interpreted as friendly rivalry.

Elliott was my host on a trip to Paris late in the war. He gave a dinner in my honor and I was seated next to René Leriche, the doyen of French surgery. During this trip I noted that Elliott placed a pillow behind his back when sitting and mentioned an arthritis of the spine which was causing some pain. This was an early symptom of a vertebral metastasis and he died shortly after the end of the war.

At the first meeting of the American Surgical Association after the end of World War II a high ranking officer of the Army Medical Corps slipped a Distinguished Service Medal into my pocket and asked me to present it to Elliott. Tracy Vorhees was the guest speaker at this meeting, still busy in the War Department with the disposition of medical supplies. I gave the medal to Tracy and told him that it might place Cutler in an embarrassing position to have me make the presentation. He agreed and said he would take care of the matter. Later, Judge Robert P. Patterson, the Secretary of War, made the presentation in the garden of the Brookline house where Elliott was surrounded by many of his former resident surgeons. Elliott had received a D.S.M. in World War I. The addition of the Oak Leaf Cluster was a memorable event.

Margaret E. Gallagher, Joseph M. Galante, and M. Margaret "Peggy" Knudson

In this chapter, Churchill describes the consultant system he developed from the ground up in the North African Theater, the role of these consultants in advising him on surgical care of wounded soldiers, and the many challenges he faced along the way. The most immediate challenges were to quickly establish himself as a competent surgeon and to ensure the competency and expertise of the consultants he recruited. He also describes the rudimentary trauma system in which he operated and of the value of surgeons supporting one another. In these respects, we see similarities between his experience and current military deployments.

Sophisticated trauma systems in the United States emerged from successes and lessons of military trauma care during the Korean and Vietnam Wars, but this chapter demonstrates that trauma systems also existed in World War II. Churchill tells a fantastic story of his diagnosis and surgical treatment of a traumatic diaphragmatic injury with intestinal herniation. He then speaks of seeing this patient again when that patient was being evacuated. How rare, both then and now, for the surgeon to care for that injured soldier and then see him again during evacuation. Churchill describes an "ends results" approach, no doubt a nod to Dr Ernest A. Codman who first emphasized the importance of monitoring outcomes. Unfortunately, it took the military until 2004 to establish the Joint Trauma System (JTS) to systematically track combat casualty outcomes from the point of injury to definitive care.

Churchill's role as a consultant resembles the position of the theater trauma consultant in more recent conflicts. Like Churchill, the JTS consultant faced challenges maintaining consistent care practices across large combat theaters, filling both operative and nonoperative positions throughout the theater, and in finding roles for surgical specialists. In Churchill's time, most specialty surgeons (neurosurgeons, urologists, thoracic surgeons, etc) had first completed a full general surgical residency prior to specialization. Early specialization in modern surgical practice now requires innovative measures to ensure that all deploying surgeons have attained the required knowledge and skills to care for combat casualties regardless of their in-garrison practice.

This chapter also reminds us of the dangers of "lessons lost." Churchill recounts that during the Tunisian campaign, wounded soldiers were dying not from their injuries but from overdoses of morphine administered intramuscularly (IM) in the prehospital setting. The initial dose would prove ineffective due to hypoperfusion; so repeated doses were administered. With warming and resuscitation, the multiple IM doses were finally absorbed, leading to toxic levels of morphine. Similarly, in Afghanistan in 2001, IM morphine was frequently used for analgesia. Through the JTS, this was replaced with the "Triple-Option Analgesia" approach: (1) meloxicam and acetaminophen for minor pain, (2) transmucosal fentanyl for severe pain without shock or respiratory distress, or (3) ketamine for severe pain with shock or respiratory distress.

Finally, Churchill emphasizes the importance of surgeons supporting each other in the theater of war. Throughout any deployment, it is imperative to talk through problems with other surgeons to truly make military medicine a continuously learning system. Only then can we successfully manage the challenges of new wounding patterns, make improvements in resuscitation and infection control, and offer the combat wounded the best chance of making a full recovery.

SUGGESTED READINGS

Butler FK Jr, Kotwal RS, Buckenmaier CC III, et al. A triple-option analgesia plan for tactical combat casualty care: TCCC guidelines change 13-04. *J Spec Oper Med*. 2014 Spring;14(1):13-25.

Cannon JW, Fischer JE, Edward D. Churchill as a combat consultant: lessons for the senior visiting surgeons and today's military medical corps. *Ann Surg*. 2010;251(3):566-572.

Military Clinical Readiness Curriculum. Accessed December 19, 2023. https://www.facs.org/mcurriculum/

National Academies of Sciences, Engineering, and Medicine. *A National Trauma Care System: Integrating Military and Civilian Trauma Systems to Achieve Zero Preventable Deaths After Injury*. The National Academies Press; 2016.

Sorbero M, Omsted S, Gonzalez Morganti K, et al. *Improving the Deployment of Army Health Care Professionals. An Evaluation of PROFIS*. RAND Arroyo Center and RAND Health; 2013. Accessed December 19, 2023. https://www.rand.org/pubs/technical_reports/TR1227.html

15

Surgery of Wounds of the Soft Parts

PRELUDE[1]

THE CLOSURE of battle casualty wounds is the most frequent operative procedure encountered by the surgical services of a general hospital in a theatre of operations. In the past four months wounds of the soft parts alone have been closed by secondary suture in eleven hundred and thirty-six patients. Wounds communicating with bones or joints are not included in this report. Although many of the wounds were small, they were usually multiple, varying from two to thirty-six per patient, so that an estimate of three thousand wound closures would be conservative.

"The following advantages of early closure and of initial evaluation of each wound in the operating room are suggested:

1. *The original dressing of the wound is accomplished under the most favorable circumstances obtainable. The air on the wards is likely to be heavily dust-laden and it is not practical to mask and gown ward personnel and patients in closely adjacent beds. Lighting facilities are often so poor that it is difficult to inspect and evaluate the wound properly on the ward.*
2. *Wounds dressed infrequently seem to do much better than those inspected often. Both time and dressing materials are conserved.*
3. *The inclusion of one or more of the senior surgical officers on these teams ensures uniform surgical judgment.*
4. *There is minimal delay in the definitive treatment of the wound. It may be sutured, more completely débrided or covered with skin grafts at this initial dressing.*
5. *The results in this sample of seventy-one wounds show that closure of the wound within four or five days after débridement can be safely done without the sulfonamides or penicillin in the large majority of cases. This results in a great saving of soldier-hospital days and means pliable, nonindurated scars with much less subsequent disability."*

DÉBRIDEMENT

The extensive application of sulfa to wounds was certainly one aspect of wound management that contributed to infection and suppuration. However, belief in the therapeutic value of sulfa led surgeons to deemphasize

---

[1]Kirtley, James A., Jr., Lt. Col. M.C., and Trabue, Charles C., IV, Major, M.C.: Report on Delayed Closure of Wounds, April 1, 1944.

the importance of adequate débridement even if they fully understood the importance of this technique in war wounds. There was a great deal of confusion surrounding the theory of treatment of wounds of the soft parts; and untangling conflicting stories, theories and practices through direct observation was an important part of my consulting function.

The teaching of wound surgery to a civilian-trained surgeon, I must repeat, is not easy. He starts with an underestimation of the severity of war wounds. A surgeon would say: "But I've worked for years at the Detroit Receiving Accident Hospital. I know how to handle wounds." But he still would have no conception of the destructive force of high-velocity missiles or the timing factor so important in treatment, and the many other elements that make wound surgery a specialty in itself. This is true today in spite of accumulated experience. When a new hospital begins to receive freshly wounded casualties, invariably the first débridements will be inadequate.

The meaning of the French word *débridement*, is to release tension by *incision*. An abscess is débrided when incised to allow pus to run out. The word *épluchage* means paring (a potato) or trimming (a grapevine). The term "trimming" has been used with reference to a wound, but in American usage débridement has come to mean incision followed by excision of dead tissues.[2] Hippocrates wrote that "contused tissues must liquefy and turn into matter." Consequently, the surgeon excises it rather than allowing it to putrefy and become a source of infection and suppuration in the human body. If one treated a wound like a malignant tumor, one might excise it ruthlessly and get rid of it completely but at the sacrifice of nerves, muscle and blood vessels; so the skill comes in excising only what is dead.

One must not mutilate living tissue or destroy functional structures. Experience teaches how to separate the living from the dead. There are well-established criteria. Experience must supplement the written word and provide the intimate, intuitive familiarity with the wound in its many and changing aspects. Layers of deep fascia are divided transversely, an exception being the strong fascia lata of the lateral aspect of the thigh. Devitalized muscle shows no contraction when pinched lightly with forceps. A knowledge of the blood and nerve supply of important muscles is necessary when they are retracted or trimmed. A characteristic earmark of an amateur in wound surgery is a short incision which provides inadequate exposure of the deeper structures. He then proceeds to carry out a "vaginal examination" with one or two fingers, instead of using sharp dissection under direct vision. Another

---

[2]To permit delayed closure and healing with minimal scar and contracture the incision is placed in flexion creases in the neighborhood of joints and parallel with Langer's lines on the trunk, neck and face. On the face, excision of tissue is kept at a minimum and incision to remove foreign bodies following the wrinkle lines. (See: Kraissl CJ, Conway H. Excision of small tumors of the skin of the face with special reference to the wrinkle lines. *Surgery.* 1949;25(4): 592-600.)

trademark of the novice is the "circumcision" of wounds of entrance and exit. The circular or oval defects are slow to heal and difficult to close by delayed suture.

A wound after débridement is never "packed" open or stuffed with gauze. Bleeding points are controlled with fine absorbable ligatures or small stitch ligatures that do not devitalize muscles. A gauze pack distorts structures and is used only as a last recourse for otherwise uncontrollable torrential hemorrhage. Fine mesh gauze can be inserted in the wound as between the leaves of a book, and the tissues brought together with a snug bandage or light plaster bandage.

Almost anything may be found in a wound, and the removal of foreign bodies is another reason for adequate exposure. Metallic foreign bodies are visualized by x-ray or fluoroscopy. Small metallic foreign bodies do not call for removal. They may be scattered widely through the tissues. That they have lodged in the body indicates a rapid decay in velocity and minimal tissue damage.

Large metallic foreign bodies require removal. Their point of lodgement often contains other foreign material not visualized by x-ray. Bits of clothing or shoe leather, splinters of wood, grass, dirt and other debris are frequent. A penetrating velocity may be given to parts of a vehicle in which the man is riding at the time he is wounded.

WOUND SUTURE

In between my trips in the field, I visited the British 94th General Hospital on the outskirts of Algiers. Here I ran across a knowing surgeon, Lieutenant Colonel Gibberd. He was a pupil of Leonard Colebrook and had the viewpoint about streptococcal and other coccal infections that had come down from World War I from Colebrook's teacher, Sir Almroth Wright. A note in my diary records that I spent considerable time discussing secondary wound suture with Gibberd and saw a few wounds in which it had been performed. Case 1, according to my notes, had been closed on the tenth day and had been carried out by undercutting the wound margins. Another wound of the same date had been closed without undercutting the margins. No oral sulfanilamide had been given and a small amount had been applied locally. The other cases are also recorded carefully in my diary, and my comment was that I was not impressed greatly by the techniques used in the secondary sutures. Gibberd grasped the skin margins with tooth forceps, a maneuver which obviously offended my surgical instincts. I comment, too, that small wounds should be excised rather than simply drawn together with sutures. Penicillin, I jotted down, should be tried as an adjuvant to secondary suture. The diary records that Gibberd is one of the few surgeons I have seen to date who does dressings wearing a face mask. He believes strongly that wounds are contaminated heavily en route to a hospital by frequent dressings. Wounds received directly from a casualty clearing station look different and are better adapted to secondary suture. Finally, I wrote that I enjoyed talking with him as he is a "surgical philosopher."

Meanwhile, I had also made a tour through the American base section hospitals under orders cut on April 18, 1943. By going back through Oran to Casablanca and visiting hospitals, I missed the closing phase of the Tunisian campaign. What I was to learn on this backward tour proved more important in the long run. First I went to Oran and to the 12th General Hospital, hoping by a talk with Mike Mason and Harvey Allen to get caught up on wound management. Interestingly enough, the deep-rooted experience of these two scholarly surgeons from the school of Kanavel and Sumner Koch had left them with too rigid concepts of wound contamination and infection to permit any experiments on wound closure. The note in my diary about my visit to the 12th General Hospital is:

E.D.C. Comments: In *cactus thorn* injuries a hemolytic staphylococcus has been recovered. The thorn itself is very long and difficult to find. I wonder if complete excision very early followed by a primary graft would not be the correct treatment.

G.H. 12 has done about 12 *secondary sutures* at periods of 3 weeks or longer after wounding. No local or oral sulphonamide has been used. Time of healing has been shortened in all.

From the 12th General Hospital I went south to the 21st General Hospital at Bou Hanifia on April 27, 1943. It was here that I first met Major Wendell S. Dove. This hospital, under the command of Lee D. Cady, was the affiliated unit organized at Washington University and was the first general hospital to arrive in North Africa.

Major Dove was Chief of the Section of Septic Surgery—a time-consuming task in the sulfa drug era of wound surgery. When I inquired as to what they were doing with the "secondary suture" of wounds I was met by incredulous looks. As I learned afterwards, steps were underway to *forbid* this procedure from being undertaken. Dove had started to do secondary closure on defects on his surgical ward. This had so shocked the other surgeons that they persuaded Lee Cady to call it to a halt. To have the Surgical Consultant of the theater arrive and ask to see secondary sutures was incomprehensible, particularly when I spent the afternoon with Dove instead of with the orthodox members of the staff. My behavior threw the hospital off balance.

I stayed with Dove and examined his patients and watched him do a secondary suture. I was fascinated by this procedure. It was a wound of the leg which had been débrided with a longitudinal incision directly through a tattoo mark. The tattoo design was that of a peacock and the gaping skin margins had separated widely the tattooed delineation of this noble bird. As I watched Dove reconstruct the peacock I had two or three ideas in mind. As a secondary suture, the operation followed an old and familiar pattern—a granulating wound with rigid margins which required undercuts was drawn together under considerable tension. I was also interested in exactly how much peacock had been excised in the débridement because a criticism of the forward surgeons was that they trimmed away too much skin, and here was a chance to demonstrate that it was the gaping of the wound that caused an *apparent* defect rather than excision of more than a narrow margin of skin. The peacock was restored nearly intact!

It can be seen from the photograph (**Figure 15.1**) that Dove carried out what was known as a secondary suture. This was a familiar procedure performed on healing wounds after fourteen to twenty-one days. Many of the great shell fragment wounds of World War I were closed in this manner.

About September 1, 1944, General Morrison Stayer, who by then was Theater Surgeon, received a letter from Major Dove in which the following paragraph is representative: "I was the first to practice and to advocate the wide acceptance of what today has become the surgical procedure performed with greatest frequency in this theater—that of the secondary or delayed closure of wounds. I began this work in septic surgery against great opposition and, in spite of success, there was reluctance in using the procedure even in clean surgery. The Army now, I feel, accepts this. It did not then."

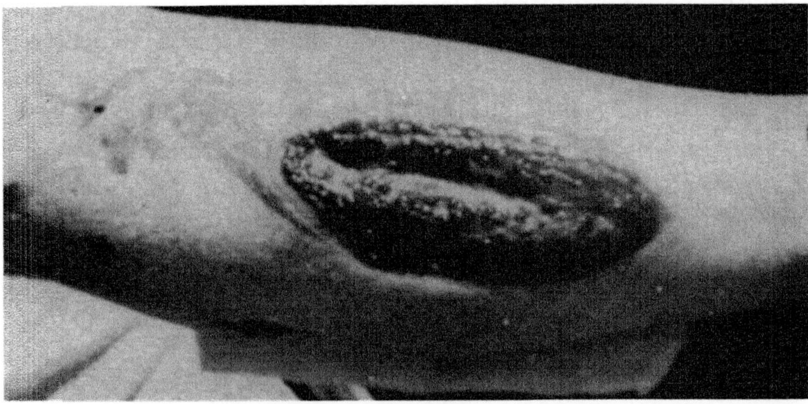

Figure 15.1 A 12- to 14-day granulating wound in the center of a tattoo of a peacock.

In a reply to General Stayer I wrote, in part, as follows: "Attention is invited to Chapter XII of Volume XI (Part I), *The Medical Department of the U.S. Army in the World War*, published in 1927.

E.D.C. Comments: With this experience of World War I as a background, it was obvious that delayed primary and secondary closure of wounds would constitute one of the most important subjects in World War II, particularly as, in line with the British experience in the Middle East, firm rules were laid down against primary suture. It was quite natural, therefore, that the consulting surgeon on his first tour of the Base Sections, should inquire into and personally examine cases in which secondary suture had been carried out."

At that time I did not urge other surgeons to do secondary sutures. I was collecting facts. My diary contains the following note, which shows why I was focusing on direct observations: "What one *sees* in this war, one *believes*."

On these early visits to hospitals, both British and American, I was learning, not consulting or teaching. I was seeing hundreds of battle wounds in all stages of healing, asking questions of the surgeons as they operated on wounds or dressed them in the wards.

I stayed several days at the 21st General Hospital and made many lasting friendships. I was also giving a great deal of thought to wounds which I was seeing in enormous numbers. The following note occurs in my diary:

OBSERVATIONS ON WAR WOUNDS

E.D.C. Comments: From time to time suture of wounds to achieve primary first intention healing appeared only to disappear. Henry de Mondeville (14th cent.) was one of the early advocates of suture. Following Lister and the reintroduction of cat gut, and later the re-use of silk, wound suture reached the apex of perfection in the Halsted school of American surgery. With this war we have suddenly swung back from this elaborate needlework to the simple procedure of opening all deep spaces and leaving everything widely open. We have rediscovered the no suture technics.

While this came in with Truetta, emphasis as usual in surgery has been placed on what is done rather than what is not done. Emphasis is placed on the closed plaster treatment or on the sulfa drugs treatment. If the picture is reversed and we look at what is *not* done, we see that no sutures and only rare ligatures are employed. In other words, today

(*continued*)

we take a wound apart as meticulously as we had learned how to sew it together. All we need is the simple kit of the Civil War surgeon—scalpel—saw—forceps—a few ligatures for large vessels. We might leave out the needles except for specialized situations and transfixion ligatures.

A foreign body in forward echelons denotes an unopened pocket of the wound. It is not dangerous in itself. In rear echelons it is without significance except for pain—interference with function—perpetuation of chronic infection—or potential hazards of infection, hemorrhage or scar formation.

A pack is a method of wound closure often as effective as a needle and suture.

Skin plaster, Orr treatment, sulfa drugs, etc. are details of after care only possible if the fundamental principle of opening the wound with trimming away of dead tissue has been observed. A looking-glass world to Halstedians!

Dedicated to the soldiers of this and countless former wars from whose torn and dismembered bodies the art of surgery continues to evolve.

From the 21st General Hospital I went to two or three of the small station hospitals and at one of them the captain at the head of the surgical service was closing wounds by secondary suture. He had about eight or ten patients whom he demonstrated to me and of whom he supplied photographs which he had taken himself. I told him I thought it was important that he continue to press this work and document his study with photographs. That was one of the first systematic attempts to perform secondary suture that I found in the theater.

In retrospect, we had gotten off the track in the emphasis on sulfanilamide therapy and overlooked older and more fundamental principles. So far as the British experience in closing wounds is concerned, there were a few instances on record but not many. There had been a comment in the Sanitary Report of the 59th Evacuation Hospital, dated April 30, 1943, (paragraph 5 d. [2]):

Two hundred and seventy-one (271) wounded P.O.W. (Prisoners of War) have been in this hospital. Twenty of these had wounds which had been débrided and closed 48 to 72 hours after débridement. On arrival at this hospital 16 of this group of 20 patients had septic wounds which were reopened and drained. Two of this group had secondary arterial hemorrhage.

The commanding officer of this hospital had added the following indorsement: "It is recommended that delayed primary suture of gunshot wounds be discontinued as 16 out of 20 such cases arriving at this hospital were septic."

When I reached Casablanca I went to the 59th Evacuation Hospital, which was acting as a station hospital, and tried to get the facts that were at the basis of this comment. I talked with the Commanding Officer, Colonel Bolibaugh (subsequently the Surgical Consultant in Korea during my visit there in 1951), and also with Carleton Matheson and Roy Cohn, two of the surgeons. They corroborated this statement and were opposed to secondary closure of wounds. In my diary is the following comment:

E.D.C. Comments: On investigation it was found that these were instances of delayed primary suture evacuated within a few days of closure. Of course, they (the closure) broke down.

I then refer to wounds closed in a hospital in Palestine that broke down after early evacuation. These wounds at the 59th Evacuation Hospital had been closed in a British hospital in Bone, by whom and why I was not able to find. I added in my diary at this time:

E.D.C. Comments: Definition should be clearly established between delayed primary suture—up to 5 days, and secondary suture—between 14 and 21 days. Assuming no contamination from dressings, I should think suture possible.

With adequate débridement, the ideal time to do "reparative suture" is the fourth day. This checks with the biologic knowledge of wound healing processes. The fourth day is just before the wound starts to become rigid through the deposition of collagen fibers. On the fourth day the wound is still flexible and the edges can be drawn together. If one waits until the tenth day this opportunity has been lost. This concept established a new "golden period," so-called, on or about the fourth day when the wounded man should be in a hospital where he can be kept at rest after having his wound sutured.

EVOLUTION OF WOUND MANAGEMENT

World War I was fought during a pandemic of the hemolytic streptococcus. The injuries sustained on the battlefields were subject to superimposed streptococcus infection, presumably from human carriers to which the wound was exposed. The chief source of contamination was the nose and throat of the attendants or of the patient himself. The great effort in World War I was to sterilize the wound in order that it might be closed secondarily and thereby minimize deformity and mutilation.

In World War II hemolytic streptococcus-superimposed infection of battle wounds was rare. If it occurred, it was controlled readily by either the sulfa drugs or subsequently by penicillin. The problem in World War II resolved itself into closure of the wound in order to prevent other types of contamination and chronic wound infection. In summary, it may be said that closure of the wound in World War II required the elimination of dead tissue by meticulous débridement. This was not always possible to attain at the initial wound débridement because of the pressure of time, the inability of the surgeon to distinguish dead tissue from living tissue, and the tendency for blood to accumulate and act like dead tissue. Consequently, the procedures involved in World War II were: (1) initial débridement; (2) leaving the wound open with textile drainage; (3) evacuation of the casualty to a hospital where he could remain during the period of wound healing; and (4) removing the initial dressing as near to the fourth or fifth day as possible and closing the wound by suture.

The evolution of this procedure not only prevented deaths but prevented untold disability and deformity in the survivors. It returned thousands of soldiers to front line duty by the prompt healing of their wounds. It eliminated completely the so-called "septic wards" of the military hospitals, thereby again breaking the chain of reinfection within hospitals. Finally, though I have no proof of this, it may have prevented a transfer of virulent micro-organisms to the civilian hospitals throughout the world, an event which in likelihood followed World War I, the Crimean War and the Civil War.

In the publications or the collections of experience that were issued to guide the surgeons of World War II, I have not been able to find any statement transmitted from the N.R.C. committees mentioning the closure of war wounds. The experience in World War I was recorded in the Surgeon General's history of that war. This was unavailable to those of us overseas and, as I have indicated, was not pertinent to our problem. The introduction of the sulfa drugs added confusion to the picture.

At the time of Pearl Harbor, as I have recounted earlier, Long and Ravdin were flown to the scene by the Surgeon General immediately after the attack had taken place. Their report was never released to the public, but was "interpreted" to the medical profession. This gave a false emphasis on the freedom from infection obtained by dusting wounds with sulfanilamide. It left surgeons believing that the new "miracle" drugs solved all problems if applied topically to a fresh wound. Because of this, the American soldier was equipped with packets of sulfanilamide powder to be dusted directly on the wound and he was provided with sulfanilamide tablets to be taken orally as a further preventive measure. This was an error which it took many months to eliminate from standard procedure in World War II, and, interestingly, it was still defended for some months after the end of the war in the N.R.C. Committee on Surgery by advocates of this measure.

In addition to the Pearl Harbor experience we have also to take account of the information transmitted to us from the British hospitals visited by

American surgeons before the United States entered the war. Many British surgeons adopted the so-called "closed plaster" treatment advocated by Truetta in the Spanish Civil War. This, again, was a trend in the opposite direction to wound closure. The wound was concealed, it is true, but left to suppurate and close by granulation and superficial contraction. Truetta's method, so-called, was misinterpreted by American surgery and confused with the Orr management of osteomyelitis by closed plaster. The principles of these two procedures, the Winnette-Orr closed plaster for osteomyelitis and the procedure proposed by Truetta as a result of his experience in handling air raid casualties in Madrid, have little in common.

Secondary closure of wounds came to my mind as a desirable procedure quite early in the North African Theater. The first official record that I recall was in Circular Letter No. 13, issued from headquarters of the North African Theater of Operations on May 15, 1943. In paragraph 2, subparagraph (c) the following statement occurs:

> Uninformed hands do unnecessary dressings. The best safeguard for the patient is an adequate and legible record that accompanies him. A receiving officer is then in a position to refer to the record instead of looking at the wound. Many wounds after débridement and arrival at the base can be closed by secondary suture. Infection arising from contamination at the time dressings are changed makes this impossible.

This paragraph follows some miscellaneous notes under the heading of "Surgical Procedures" in which I was urging the medical officers of the theater to avoid looking at dressings on the way from the forward area to the rear. I used the following slogan in paragraph 1, which ultimately was reused by the Surgeon General in Washington:

> The evacuation line (paragraph 1, sub-paragraph [e]) is *not an assembly line* in which each surgeon does his bit to the patient. It is a *conveyance line* along the course of which the progress of the patient may be halted to save life or limb or render him transportable.

This circular letter was the result of seeing the freshly injured at the front and also from preliminary observations in the base. We had already come to appreciate that the excision of dead tissue could not be minimized or delayed even though sulfanilamide was given orally and topically. Ogilvie had tried to reduce the magnitude of tissue excision, feeling that some reliance could be placed on sulfanilamide therapy. This concept of wound "trimming," which originated in the Middle East under his direction, was well expressed in his *Surgery Under Two Commands* and will not be repeated here because the concept of a limited débridement that came into the North African Theater with the British Eighth Army led to confusion in the United Kingdom forces in Sicily. The British Eighth Army trained by Ogilvie then came under Weddell's teaching of the British First Army. It was this confusion that Brigadier Donald had to resolve because the First Army surgeons were criticizing the Eighth Army surgeons for doing inadequate excision of dead tissue.

In the Sanitary Report of the 21st General Hospital, dated April 9, 1943, is the recommendation "that sulpha drugs not be used in any sense in lieu of careful and complete débridement." The comment in my diary which follows the transcription of this item is as follows:

E.D.C. Comments: The common error has not been due to reliance on sulfa drugs but ignorance re débridement. The tendency (to rely on sulfa drugs) in a very few cases has been noted and almost invariably secondary infection has delayed return to duty or evacuation to the Zone of the Interior.

Ian L. Valerio, L. Scott Levin, and Stephen J. Kovach III

Hippocrates once asserted: "If you want to learn surgery, go to war." Soft tissue wound reconstruction with secondary suture, that is, early delayed wound closure performed 4 to 5 days after initial war-related injury, has been shown to be a resourceful, useful technique. As referenced by Lieutenant Colonel Kirtley and MAJ Trabue in the prelude to this chapter, "Closure of battlefield wounds was the most frequent operation encountered by the surgical services of a general hospital in the theater of operations." Delayed closure within 4 to 5 days postinjury proved to be a resourceful technique during World War II, and its application to wounds treated during Vietnam through the Iraq and Afghanistan Wars remains true.

War-related soft tissue wounds consist of high-velocity ballistic injuries and large defects from blast events. The resulting wounds are often heavily contaminated, possessing variable amounts of devitalized, dysvascular soft tissues. Furthermore, the primary and secondary effects from pressure wave transmission elicit cavitation and additional adverse effects on the surrounding soft and hard tissues.

The surgical treatment of the battlefield wound is ideally performed in an operating theater with good lighting and optimal positioning. The surgeon performing the index debridement should ideally define plans for timing of reexploration and/or definitive closure. A "second look" procedure may be indicated to reassess tissue viability, but unnecessary delay in closure due to too frequent wound inspections increases infection risk and promotes the inflammatory and scarring processes. These principles were true in 1944 and still remain valid today.

The introduction of negative pressure therapy (NPT) decades after World War II has advanced soft tissue injury care in war-related wounds. NPT has been shown to decrease bacterial proliferation and edema, while maintaining the physiologic environment and properties of the open wound. NPT also does not preclude the surgeon's ability to perform early secondary closure, and it can be utilized to aid in the surgical healing of the incisional closure as well. An upcoming clinical trial will evaluate the role of biomarkers from NPT effluent to inform optimal closure timing.

The most critical aspect of war-related wound care remains effective surgical debridement. Extensile exposure of entry/exit wounds is mandatory. Systemic antibiotics are adjunctive and not a replacement for surgical wound bed preparation. The so called "wet-to-dry" dressings are archaic; they should not be utilized for prolonged periods, and they are not a substitute for the need for excisional debridement of devitalized tissue. Finally, inadequate debridement and wound desiccation are recipes for further bacterial colonization and/or infection, further harming definitive wound healing.

In cases when early secondary closure cannot be performed and when white structures (bone, tendon, nerve) and/or vessels have been preserved yet remain exposed, an extensive armamentarium of vascularized tissue transfer techniques can be employed. Subsequent advances in local, regional, and distant flaps and the development of the microsurgical reconstructive ladder/elevator have dramatically changed surgical wound care over the last four decades. Additionally, the concepts of perforator flaps, propeller flaps, and free tissue autogenous transplantation (free flaps), coupled with the concepts of orthoplastic surgery, that have evolved following World War II have become critical advances in surgical treatment of war wounds.

Beginning with principles extolled by Sir Harold Gillies during World War I, the concept of replacing "like in kind" holds true through today's modern treatment of war wounds. Early secondary wound closure ascribes to this concept as long as one masters the utmost doctrine of proper surgical debridement in preparing a wound for definitive closure.

SUGGESTED READINGS

Dente CJ, Styrmisdottir E, Shi A, et al. Driving biology: The effect of standardized wound management on wound biomarker profiles. *J Trauma Acute Care Surg.* 2020;88(3): 379-389.

Klifto KM, Azoury SC, Othman S, Klifto CS, Levin LS, Kovach SJ. The value of an orthoplastic approach to management of lower extremity trauma: systematic review and meta-analysis. *Plast Reconstr Surg Glob Open.* 2021;9(3):e3494. Erratum in: *Plast Reconstr Surg Glob Open.* 2021;9(5):e3642.

Maurya S, Bhandari PS. Negative pressure wound therapy in the management of combat wounds: a critical review. *Adv Wound Care (New Rochelle).* 2016;5(9):379-389.

Sabino JM, Slater J, Valerio IL. Plastic surgery challenges in war wounded I: flap-based extremity reconstruction. *Adv Wound Care (New Rochelle).* 2016;5(9):403-411.

Shin EH, Sabino JM, Nanos GP III, Valerio IL. Ballistic trauma: lessons learned from Iraq and Afghanistan. *Semin Plast Surg.* 2015;29(1):10-19.

16

A Time for Reassessment

THE ENDING of the Tunisian campaign and planning for Sicily was a time for reassessment and a time for gathering the information collected in North Africa to help us avoid past errors. The following is a circular letter that was sent out from II Corps:

RESTRICTED HEADQUARTERS II CORPS
Office of the Surgeon
APO 302

12 May 1943

Subject: Treatment of Casualties.

To: All Unit Surgeons.

    1. *a.* Medical service in the recent campaign has been extremely commendable.

    b. Experience gained will allow us to progressively improve this service.

    2. *a.* The date and hour of wounds incurred (even though approximate) should be entered on the EMTs and the Field Medical Records.

    b. The recorded diagnosis should always include the type, severity and location of the wound and whether WIA, self-inflicted, accidentally incurred, etc.

    c. The agent producing the wound (rifle bullet, high-explosive, shell, mine, hand grenade, etc.) should be recorded when it is known.

    d. The date and hour of admission to any installation and of all operations should be recorded on EMT or Field Medical Record.

    e. Morphine must not be given in excessive dosage and every dose of morphine must be recorded. It should not be given in head injuries and should be used sparingly when a chest wound exists.

(*continued*)

f. As long as plasma is available, intravenous glucose and saline solutions should not be given to the patient who is in shock. Plasma should be administered in large quantities and rapidly until shock is controlled. If hemorrhage has been a major factor, whole blood transfusion is indicated.

g. Fluid should be restricted in head injuries except plasma or blood necessary to control shock.

h. Burns will not be treated with tannic acid or other coagulants. Sterile dressings of surgical gauze or sulfanilamide ointment, covered with plain gauze well beyond the wound, snugly and securely held in place, constitute the preferred dressings. Sulfonamides should be given by mouth and plasma given intravenously as indicated.

i. Penetrating wounds, particularly from high explosive fragments, should have fluoroscopic study whenever possible before débridement. The débridement should be thorough and all foreign bodies removed. Skin should not be needlessly sacrificed. For adequate exposure or drainage, incision rather than excessive excision of skin is indicated. Wounds should not be sutured (except certain wounds of the skull, face, chest, and abdomen). Close mesh surgical gauze should be placed on the wound (do not plug drainage with a tight pack). Large flesh wounds should be snugly bandaged with an elastic bandage or stockinette.

j. Circular plaster casings should be padded and split shortly after application. They should be strong enough to withstand ambulance transportation without breaking.

k. The hanging plaster cast has been found unsatisfactory in the treatment of fractures of the humerus in patients that must be transported.

l. The Tobruk splint has been quite satisfactory when properly applied.

m. In some instances the halfring log splint has been improperly applied. Five triangular bandages or muslin bandage slings should be used in its application. The foot hitch should always be applied over the shoe. Padding between shoe and hitch over dorsum of foot and tendon achilles adds to the comfort of the patients and reduces the likelihood of pressure sores. If the patient is to travel far or long behind the clearing station, adhesive or elastoplast skin traction should replace the foot hitch. The splint should be bound to the litter. Further instruction of medical officers as well as enlisted personnel seems indicated.

n. Patients who have had abdominal operations do not stand transportation well until 7 to 10 days after operation. If a hospital installation is not too far behind a clearing station, it is best to evacuate such patients to the hospital before surgery is performed.

3. The data contained in this circular will be made a subject for instruction during the forthcoming training period.

RICHARD T. ARNEST
Colonel, Med. Corps.
Surgeon

POINTING OUT ERRORS

We realized that we had many lessons to learn and also that we had the problem of getting the knowledge across to our forward surgeons and those in the rear areas as well. At the end of the North African campaign in May 1943, I invited Frank Berry to come to Algiers and help prepare a circular letter designed to summarize the experience in the management of wounds.

It is impossible to overemphasize the sensitivity of the surgeons of the combat zone to criticism about what they were doing. I decided that we would put out a circular letter entitled "The Tunisian Campaign. Comments by the Hospitals of the Zone of Communications on the Treatment of Battle Casualties in Forward Areas." This, therefore, was not to be a comment from somebody sitting on his fanny in a swivel chair, but the comments of surgeons who had taken care of the wounded after they had been evacuated from the forward hospitals. The rear echelon was to point out errors that were prevalent in the forward area. Frank and I worked over this circular in Algiers and it was issued as Circular Letter No. 20 on June 22, 1943.

The circular letter was not composed of criticisms but of collected comments. We wrote to the chief of surgery of each hospital in the base sections which had received casualties, asking for these comments. It was a bona fide study and the circular letter was documented by an appendix containing case records. The forward surgeons were very shrewd in recognizing their cases, although these were not identified. They were related as case histories with no hospital or surgeon identified. We received one irritated letter from a surgeon about a patient of his whom he had recognized, but on the whole the surgeons took the comments in good grace because they were well documented. It soon got around that Frank Berry had helped in the compilation and he had been in the forward area and was greatly respected by the surgeons there.

This circular letter came out as our first comprehensive advice on what to do with wounds. Previous to that I had issued a circular letter on sulfanilamide which Perrin Long had prepared and held up until I arrived. I made some alterations but not many. Also, I had issued the brief admonition not to close wounds by suture and included a few other simple technical matters. Wound healing was covered extensively. We selected the criticisms about the so-called "packing" of wounds—the stuffing them with gauze. We recommended the term "pack" be dropped from usage and reserved specifically for a temporary use of gauze to control hemorrhage. We were, however, still transmitting the advice of a rear hospital that sulfanilamide be sprinkled into all crevices of the wound and the surgical gauze be inserted loosely. There was no way to challenge the use of topically applied sulfonamide at that period in the war.

MANPOWER

During lulls in combat, it was difficult to dissuade the enthusiastic surgical specialists from undertaking elective operations that had little or no chance of returning a soldier to duty in an overseas theater. The term "elective" means that both the time and the place of an operation are open to selection, and other considerations such as prolonged supervision of aftercare, special exercises and physical therapy may play as important a role as the operation itself in effecting partial or complete recovery. The mobile hospitals, usually under canvas, were the chief offenders. At times their commanding officers permitted these operations, either from ignorance or to keep up the morale of eager and restless surgeons. Line officers not infrequently urged operation to enable them to retain a valuable mess sergeant or other soldier.

Circulation Letter No. 19, issued from the Office of the Surgeon, NATOUSA on June 26, 1943, dealt with this subject in no uncertain terms.

HERNIATED NUCLEUS PULPOSUS

When a diagnosis of herniated nucleus pulposus (ruptured intervertebral disc) is made in Army personnel, the patient is to be transferred to the Zone of the Interior without operation, provided he is unable to maintain limited or full duty status in this theater. In exceptional instances operation may be performed but only on written recommendation of a Disposition Board of a General Hospital.

OPERATIONS FOR DISLOCATION OF THE SHOULDER

Open operation for dislocation of the shoulder is to be undertaken only on the recommendation of the Disposition Board of a General Hospital.

OPERATIONS ON THE KNEE JOINT

Careful surgical judgment is to be exercised in the selection of cases for excision of semilunar cartilages. A history of locking is essential.

Instability of the knee joint is a contraindication. Postoperative care in the form of early weight bearing without crutches and exercise of the quadriceps muscle groups instituted early under supervision is essential to recovery.

Operations for major knee disabilities such as repair of collateral or cruciate ligaments or removal of both cartilages are to be undertaken only on recommendation of a Disposition Board of a General Hospital.

A Disposition Board had senior officers representing the field of surgery, medicine and psychiatry. They were kept informed of the needs for service troops and combat replacements; and they had the authority to recommend sending a soldier to the Zone of Interior if in their judgment he could not be rehabilitated within the period set as the "evacuation policy" of the theater. This was 90 days or 120 days, for example, and represented an informed estimate of the period required before a patient in hospital could be returned to duty. Disposition Board meetings were a heavy workload for the senior officers of the general hospitals and took them away from individual patient care and operative surgery.

Secretary of War Henry Stimson said that in World War II the country came into sight of the limits of its manpower. This was illustrated by some of the replacements sent overseas as combat soldiers. In many instances they were unfit for any kind of army duty. I found Lieutenant Colonel C. W. Christenbury, Commanding Officer of the 1st Replacement Depot in North Africa, thoroughly discouraged with both the morale and the physical condition of men who were arriving from the States as replacements for general duty service. Many had physical defects that disqualified them for any useful service in the theater. The most common were third-degree pes planus, symptomatic deformities and old fractures of the feet, varicose veins, hypertension, asthma, and chronic bronchitis. Soldiers with inguinal hernias were sent over with the assurance that the hernia would be repaired in North Africa.

A single illustration recorded in my diary will suffice:

E.D.C. Comment: R.J.S., a North Carolina farmer, was inducted into Army Service in November, 1941, and had just arrived in North Africa as "Grade A Combat Troop Replacement." Several years ago he was in an auto accident, injuring lower cervical region and left elbow.

(continued)

Examination shows stiff and painful upper dorsal and lower cervical spine with extreme limitation of motion. There is a scar over ulnar nerve at left elbow with classical complete ulnar paralysis. When asked to remove his coat so I could see the scar, he had to be helped off with it. Any child could see that he couldn't even shoot squirrels with his paralyzed hand.

I was so disturbed by this case that I entertained the idea of deliberate psychologic sabotage for the effect on the morale of other troops. After seeing and hearing of the physical defects in Replacements, I am ready to concede carelessness rather than sabotage. How it could have been missed, however, is still beyond my comprehension.

A replacement sent to any organization is at a disadvantage for several weeks. He may overcompensate for his loneliness by boasting of his prowess or stay by himself and suffer from nostalgia. The men who have trained and lived together for months are slow to receive him into the group until he has proven his merit. This is particularly true in combat units in which a soldier's life may depend on the loyalty of a comrade.

Hospitals and other service units had heavy drains made on their enlisted detachments for able-bodied soldiers to be trained for combat replacements. Patient care suffered correspondingly, because if replacements were sent to fill their places, they were inexperienced in hospital work and unaccustomed to meeting the needs of sick and wounded patients. They were assigned to guard duty, working on tents and simple housekeeping tasks. Prisoners of war and civilians were used in increasing numbers during the course of the war. We were, indeed, "in sight of the limits of our manpower."

On June 10, 1943, I submitted a report to the Surgeon, NATOUSA, on the subject of: "Surgical Lesions in Replacement Personnel from the Zone of the Interior." The figures obtained from Colonel Christenbury gave an estimated percentage of replacements arriving in Convoy UGF-7 as 38.2 ultimately available for general duty assignment. The total number of arrivals was 2,710. All but three of these had been classified, in the states, for general duty.

Valerie G. Sams, Miguel A. Cubano, and Nigel R. M. Tai

This chapter provides a window into the challenges, observations, frustrations, and solutions faced by the surgical teams assigned to the North African-Mediterranean Theater of Operations during World War II. In his role as Chief Surgical Consultant, Colonel Churchill was a tireless proponent of the use of whole blood and standardization of wound care for the soldiers in theater.

Churchill addresses the concept of documenting and heeding the lessons learned from previous battles to mitigate what we commonly refer to as the Walker Dip. He also addresses the delicate business of communicating medical errors. To gain credibility, he encouraged real case presentations and commentary from those caring for the patients in the battlefield. Surgeons in combat hospitals developed best practices by learning from prior medical errors and practices leading to poor outcomes. The cases were compiled in a de-identified way to avoid overt attribution and to encourage open discussion. In a similar fashion, while deployed to Iraq in 2003, Colonel John Holcomb recognized there was no system connecting those providing care to combat casualties throughout the chain of evacuation. In response, he and other military trauma leaders established the Joint Trauma System (JTS) and the DoD Trauma Registry (DoDTR). A weekly Combat Casualty Care Conference was central to this new initiative. In this forum, challenging cases could be reviewed to identify opportunities for improvement. These conferences motivated the development of Clinical Practice Guidelines (CPGs) to establish quality care standards and provide deployed surgeons with a roadmap to success.

Churchill's second point in this chapter focuses on challenges that impact medical manpower. Personnel gaps, inappropriately trained individuals, or backfills with disqualifying conditions significantly degrade care on the front lines of battle. He also highlights the resources required to evacuate surgical patients who cannot be quickly returned to duty. These members must be replaced, and the new personnel are certainly not immediately up to speed upon arrival. The idea of immediate return to duty without evacuation is relatively foreign to those of us who have served for the past couple of decades during the Iraq and Afghanistan conflicts. There are four categories of casualty outcomes for commanders to consider based on operations: immediate return to duty, delayed return to duty, highly functional survival, and survival with potentially profound dysfunction. Immediate return to duty is designated for those casualties with an injury that can be managed in theater. The concept of returning as many to the fight as possible will require a significant shift in our thinking and practices, but they bear consideration for future peer conflicts.

Now, 80 years later, we still face manpower issues, bureaucratic barriers, and training challenges, all of which degrade the quality of care we can provide to our combat wounded. Was Colonel Churchill ahead of his time, or are we just 80 years behind? To succeed in future conflicts, we need visionary thinkers like Churchill to internalize these thorny problems and deliver real solutions for the benefit of our warfighters and our nation.

SUGGESTED READINGS

Beldowicz BC, Modlin R, Bellamy M, Hiller H. Situational triage redefining medical decision-making for large-scale combat operations. *Mil Rev.* 2022 Jul-Aug:115-122

Jensen G, van Egmond T, Örtenwall P, Peralta R, Aboutanos MB, Galante J. Military civilian partnerships: international proposals for bridging the Walker Dip. *J Trauma Acute Care Surg.* 2020 Aug;89(2S Suppl 2):S4-S7.

Spott MA, Kurkowski CR, Zsolt Stockinger Z. The Joint Trauma System: history in the making. *Mil Med.* 2018 Oct;183(suppl_2):4–7.

Spott MA, Kurkowski CR. The Joint Trauma System teams dedicated to optimizing combat casualty care. *Mil Med.* 2018;183(suppl_2):190-192.

Steckel FC. Morale problems in combat: American soldiers in Europe in world war II. *Army Hist.* 1994;31;1–8. http://www.jstor.org/stable/26304183

17

Prostitution and Venereal Disease

PRELUDE

(The great earthquake of Lisbon took place on November 1, 1755.)

PANGLOSS MADE an answer in these terms: "Oh, my dear Candide, you remember Paquette, that pretty wench who waited on our noble Baroness; in her arms I tasted the delights of paradise, which produced in me those hell torments with which you see me devoured; she was infected with them, she is perhaps dead of them. This present Paquette received of a learned Grey Friar, who had traced it to its source; he had had it on an old countess, who had received it from a cavalry captain, who owed it to a marchioness, who took it from a page, who had received it from a jesuit, who when novice had it in direct line from one of the companions of Christopher Columbus."

. . . the sky darkened, the winds blew from the four quarters, and the ship was assailed by a most terrible tempest within sight of the port of Lisbon. . . . The sheets were rent, the masts broken, the vessel gaped . . . The ship foundered; all perished except Pangloss, Candide and that brutal sailor . . . The villain swam safely to the shore, while Pangloss and Candide were borne thither upon a plank.

Scarcely had they reached the city . . . when they felt the earth tremble under their feet . . . Whirlwinds of fire and ashes covered the streets and public places; houses fell, roofs were flung upon the pavements, and the pavements were scattered. Thirty thousand inhabitants of all ages and sexes were crushed under the ruins. The sailor, whistling and swearing, said there was booty to be gained here.

The sailor ran among the ruins, facing death to find money; finding it, he took it, got drunk, and having slept himself sober, purchased the favours of the first good-natured wench whom he met on the ruins of the destroyed houses, and in the midst of the dying and the dead. Pangloss pulled him by the sleeve.

"My friend," said he, "this is not right. You sin against the universal reason; you choose your time badly."

"S'blood and fury!" answered the other; "I am a sailor . . . a fig for thy universal reason."

VOLTAIRE in *Candide*

THE CONTROL OF VENEREAL DISEASE

Prostitution flourished in North Africa as it had for centuries. The influx of troops—American, British and French—fanned this activity into flames. Harlots were waiting on the beachheads, solicited patrons openly on the streets and clustered like flies around troop rest areas. The prostitutes ranged from high-class French women who fled to North Africa to escape the Nazi invasion to native girls straying down from the mountains to the coastal cities where they were caught by procurers and held as virtual captives in houses of prostitution.

Every headquarters and large hospital had its venereal disease control officer. Prophylaxis stations were set up along the streets and hospital beds grouped in wards were filled with the acute complications of gonorrhea and fresh syphilis. Although the patients were classified as surgical, fortunately I escaped all responsibility for supervision of treatment or the enforcement of control measures.

Some estimate of the magnitude of the venereal disease incidence can be found in a census of patients admitted to the 77th Evacuation Hospital in II Corps. This large tented hospital was in support of combat in southern Tunisia and moved back to Meskiana at the time of the threatened breakthrough at the Kasserine Pass. The first 1,000 surgical patients admitted numbered: 258 battle casualties, 120 with venereal diseases, half of whom were new cases of syphilis. The others were injuries from accidents, hemorrhoids, infected pilonidal cysts and minor infections.

Punitive measures failed to control venereal disease. A threat of court-martial for those failing to take prophylaxis did not shorten the crucial period between exposure and prophylaxis. So long as a soldier signed the "jit book" on his return from a few hours off duty, he was safe. Restriction of leave passes in units that had a venereal disease rate above an arbitrary level was more effective because the nonoffenders assumed the responsibility of looking after the others.

There was also an ostrich-like policy of some of those in authority who refused to publish educational posters and pamphlets because they considered them "derogatory" to the American soldier.

It was not necessary to leave Algiers to see the many ways in which prostitution was carried on in North Africa. Some of these will be described briefly.

Individual Solicitation: One or two prostitutes "worked" a circumscribed area which usually contained a few restaurants or open-air cafés with sidewalk tables. The Aletti Hotel area was the hunting ground of a familiar character whom we christened "Big Bertha." She had at least one associate. Big Bertha's sobriquet—originally, of course, that of an enormous German gun in World War I—came from the name given an antiaircraft mortar installed among the hills that surrounded the harbor. During an air-raid this mortar was fired with a deafening blast to fill the sky with exploding bombs and parachuting magnesium flares.

Big Bertha was swarthy and powerfully-built, and, it was claimed that she could serve many squads of GI's in a single evening. When she paused at a table, her dark eyes swept constantly around the restaurant in search of prospective patrons. I remarked on the good looks of her associate one evening, and Bertha asked quickly whether I would like to have her.

Cribs: The fringe of the Casbah in Algiers was sprinkled with small rooms on the level of the sidewalk, oftentimes with a window fitted with a curtain. If the curtain was pulled and the door closed, it indicated that the inhabitant was "busy." At other times she sat at the window on rainy days and in fair weather solicited trade in front of her crib. One, I recall, wore a tattered, bright blue nightdress and attracted attention with a tambourine.

Brothels: These were numerous in all North African cities. A patron could enter, be seated at a table, order a bottle of wine and the girls would join him at his table until it was time to be taken upstairs. "Runners" solicited customers in the street and guided them to the nearby house. There was at least one of these in Marrakesh that specialized in children—both boys and girls under twelve years of age.

The strong odor of musk and of perfumes made in the Casbah from the essential oils of flowers and attar of roses permeated most of the brothels. To this aphrodisiac atmosphere was added the acrid odor of sweaty bodies and the pungent smells of stale wine and beer (**Figure 17.1**).

Prostitution on a large scale took place in Algiers and in Casablanca in two very large installations—the "Sphinx" and the "White City."

The Sphinx was in the lower reaches of the Casbah. A large multicolored effigy of a sphinx with bare breasts was suspended above the front door. There was a side door for exit. The Sphinx had a bar and a large open floor for the milling crowd of patrons and busy prostitutes. A harlot did not drink when at work but the patron was expected to buy one for her. This added to the income of the establishment since the same glass of wine or liquor the harlot supposedly "drank" was used repeatedly.

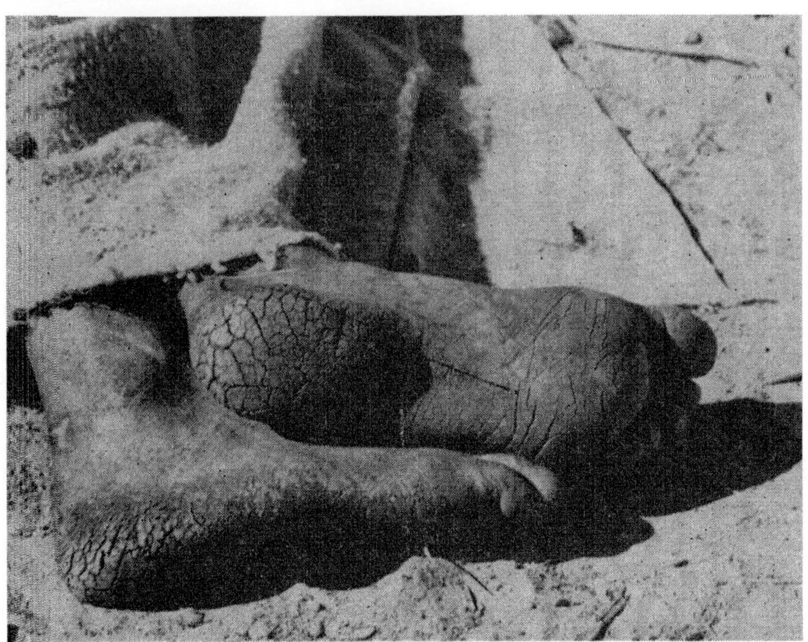

Figure 17.1 Seen in the bend of a stone stairway in the Casbah.

Tiny rooms were on the balcony which extended on three sides of the large central floor. When a patron had spent money at the bar, a girl would seize him by the hand and hurry him up to the balcony. There they would enter a vacant room and the door would close. The girl lost little time during the rush hour and the patron would reappear buttoning up his trousers and be guided to the exit door. I recalled the old P. T. Barnum sideshow in which the gullible were guided by signs: "To the Egress" and finally found themselves out on the street again.

I visited the Sphinx with a small group that included the Theater Surgeon and an M.P. We entered a side door and went up to the balcony to view the scene below.

The White City on the outskirts of Casablanca was a large area laid out in streets lined with brothels of all sizes and descriptions. Built originally as a housing project, it was not successful as such and so was converted into its present function. The inmates were said to be used by the French police as stooges to obtain information, particularly from U. S. Army officers. Servicemen's mistresses living in Casablanca were said to be blackmailed by the threat of being sent to the White City. Once an inmate, the girl was held in slavery by the inability to pay the original fine and by pyramiding expenses charged against her for board and lodgings. She could be redeemed only by payment of the amount due. The "city" was surrounded by a wall with a gate kept closed until three or four o'clock in the afternoon. French doctors carried out inspections of the inmates, supposedly weeding out fresh cases of syphilis and acute gonorrhea. The girls were provided with certificates of inspection. I visited the White City accompanied by the urologist and venereal disease officer of the 6th General Hospital—Sylvester Kelley—and an M.P. The visit was in the morning but a large crowd of French Moroccan soldiers was already gathered at the gate.

Visitors to the North African Theater were eager to see the sights of the Casbah in Algiers. When Elliott Cutler came on a tour, I went with him as his personal escort and selected a brothel with mural paintings after the style of the murals in Pompeii that are not shown ordinarily to visitors. They were cruder and more garish. As we were walking through, I said casually to Elliott, "Look at the murals in that side room." He came back in excitement, saying "Pete, you have been here before!" Of course I had. It was one of the "sights" for visitors.

My role has been described as that of a bystander insofar as venereal disease was concerned. Only rarely did I become concerned as Surgical Consultant. As escort to the Secretary of War, Henry Stimson, it was protocol to follow him through the surgical wards of our hospitals. Despite diplomatic attempts to steer him away from the tents occupied by venereal disease patients, he entered one and paused by a cot. Fortunately, I managed to alert Secretary Stimson before he asked his usual question: "How were you wounded, soldier?" (see Chapter 29, V.I.P. Visit).

When the first sizable shipment of penicillin arrived in the theater, we were eager to use it as an adjunct to the planned closure of battle fractures. The hospitals were loaded with sulfonamide-resistant venereal disease. The penicillin was used to treat those "wounded" in the North African and Italian brothels—and those wounded in combat with the enemy had to wait.

This episode is truthfully and cryptically recorded in *Medical Service in the Mediterranean and Minor Theaters*, page 253, Department of Army, Washington, D. C., 1965. It states: "The Italian campaign included the wider use of penicillin, which had been allocated for specific treatments in the closing months of 1943, but became relatively plentiful early in 1944."

Martin M. Abbrecht, of the Department of Preventive Medicine, New Jersey College of Medicine, is quoted in an AMA publication of January 23, 1967, as estimating that some 120,000 new cases of syphilis and more than one million cases of gonorrhea are discovered yearly in the United States. Four thousand Americans die each year of syphilis and 3,000 infants are born with the disease.

Richard R. Leger, in *The Wall Street Journal* of June 18, 1968, reported: "More Americans contracted gonorrhea last year than caught the measles. 'Gonorrhea is now out of control,' warns Dr. William Brown, chief of the venereal disease program of the National Communicable Disease Center. Officials of the center predict 1.3 million Americans will become infected with gonorrhea this year, up 25% from two years ago and double the number of a decade ago."[1]

MEDICAL INSPECTION AND TREATMENT

Here is a report that was issued by Perrin Long:

ALLIED FORCE HEADQUARTERS
Office of the Surgeon
A.P.O. # 512

7 February 43

Subject: The Medical Inspection and Treatment of Registered Prostitutes in Algiers.

To: The Deputy Surgeon, Medical Section, AFHQ.

1. The Centre de Salubrite (prophylactic center) and hospital for the inspection of and treatment of venereal disease in registered and certain unregistered prostitutes is located at the Place D'istree, off the Rue de Verdun, on the edge of the Casbah in Algiers. The building in which it is housed consists of a three story masonry building having a central open court which is about 70 by 40 feet in size. The director of the prophylactic service is Dr. Colonieu who is a dermatologist and a venereal disease specialist in Algiers. He is part-time and has six part-time physicians working under his direction. The Centre de Salubrite is utilized solely for the medical inspection and treatment of prostitutes or suspected prostitutes, there being six other public dispensaries dealing with the treatment of venereal disease in Algiers.

   a. The Prostitution Problem in Algiers. There are 600 prostitutes registered as such with the police in the city of Algiers. About 450 of these women are in houses of prostitution or "magasins" (cribs in native quarters), and 50 on the streets. The number of clandestine prostitutes or occasional offenders is unknown, but is said to be large and probably increasing since the arrival of the armed forces of the United Nations in Algiers. Roughly 450 of the prostitutes are of native origin while 150 are Europeans. The incentive for prostitution is largely a financial one. Domestic servants in this area earn about 800 francs per month while

---

[1]Reprinted with permission of *The Wall Street Journal.*

typists, etc. earn about 2,000 to 3,000 francs a month. An able prostitute in a house such as the "Sphinx" can earn more than 1,000 francs a day, and most of the registered prostitutes earn 500 or more francs a day. These women retain 50% of their earnings and in addition receive 50% of the profits made from the sale of alcohol, etc. to their patrons. Hence it is obvious that their incomes are relatively large. The system of registration is interesting. A woman who decides to enter the profession may go voluntarily to the police and request to be registered. Not very many do this. The greater part have enforced registration as the result of being picked up by the police for examination and questioning two or more times. The first time they are picked up by the police they are not questioned or investigated but are sent to the Centre de Salubrite for examination. There, if they are found to have a venereal disease, they have two choices, the first being that they can be put into the first offenders' ward which is distinct and away from the registered prostitutes' ward and be treated, or they can go to the Mustapha hospital and be treated as a civilian patient. However, if they are picked up a second time, they are then questioned and examined by the police who then send them to the "Centre de Salubrite" where they are examined and where a social worker goes into their social status. If it turns out that they have no job and prostitution is considered their main source of livelihood, the director recommends to the Prefect that they be registered as prostitutes, and if the latter concurs, the police issue them a card of registration. When registered, it is necessary for them to report twice a week at the "Centre de Salubrite" for medical inspection, for which they pay 10 francs a visit. Each visit is recorded on the back of their card by symbols, A (free to work) and I (interdite or diseased). When dismissed they have enforced free treatment and if they don't cooperate they are arrested and put into two dungeon-like cells in the Centre de Salubrite. Another interesting angle is that they may ask to be removed from the register of prostitutes, and if social service investigations prove their request to be worthy of consideration they are stricken from the register. Last year five native and three European prostitutes were taken off the register.

b. Medical inspection and treatment of prostitutes. At each visit the prostitute strips completely and her skin is inspected for scabies, ring worm, lice, etc. The external genitalia are examined, a speculum is introduced into the vagina and an inspection of the vagina and cervix is made with a smear being taken from the latter. This smear is stained with methylene blue and examined immediately. If an abnormal mixture of bacteria is noted or if gonococci are present, the patient

(continued)

is held for treatment. Wassermann and Hinton reactions are done on blood samples every three months. Each examining physician always examines the same prostitutes and in groups of 100. There are two groups examined each day, one at 8 AM, the other at 2 PM. *About one hour and thirty minutes are required to examine one hundred prostitutes.* If a prostitute is found infected, and in an infectious stage of her disease she is immediately brought into the hospital and treated until she is considered noninfectious. The treatment for gonorrhea is based on the use of sulfathiazole or sulfapyridine in fairly large doses over a period of three days with the test of cure being a smear stained with methylene blue on the fourth day. Syphilis is treated with neo-arsphenamine, sulfarsphenamine, and bismuth. A large outpatient clinic for the treatment of syphilis among the prostitutes is in existence. The majority of the registered prostitutes have syphilis. It was Dr. Colonieu's opinion that practically all of the prostitutes were infected with one or the other venereal disease and that gonorrhea was rampant among them.

c. Analysis of the effectiveness of the inspection and treatment of registered prostitutes. It is obvious that an examination consisting of a cursory physical inspection, a smear stained with methylene blue, and a Wassermann test performed every three months, does not offer much protection against the chances of being infected with gonorrhea or syphilis from these prostitutes. Only gross infections with gonorrhea will be diagnosed and syphilis may possibly be existent for two and one half months before the Wassermann test will reveal its presence under the system of taking Wassermanns every three months. While Dr. Colonieu seemed quite enthusiastic over his three day treatment of gonorrhea, one must conclude from the experience of others that the treatment prescribed is not sufficient, nor is the cure adequate.

d. The hospital was extremely well kept and the records of the patients were neat and complete.

2. Conclusions: In North Africa we have heard about the effectiveness of the medical inspection of registered prostitutes in respect to the control of venereal disease but an analysis of the facts reveals:

a. The inspection is by necessity cursory, and because of the methods employed the existence of gonorrhea may be entirely missed and that of syphilis not noted for three months.

b. While undoubtedly the medical inspection in the Centre de Salubrite is superior to that carried out in St. Nazaire, France, in 1917 (smears for gonorrhea are made and Wassermann tests are done every three months), the procedures witnessed this morning are strongly reminiscent of those described by Dr. Hugh Young as occurring in St. Nazaire during World War I.

    c. The treatment used for gonorrhea is inadequate.

    d. The treatment used for syphilis is adequate and it is highly likely that inasmuch as the majority of the registered prostitutes are undergoing treatment for syphilis, the chances of contracting syphilis from them are less than they would be from clandestine or occasional prostitutes.

PERRIN H. LONG
Lt. Col. M.C.
Consultant in Medicine

Prostitution and Venereal Disease
COMMENTARY

Jeremy W. Cannon, Emily Mayhew, and Clinton K. Murray

The concluding chapter of "Part Two" of *Surgeon to Soldiers* addresses a topic that may seem unusual for a surgical monograph: venereal disease. Dr Churchill frames this chapter with a series of vignettes from Voltaire's classic satire *Candide*, set against the backdrop of Lisbon's destruction in 1755. In the final vignette, an unnamed sailor reveals his priorities in a burst of egocentric hedonism. Yet, as Churchill's observations confirm and history has demonstrated time and again, such high-risk behavior erodes the fighting force and offers a strategic advantage to the enemy. Although there may be debates on the merits of General Order Number 1 in modern US combat commands (order detailing prohibited activities including sexual contact with host nationals, among many others), its pragmatic aim to preserve a sober, fit, and healthy force remains an unassailable exercise in common sense.

It can be inferred that Churchill has included this topic because of the significant implications sexually transmitted infections (STIs) have for other patients with physical injuries. **Table 17.1** underscores the scourge of these preventable, self-inflicted wounds on deployed units by depriving the front line of essential personnel while also consuming critical medical assets needed for combat casualty care.

In the conclusion of this chapter, Medical Consultant LTC Perrin Long notes, "the treatment used for gonorrhea is inadequate." While this statement held true in February 1943, it did not remain so for much longer. The high rates of STI and the inadequacy of their treatment were partly due to French physicians administering small doses of sulfa drugs to the sex workers they were due to inspect. This approach masked symptoms so that certification could be issued, but it led to incompletely treated STIs and likely increased resistance at the same time. However, with the arrival of penicillin in 1943, ten British soldiers in North Africa with severe gonorrhea were treated with penicillin manufactured in Britain. These pilot subjects were completely symptom-free within forty-eight hours, "like turning off a tap." Treatment of gonorrhea was suddenly very much adequate, astonishing even. Yet, limited penicillin supplies and meager production rates created a new dilemma: antibiotic triage. Churchill's wry remark touches on both the patients "wounded" in North African and Italian brothels and the decision to prioritize their treatment over combat casualties. But, as the Allied campaign moved to Italy, every soldier became needed; thus, returning STI-infected

TABLE 17.1 ■ Burden of Sexually Transmitted Infections (STIs) in World War I (April 1917–December 1918) and World War II (1942–1945)		
Measure	World War I[a]	World War II[b]
STI admissions	357,969	1,250,346[c]
STI-related days lost	6,804,818	23,265,736
Disease-related admissions for STI[d]	10.2%	8.3%
Cost of STI treatment	$45 million[e]	
Medical personnel needed for STI care	3,200	

[a]Data from Pappas JP. The venereal disease problem United States army: an outline of its history, legislation, and points of attack, with a summary of the current methods of control. *Mil Surg.* 1943;93(2):172-183.

[b]Data from Chapters I and III including Tables V and XXI, *Medical Statistics in World War II.* Office of the Surgeon General: Department of the Army; 1975.

[c]Compared to 723,560 battle injury admissions.

[d]Proportion of hospital admissions for STIs relative to all other noninjury, disease-related admissions.

[e]Equivalent to approximately $1.1 billion in 2023 according to the Bureau of Labor Statistics (https://www.bls.gov/data/inflation_calculator.htm).

men quickly and cleanly to the front lines became a priority. Fortunately, US industrial production of penicillin soon ramped up dramatically and filled the gap once British supplies were exhausted.

Today, nearly eighty years after the end of World War II, poly-resistant STIs have once again rendered most of our treatments inadequate. In the words of the Centers for Disease Control and Prevention (CDC) regarding gonorrhea, "We are currently down to one last recommended and effective class of antibiotics, cephalosporins, to treat this common infection." Thus, this chapter not only provides a glimpse into the past but also serves as a clarion call for future deployed surgeons who will face aggressive multidrug resistant infections of various types. These infections pose a grave threat to our fighting strength and may claim the lives of otherwise salvageable combat casualties—who will bring about the next penicillin miracle?

SUGGESTED READINGS

Aldous WK, Robertson JL, Robinson BJ, et al. Rates of gonorrhea and chlamydia in U.S. military personnel deployed to Iraq and Afghanistan (2004-2009). *Mil Med.* 2011;176(6):705-710.

Helfand WH, Woodruff HB, Coleman MH, Cowan DL. Wartime industrial development of penicillin in the United States. In: Parascandola J, ed. *The History of Antibiotics: A Symposium.* American Institute of the History of Pharmacy; 1980.

Ljungquist O, Nazarchuk O, Kahlmeter G, et al. Highly multidrug-resistant gram-negative bacterial infections in war victims in Ukraine, 2022. *Lancet Infect Dis*. 2023;23(7):784-786.

Pappas JP. The venereal disease problem United States army: an outline of its history, legislation, and points of attack, with a summary of the current methods of control. *Mil Surg*. 1943;93(2):172–183.

Smallman-Raynor M, Cliff A. *War Epidemics: An Historical Geography of Infectious Diseases in Military Conflict and Civil Strife, 1850-2000*. Oxford Academic; 2020.

PART THREE

Sicily

18

Preparation for Sicily—Operation Husky

On June 9, 1943, I prepared Circular Letter No. 16 with subject: "Memoranda on Forward Surgery Especially Applicable to Amphibious Operations." *Some of the high points of this circular were:*

> MEMORANDA ON FORWARD SURGERY ESPECIALLY
> APPLICABLE TO AMPHIBIOUS OPERATIONS
>
> June 9, 1943
>
> 1. a. Surgical operation performed under unfavorable conditions without facilities for proper aftercare is often more hazardous than prompt evacuation if the patient is transportable or can be made so.
>
> b. Wounded evacuated by water should, particularly during early phases of combat, be so bandaged and splinted that they can swim or at least remain afloat should emergency require it.
>
> c. Overdosage with morphia produces dangerous coma and respiratory depression that may delay the administration of an anesthetic or render evacuation transport hazardous.
>
> d. All wounds are left open after débridement, frosted with sulfanilamide and loosely filled with surgical gauze. *There are no exceptions.* (See below for specialized regional situations.)
>
> e. Only bruised and devitalized skin need be excised, and this with narrow margin. Avoid circumcision of wounds leaving circular defects by using linear extensions to gain exposure.
>
> f. During débridement open all deep pockets and transversely divide fascial planes.
>
> g. Do not *pack* wounds with gauze or sulfonamide.
>
> h. Immobilize site of extensive injury even if fracture is not present.
>
> i. Continue oral administration of sulfonamide. . . .

(continued)

2. *Plaster Casts*

   a. *Split or bivalve all casts as soon as dry. There are no exceptions....*

3. *Compound Fractures*

   a. Objects to be achieved in initial surgery are control of infection and safe, comfortable transportation. Reduction and rigid fixation of fractures can be accomplished at the base....

   b. *Knee Joint:* In débridement minimize incisions that compound synovial membrane. Loosely fill débrided wound with surgical gauze. Evacuate early, immobilized in plaster or preferably Tobruk splint.

   c. *Leg:* Careful débridement [of] *all* wounds in multiple injuries, as circulation frequently impaired and gas gangrene likely. Penetrating wounds of calf may require incision for hemostasis as deep hematoma impedes circulation. Bivalve rather than split casts so inspection of dressings may be possible without losing position in compound fractures. Hold patient if circulation is questionable....

4. *Chest*

   a. Temporarily close sucking wounds by pad of surgical gauze held firmly by adhesive strapping. Insert small catheter 2nd interspace to relieve pressure pneumothorax....

   b. Initial definitive surgery limited to débridement and closure of wound of chest wall without complete suture of superficial layers and skin. Local anesthesia is often satisfactory and avoids hazards of asphyxia....

5. *Abdomen*

   a. First priority for emergency surgery. Close abdominal wall with stay sutures.

   b. Exteriorize large bowel and rectum perforations or perform proximal colostomy. *There are no exceptions.*

   c. Examine carefully for evidence of abdominal penetration all casualties with entrance wounds in buttocks or chest.

   d. Perforation of intestine, particularly ileocecal region and multiple, is caused by hydraulic blast wave from bomb exploding in water. No external evidence of injury....

6. *Burns*

   a. Cleansing may be limited to removal of gross debris and thick coating of oil by mechanical means.

   b. Apply boric ointment or surgical gauze, cover with sterile mechanics waste and bandage firmly. Burns damaging eyes require closure by bandage.

c. For emergency transport by water do not obstruct vision or respiration by bandaging. Leave jaw free for possible vomiting.

d. Shock in burns is often delayed for 4 to 6 hours. Use this period for evacuation when possible. Otherwise extensive burns must be held until equilibrium is established. Most flash burns are partial thickness injuries with small patches of full thickness loss. Life endangering shock not common unless surface area is unusually extensive or unless environmental temperature is immoderately high....

No sutures. There are no exceptions.

An appendix provided detailed directions for a plaster transportation splint recommended for fractures of the femur, wounds involving the knee joint and fractures of the leg near the knee.

Three thousand six hundred and fifty copies of this circular letter were mimeographed and circulated to all medical officers in the theater.

I persuaded the surgeon in charge of the amphibious landing in Sicily to issue a circular letter because he had new troops and new doctors who had no experience in North Africa. This circular letter told them how to handle casualties, and I tried my best to indoctrinate the hospitals that were going to Sicily. Some came into the theater and were kept "in moth balls" until they were combat-loaded so that there was no opportunity to meet with them. The chief thing I was able to accomplish for the Sicilian campaign was to get ready to receive the casualties that were to come back to the near shore from the amphibious operation. From G-2, I obtained the number of casualties that were expected. This number was separated into the proportion of killed and wounded which had prevailed in North Africa—our only experience to date. Then we had a predicted number of wounded as a basis for calculation. Next I took the distribution of the wounds and injuries: How many would have burns, how many extremity wounds, how many would have head wounds and so on. In the Bizerte-Tunis area, we set up the hospitals which were available and reinforced them with surgical teams. I tried to get a system established to sort the wounded as they came back from Sicily and distribute them among these hospitals.

Fortunately we did not have the number of casualties that G-2 had estimated. Our distribution system worked only in part. Again, I came up against one of the doctrines of the Army as it existed at the outset of the war; namely that *one could not set up specialty centers.* This idea had been carried over from World War I when the setting up of specialty centers had so irritated the regular Army. The Medical Corps between the wars was out of touch with the increasing specialization of civilian medicine. My colleagues in the regular Army also knew little about the professional work of the R.A.M.C. in the Middle East.

SPECIAL CENTERS

In the establishment of special centers, I had two thoughts in mind. The hospitals set up in Bizerte and Tunis were for the greater part newly-arrived station hospitals. They were neither staffed nor equipped to care for the wounded. The attachment of auxiliary group teams gave them surgical manpower and specialized instruments. Also, I subscribed wholeheartedly to the advice of Heneage Ogilvie based on his experience in the Middle East. An extract from a report by Ogilvie had been copied into my diary in Washington. The report in full was loaned to me by Colonel Gillespie.

> The most productive use of specialized surgical skill in the medical services of an army is to provide Centres where work of one type is done under ideal conditions and to an exacting standard. These Centres should set a level of performance and of results by which others are judged and should receive and treat all unusual and difficult cases in their specialty, or those where a bad result may be feared. But they should not sweep every case, large or small, directly or indirectly connected with their cult, within their walls, nor employ gestapo methods to prevent good work by members of the wrong union.

In Bizerte we had established the beginning of special centers. For example, neurosurgery centered in the 33rd General Hospital with Eldridge Campbell. He was beginning to develop simple and effective procedures for head wounds. I spent a great deal of time in the Bizerte area talking to the staffs of the new hospitals as they were setting up. The 37th Evacuation Hospital (Texas) had arrived, with General Blesse's brother Harry as Commanding Officer. The 3rd General Hospital was from Mt. Sinai in New York. The other hospitals that were not going on the assault were cluttered in an area north of Tunis. As we were setting up this area we had a visit from Dr. Allen Whipple, who came under travel orders from the N.R.C., and his presence was an inspiration to everyone. A thoughtful, scholarly surgeon.

The hot wind from the Sahara (hamraseen) enveloped the Tunis-Bizerte coast of North Africa during the early days of Operation Husky. On July 6, 1943, I left Algiers and arrived in Mateur via Telergma at 11:15. At the brief stop in Telergma the heat was intense and fine sand from the desert, carried by the southerly wind, filled the air and grated between my teeth. D-day was July 10 and my primary task was to set up on the near shore (Bizerte-Tunis region) some sorting of the wounded as they arrived from Sicily.

This seemed essential if the station hospitals in process of setting up along "hospital road" were to be utilized to admit and care for the seriously wounded. The 2nd Auxiliary Surgical Group was moving its headquarters to a grove nearby and its teams were available to reinforce the small and inexperienced staffs of the station hospitals.

This attempt to improve the surgical care of the wounded was opposed by the Surgeon of the Eastern Base Section (E.B.S.). He was not going to have his ambulances "peddling milk bottles along a road," meaning that an ambulance could go from the dock to one hospital only. I then suggested that sorting be done before the ambulances were loaded, but this was considered impossible.

That I was not alone in the attempt to bring more order into the distribution of casualties is attested by the following extract from a letter written by Frank Berry on August 10, 1943.

> Colonel Forsee and I are extremely discouraged with the triaging and evacuation of patients in this area. Apparently no attempt is made to allocate the patients properly. One night without notification we received a load of 350 of all sorts and of course had only 100 beds. The trucks would not wait but insisted upon unloading, and then we had to call them all back after authorization from E.B.S. Another time we had 200 sent us, about 150 of which were N.P.'s and no attempt had been made to send them to the 43rd (a station Hospital designated for neuropsychiatric cases).
>
> Colonel Rudolph (a very able and cooperative officer of the regular Army Medical Corps who had succeeded the Surgeon of E.B.S. who opposed the sorting) has such a big job on his hands that he should not be bothered with simple things like this. Still nobody seemed to be interested. An evacuation is a most hit or miss and uncertain proposition. Except for a brief period in the Tunisian campaign, this has been so all along. No one seems to be really interested in the prompt and proper evacuation of the patient nor to have the adequate authority and cooperation to accomplish it smoothly. Our idea is that there should be some top M.C. officer in charge of evacuation. He must have complete authority from NATOUSA over all the local sectors. He should have as assistants and coordinators a representative from the Air Force and one from Transportation, and one or two competent junior officers. This group should know the plans, work out their own plans and coordinated action, and should spend a good part of their time in travel so as to know the problems of the hospitals and air, rail, port and motor facilities.
>
> Give this a thought or two and maybe you could put something across through General Blesse and NATOUSA. It would be a blessing for the patients and a great contribution to the efficiency of the Medical Department.
>
> Sorry to bother you with all this but these troubles and flights of ideas often arise in these bucolic atmospheres. Or maybe it's just the heat and this eternal wind.

The struggle of the professionally-oriented medical officers to enlighten the administrative officers continued throughout the war. The former were responsible for the care of the patients—the latter for the movement of patients. An official report from the Fifth Army later concluded: "The fundamental errors in field service are apparent: (1) Failure to divert the first

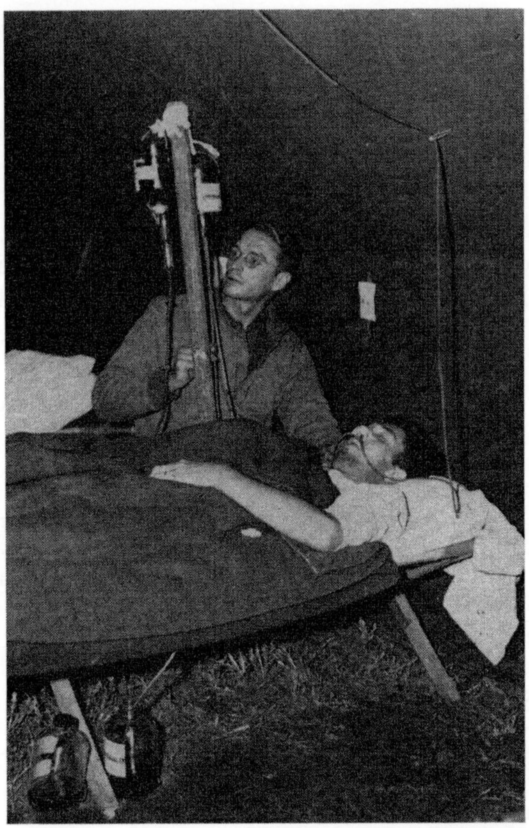

Figure 18.1 Postoperative care of a severely wounded soldier.

priority cases to Field Hospitals, and (2) overloading Evacuation Hospitals by large numbers of consecutive admissions when this is not necessary" (**Figure 18.1**).

Nine station hospitals were grouped near Bizerte and five in or near Tunis. Six general hospitals—Mt. Sinai, Tulane, Albany, Louisiana State, King's County and Vanderbilt—were unpacking and getting ready to receive patients. At least two 750-bed evacuation hospitals were in the area. The 48th Surgical Hospital, which had carried a heavy load in southern Tunisia, was being reorganized and reequipped as a 400-bed Evacuation Hospital—the 128th. A hospital ship—the *Seminole*—was standing by in the Bay of Tunis. I took a picture of her with my Leica but a small group of GI's, believing they had found a German spy, raised a clamor and called a nearby guard. Fortunately, I was able to produce identification and a written permit from A.F.H.Q. to photograph medical subjects. Nerves were on edge and excitement mounting as D-day approached. The North African campaign was over and the theater was moving toward Italy.

DIARY

Extracts from my diary record those exciting days:

July 6, 1943
In afternoon to hospital road to see station hospitals in process of setting up. To the French Marine Hospital buildings that successively have been a German hospital, the 9th Evac. and now with the 3rd General moving in. Temperature in the evening in Mateur 95°.

July 7
To 114th Station with Long, Forsee and Sampson. Explained burn center with itemized listing of personnel and supplies. Said to have good ophthalmologist. To 56th Evac. urging on Col. Blesse and Lt. Col. Carter importance of triage and necessity of not filling large numbers of beds by holding cases for surgery that can be sent along to other hospitals, particularly heads, chest and burns that require special post-operative care and long average duration of stay.

July 8
Major Haynes now ordered from No. 58 to No. 54. This would balance the two—centering general surgery and neurosurgery at No. 54 and general surgery and thoracic at No. 58 . . .

July 9
To Tunis. Thirty-eight Evac. well sited. Number 54 in building in city. Number 58 in the desert outside the city. Windy and dirty.

July 10
More evangelistic work in selective evacuation. E.B.S. will not admit possibility and shows sign of impeding evacuation jitters. In preparing for influx of battle casualties not enough allowance was made for the number of patients in hospital in area that results from concentration of a strong assault force. This comes from normal incidence of disease, increase in road accidents and explosives with concentration of traffic and bombing.

In forward area E.B.S.
    4,222 empty beds
    2,245 full beds
    6,467 Total

(continued)

In rear area E.B.S.
   2,195 empty beds
   1,716 full beds
   3,911 Total

July 10
D-day.

July 11
Down to the docks to inspect the "hards" where LST's are to unload casualties. Visited Naval Hospital and Dispensary. In afternoon with General Blesse to inspect the *Seminole*, just arrived from the States and here to evacuate E.B.S. to Algiers. Good meal on board. Surgeons anxious to do bone plating for battle fractures on ship between ports. A few naval casualties from a mine sweeper came in at 3 o'clock in the morning.

Evacuation fever rising!

To E.B.S. Headquarters for lunch. A batch of patients chosen for evacuation by *train* were being loaded on planes. Several of these picked out as unsuitable—either untreated malaria or minor complaints.

July 13
To hospital road. Came down with fever in afternoon.

July 14-15
Lying up with dysentery at 56th Evac.

July 16
To 9th Evac. to see McKittrick and also to meet Stricker (French surgeon whom I knew in Algiers).

July 17
Slight return of dysentery so laid up again today. The weather is monotonously fine. Clear, hot sun all day with temperature around 80°. Cool evenings with steady wind off the sea. The country is dry as a bone and far from attractive. It has been so thoroughly lived in for centuries that it resembles the bear grotto in a zoological garden—all slightly unclean. Occupation by armies recently has not helped. Every olive grove has been converted into a dusty bivouac.

Success in the assault on Sicily has led to optimism regarding the cumulative effects of bombing, Russian offensive and loss of the Mediterranean on Germany.

July 18
Down to the grove with 2nd Aux. Group for Sunday dinner.

July 19
Striker, Forsee and I to 54th Station Hospital in Tunis. Very few patients. In afternoon to Carthage. Visited Musée Lavigerie part of Lapeyre des Peres Blancs. Most of their rare treasures are in storage but many are still on display especially a collection of Roman clay lamps. Dinner at French Officers' Club.

July 20
In morning to Station Hospital #58 which is reinforced with teams. Reeve Betts and Longacre and others but very few patients. Station Hospital #60 just setting up and will be ready in a week. To British G.H. #97. Case of anthrax. Also bad burn. Some burns have died with hyperpyrexia on seventh and eighth day.

Sirocco temperatures. Have also had heat stroke with body cast for spine injuries and now treat only by plaster bed. The excellence of British tentage with double walls and fly in this climate, compared with ours. Also when they choose a site in an emergency they get busy with plans for change. General lack of imagination and intelligence at operations level in U.S.M.C. outstanding.

Special dinner in evening to Col. E. Hume on his way to AMGOT in Sicily.

July 21
Short talk to staff of #54, then to Tunis where I bought Roman lamps, a bowl from Pichon and a figurine probably of Cretan origin. (The bowl turned out to be a fake.) Then to Mateur and lunch at E.B.S. Spaulding low because yielding E.B.S. Surgeon post to Col. Rudolph. Met Holmes, Ginn and Hicks. Discussion of confusion in carrying out plans.

Dropped Striker at 2nd Aux. Group with Forsee and on to 56th. Possibly will go to Sicily tomorrow. Medical meetings on malaria this evening. Fifty-sixth Evac. has had approximately 400 cases in past month.

July 22
To Tunis with General Blesse and Long. Lunch at #54. To see Major Guilford at Foch Field. Back to 38th Evac. for night.

Renford Cindass, Jr, John D. Horton, and Hasan B. Alam

As "Part Three" of *Surgeon to Soldiers* starts, the Allies are moving from first contact with the enemy in North Africa to the invasion of Italy through Sicily. For context, Operation Husky (July 1943) is the Allies' second large-scale amphibious landing operation involving 450,000 ground forces and produced about 25,000 Allied casualties. This operation followed the landing in North Africa (Operation Torch, November 1942) of 100,000 ground forces and preceded the D-Day invasion at Normandy (Operation Overlord, June 1944) with over 2 million troops. Churchill describes his steps to influence care at both the tactical level (eg, close to the point of injury) and the operational level (eg, after patient evacuation to hospitals on the North African coast).

Providing optimal care in a suboptimal environment is a challenge inherent to military medicine. Churchill starts this chapter with what modern surgeons would recognize as a clinical practice guideline (CPG). There were "new doctors who had no experience in North Africa," and he wanted to get forward surgeons up to speed as quickly as possible. This memorandum was the culmination of lessons learned during the North African campaign neatly summarized for the non–battle-tested surgeon. Among many other instructions, he unequivocally made it clear that the treatment in his memorandum is the standard of care by stating 4 times that "there are no exceptions."

Churchill next highlights the disconnect between medical and administrative officers, a sentiment that can be felt still today. Often, there is a difference between what clinicians think is best for patients and what administrators believe is logistically/financially more desirable. For a while, Churchill attempted to reestablish specialty centers, which the Allies widely used during World War I. In this system, patients would first evacuate from a casualty clearing station to a base hospital. From this central hub, patients would then be transported to hospitals with specialized physicians, nurses, and wound care management for surgical, orthopedic, ENT, maxillofacial, and neuropsychiatric care. Such a system created complex patient movement logistics; so the Army banned specialty hospitals. Instead, patients were quickly triaged and dropped off at a hospital to prevent ambulance drivers from "peddling milk bottles along the road." This lack of coordination led to overwhelming casualty loads at proximate hospitals, further delaying definitive patient care.

Much has changed since Churchill's time, but many of the problems he faced persist today. The concept of circulated memorandums has now taken the form of CPGs published by the Joint Trauma System (JTS). As for patient evacuation, Dr Frank Berry noted the need for a "top MC officer in charge of evacuation." During the Global War on Terror, a patient movement cell, headed by a physician, coordinated all theater evacuations to balance how, where, and when patients should be evacuated using the guiding principles of early surgical stabilization with damage control surgery followed by evacuation to higher roles of care for definitive treatment and specialty care. Current Army doctrine implements modular field hospitals. If specialists are needed in an area, augmentation units can be attached to these hospitals, allowing for multidisciplinary care for patients with polytraumatic wounds. A near peer engagement with overwhelming casualty numbers will no doubt stress our current system just as Churchill experienced. Future generations must continue to innovate and design even better solutions.

SUGGESTED READINGS

Atkinson R. *The Day of Battle: The War in Sicily and Italy, 1943-1944.* Henry Holt; 2007.

Department of the Army. *Army Health System. FM 4-02.* Department of the Army; 2020.

Joint Trauma Systems. Clinical practice guidelines. https://jts.health.mil/index.cfm/PI_CPGs/cpgs

Mayhew ER. *Wounded: A New History of the Western Front in World War I.* Oxford University Press; 2013.

19

The Sicilian Campaign

I Left Foch Field near Tunis, on July 23, 1943, in a M-47 loaded with litters and blankets. We circled Pantelleria until a fighter escort arrived from Sousse and then, after a stop in Licata, arrived in Agrigento. A car from Seventh Army Headquarters took me to the 11th Evacuation Hospital north of Agrigento. The following morning I went on to Palermo—a deserted and badly bombed city.

Colonel Franklin was the Surgeon of Seventh Army and his office was moving into the palace. I spent the night at the Excelsior Hotel where I cooked my own breakfast in the hotel kitchen in the morning.

In Sicily I saw for the first time the wreckage caused by Allied bombing and long-range Naval shelling. The narrow streets were impassable; the main routes had been cleared by the engineers with their bulldozers. I recall pulling to the side of the road to allow a convoy of amphibian trucks (DUKW's) loaded with 3rd Division soldiers to pass. These monstrous DUKW's were winding their way through the blasted villages. Some houses had lost the outside walls and looked like doll houses in which the rooms are exposed to view with furniture and pictures in place. Bodies still were buried beneath the rubble and the slightly sweet, nauseating stench of decomposing corpses filled the air with the odor of death.

As the "ducks" wended their way to Palermo, children ran alongside, holding up their hands and screaming: "Caramelli, caramelli!" The soldiers tossed them candy and chocolate bars. Hijacking GI's for caramelli and singing arias from Verdi were the two great arts of the Sicilian boys. We spent a night at the headquarters of the 3rd Division Medical Battalion with Commanding Officer McCarthy. Pugsley was the 3rd Divisional Surgeon.

By July 26 we were back in Palermo, which had been occupied by the 3rd Division on July 23. The Seventh Army was moving its headquarters into the new postal and telegraph building which was in a state of complete confusion.

The postal and telegraph systems of a country are comparable to the network of the central nervous system. They not only symbolize, but make possible, integrated social life—and civilization itself. To see a post office in a state of complete disintegration comes as a shock. The postal service only functions with orderly government and strict federal legal control.

In the post office at Palermo, records, archives, files and documents dear to the hearts of postmasters were strewn about the corridors in complete disarray. I picked up a little box bearing an indecipherable address. Inside, carefully wrapped in tiny tissue paper parcels, each marked with an order number, were repair parts for watches. There were springs, wheels, parts of the casing. Even time itself, the regulating medium of the civilized world, falls with the devastation and wastage of war.

Dick Arnest, Howard Snyder and Bill Anspacher, the North African triumvirate of II Corps, were at their headquarters near Petralia. The Corps was then under command of General Omar Bradley, and we paid him a call. The 93rd Evacuation Hospital was nearby with Don Currier, of Cambridge, as Commanding Officer and Eddie Harding, of the Boston City Hospital, as Chief of Surgery.

Night driving, with just slit blackout lights, was difficult on the narrow crowded roads. We reached the 15th Evacuation Hospital, where Charlie Wasden was Chief of Surgery, late in the evening on July 29. He was able to produce a chicken dinner before finding cots for a night's sleep.

After a quick return trip to North Africa, I started back to Sicily on August 3, spending the night at the 38th Evacuation Hospital near Tunis. Paul Sanger provided ice-cold draft beer from his new refrigerating system. Perrin Long showed up about mess time. George Wood had taken over as Commanding Officer following the transfer of Bachspies elsewhere.

Arriving in Gela, I borrowed a jeep and drove to Castle Farano, now converted into headquarters for an engineer outfit and also for Lieutenant Colonel Smith, Commanding officer of the 261st Medical Battalion (**Figure 19.1**). The 1st Engineer Special Brigade moved 104,134 dead-weight tons of supplies over the beaches of Sicily between the tenth and thirty-first of July. The Castle Farano was a pretentious but somewhat threadbare baronial castle on the rocks of the coast line. To my amazement the kitchen was well equipped with copper cooking utensils. Some needed retinning but otherwise they were ready for service. Colonel Smith provided me with a jeep and driver for the trip north.

When we arrived at II Corps on August 5, the 3rd Division was engaged near San Petrillo. The battle of Troina was nearing its end. This battle was referred to later as the toughest battle in which American troops have been engaged since World War I. Shelling was going on when we arrived. Troina was being evacuated by the Germans but was not occupied by our troops because of a bombing mission scheduled for 7:30 the next morning. The next evening Troina was clearly visible from our tent at II Corps. It was a typical Sicilian skyline city on a mountain top.

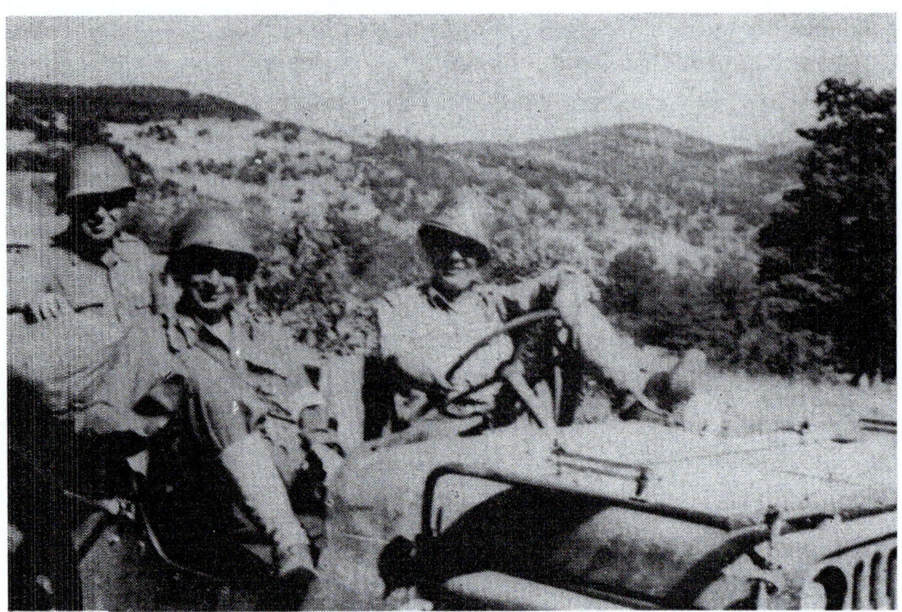

Figure 19.1 Left to right: Major Howard Snyder, the author and Lieutenant Colonel Perrin Long.

UNUSUAL CASES

After mess that same evening I went over to the 11th Evacuation Hospital east of Nicosia. Some of the unusual cases examined were described in my notes as follows:

Case 1: Abdominal Wound.
German P.O.W. 36 hours after apparently trivial wounds of abdominal wall. Exploration advised. Advisability of managing late cases of abdominal wounds by nonoperative peritonitis regimen continually being raised by surgeons, particularly younger officers schooled in this type of treatment for appendiceal peritonitis. Unless patient is *in extremis*, I believe operative treatment indicated. Undoubtedly a number of small perforations would seal themselves off and spontaneously bring the peritonitis under control. Large perforations, complete division of the bowel, penetration of urinary bladder, penetration of gall bladder and other unpredictable results of wounding are so frequent that exploration is essential. Also, in the forward areas facilities are not present for skilled and prolonged management of the complications of uncontrolled peritonitis—residual abscesses, intestinal obstruction, ileus, disturbance

of electrolyte balance and dehydration. Maintenance of fluid balance with measured intake and output, chloride determinations, Miller-Abbott intubation, and other adjuncts to skilled management of peritonitis available in civilian hospitals are nonexistent. Even maintenance of adequate Fowler position on a cot is impractical, although a box placed under the head of the cot gives an inclined plane that is more comfortable than many head rests that have been used for years.

In this case a perforation was found in the small bowel—walling itself off with a plastic peritonitis. While the peritonitis was localizing, a residual abscess with obstruction was likely.

Case 2: Question of Cerebral Malaria.
Penetrating wound of left shoulder. Patient in deep coma. Being treated as a head injury with concussion, although no evidence of external trauma to the head. Temperature 103.8°. (Rectal temperatures should be recorded more frequently in shock wards.) Divergent strabismus—fixed pupils—diminished or absent reflexes. Said to be in "shock"—although blood pressure was 100/70; extremities hot, veins full and respiration depressed often of Cheyne-Stokes type.

A tentative diagnosis of cerebral malaria was suggested and blood film requested. The blood smear was negative, but nevertheless intravenous quinine advised. This was about 20:00. He died at 02:15 August 7 of respiratory failure. Autopsy showed a downward course of a rifle or machine gun bullet that fractured 4th and 5th ribs and passed through the lower part of the upper lobe. The missile struck and fractured the 7th rib and lay free in the pleural space. A total of 1,500 cc. blood and fluid in pleura. No pneumothorax. There were no gross signs of cerebral concussion. No edema of the brain, and no petechial hemorrhage. As both thick and thin smears for malaria were negative, the final diagnosis is left in doubt. He was given 2 cc. quinine i.v. at 2300 hours and 100 cc. sodium sulfadiazine at 0100.

Possibilities remain: cerebral malaria—cerebral fat embolism, unlikely because lack of fracture of long bones—cerebral anoxia during period of initial shock, producing irreversible cerebral damage.

Case 3: Hemorrhage from Fractured Rib
"L.F." Tagged 2 Bn. 39 Inf. Aid. Post. August 6 0100. W.I.A. Diagnosed N.V.D. 250 cc. plasma, ½ gr. morphia. Arrived Col. Co 5 @ 0220. Diagnosis ruptured viscus. To Cl. Co. @ 0230. Admitted Cl. Sta. 9 Med. Bn. August 6. Diagnosed W.I.A. Wound of head, severe, bullet, pen. T.A.T. 1 cc.

(continued)

Admitted 11 F.H. August 6. 0340. G.S.W. head.

0500	500 cc. plasma
0615	500 cc. plasma
1000	1000 cc. 5% glucose
1500	500 cc. plasma

Trans. 11 F.H. 1300. Diagnosed W.I.A. (1) G.S.W. head contused, severe right temporal; (2) concussion, pulmonary, left severe due to blast. X-ray said to show long linear fracture right temporal bone. Left lung field hazy throughout with slight displacement mediastinum to right. Seriously ill. Diagnosed shock, traumatic, severe, due to blast.

Examined at 2200 hours. Conscious—breathing rapid—pulse weak and thready. Cool extremities. Displacement trachea to right. Left chest dull laterally and posteriorly—absent B.S. Anteriorly showed tympany with absent B.S., interpreted by Long as pneumothorax, by Snyder as Skodaic resonance, and by me as possibly air-containing viscus with rupture of diaphragm.

Thought wise to fluoroscope before aspirating chest. This was done demonstrating stomach below diaphragm. Then preparations to aspirate chest made, but as novocain being injected, patient died. He had received no O$_2$ therapy. Died 0020 hours August 7.

Autopsy August 7 at 1100 hours showed 4500 cc. blood filling left pleural cavity. Source of hemorrhage was fracture of 6th rib in midaxillary line with complete severance of neurovascular bundle of 5th interspace. Sharp fragment of rib had penetrated lung, but this small puncture was sealed with blood clot. Some extravasation blood under parietal pleura around site of fracture indicating source of hemorrhage was intercostal vessels.

There was no evidence of external trauma over site of fracture or elsewhere on chest. The wounds of head were trivial, nonpenetrating. No evidence of brain injury, and fracture of skull described by x-ray unconfirmed at autopsy.

Additional observations recorded during this death from hemorrhage:

1540 hours	B.P. 60/40	250 cc. plasma
1620 hours	B.P. 60/40	
2200 hours		500 cc. plasma

This man bled to death (4,500 cc.) into his pleural cavity under careful (?) supervision and repeated plasma administration.

Just how the localized fracture of the 6th rib was sustained is unknown. Possibly he fell on a rock or his rifle. Being admitted as a head wound, he had been turned over to the neurosurgeon, who was content to accept diagnosis of blast injury to lung.

VISITS TO MEDICAL FACILITIES

Howard Snyder felt we should distribute another circular letter calling attention to the basic principles of wound management. Surgeons brought to the forward area for the first time were making the same old mistakes. So we started to work on: "The Care of the Wounded in Sicily."

August 7 was spent at II Corps completing this letter, but we still had time to visit the 11th Field Hospital and the 11th Evacuation Hospital. At the 11th Field Hospital there was a group of badly injured casualties admirably managed by the surgical teams. This seemed to be the solution to forward first-priority surgery—a well-equipped field hospital platoon staffed by surgical teams (**Figure 19.2**).

It also clearly showed the advance in the surgery of the wounded made in Sicily—the adaptation of the so-called field hospital for this purpose. This hospital spanned the gap between the 48th Surgical Hospital of southern Tunisia and the mobile Army surgical hospital of Korea.

The following day, Perrin Long, Howard Snyder and I drove up to San Stefano. After a stop at the 15th Evacuation Hospital, we arrived at Mistretta,

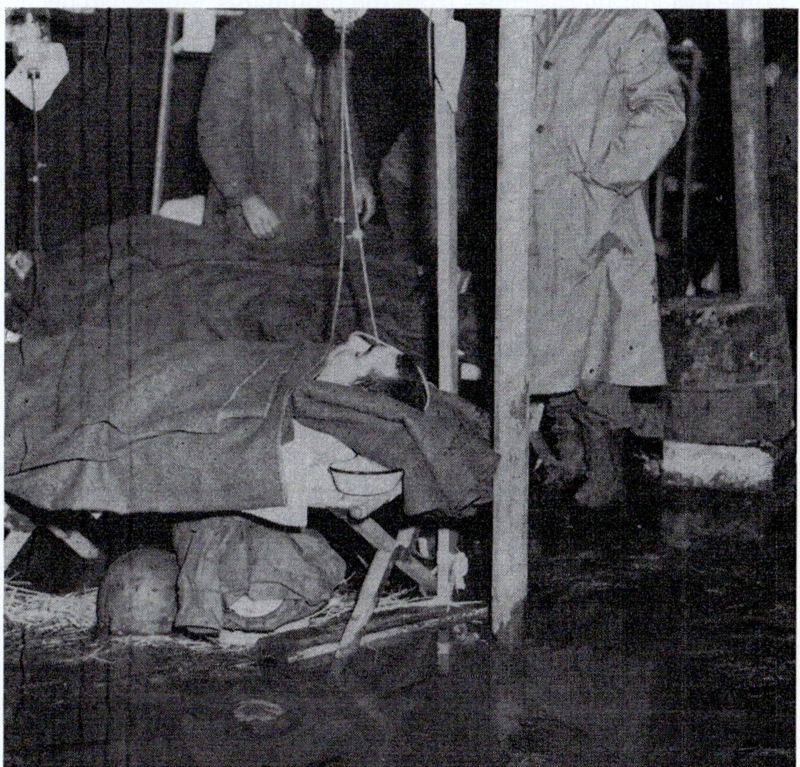

Figure 19.2 Resuscitation tent in the mud.

a clean little city, late in the morning. We drove into the courtyard of the 304th Italian Field Hospital, now under charge of Lieutenant Gregorie of the 54th Medical Battalion—a Boston doctor. The place was in good shape, with a staff of Italian medical officers taking care of the patients. I saw a case of probable cord tumor that I advised sending to the 128th Evacuation Hospital. Later this turned out to be a lipoma, according to Haynes, who took it out.

The Italian staff insisted we have lunch with them, so we crossed the street to their quarters, where a congenial lunch party was held. We had grayish spaghetti with tomato paste sauce—and then some fresh beef. A bottle or so of wine was produced. The Italians were mostly local doctors from Sicily, and anxious to have news from their homes. Autographs were exchanged, pictures taken and I departed with a bottle of marsala under my arm.

McCarthy and his 3rd Medical Battalion headquarters were set up between the road and the sea just east of San Stefano. A platoon of the 11th Field Hospital with surgical teams (Haggerty and Partington among others) was adjacent to his clearing station, and the 93rd Evacuation Hospital was down the beach about a kilometer. The 3rd Division had been having a tough time evacuating casualties from the mountains. Mules had been used for sitting cases but not for carrying litters.

After supper we went to the clearing station where some of the casualties were just coming in from an aid station that had been isolated for a day.

ADDITIONAL CASE HISTORIES

Fracture of Femur: "H.K." wounded 1700 hours August 6. Tagged 3rd Bn. Aid. August 7 at 0530. Arrived clearing station August 8 at 2200 hours.

He had a compound fracture of the lower third of the left femur. After they got him into the aid post he stayed in a foxhole with one small meal a day. A two hour litter carry, then long ambulance ride through San Fratello and down the coast road. No splinting of any type. He was perfectly well on arrival at the clearing station with pulse of 100 and B.P. of 130/64, chatting and smoking a cigarette. His leg was not causing pain, although felt better when it was put into a Thomas splint for transfer to the field hospital next door. The doctors on duty did not think it necessary to splint him for such a short distance but I insisted upon it as an object lesson—also he would have to have x-rays taken and might face a delay of three hours.

Soft Part Wound: "G.S." wounded August 7 at 1200 hours. Tagged and given 1/2 gr. morphine at 0112. Apparently it was thought he had a fracture as the right leg was splinted with a signal flag stick on the outer side and a bayonet on the inner. After wounding, he was carried downstream on a litter made from his shirt and two rifles. Then supported on the shoulders of two men, he jumped along on his uninjured leg. The wound bled but not a great amount. During the last three days he has had one K-ration supper unit and a little water.

He arrived at the clearing station August 8 at 1210. Good spirits—B.P. 132/70 and pulse of 90.

This story was taken, thinking he had a compound fracture because of the splinting but it was only a flesh wound.

Fracture of Leg: "A.S" aged 28. Tagged Bn. Aid. August 7 at 1000. Wounded in right leg with compound fracture on August 6 at 1945 hours. Bandaged and splinted with two sticks as soon as the medic got to him. The sticks are still on serving as the only splint. The delay in reaching the aid post was because of a counter attack.

He was brought down from the hills over a mile litter carry. On the way down a German P.O.W. carrying the litter was killed and the patient received a second wound in the left thigh.

Had C-ration to eat and some water. Arrived clearing station August 8 at 2215 (48 hours after injury). B.P. 114/48, pulse 100. Excellent condition.

Comment: These wounded were from the 3rd Division San Fratello action. There was no evidence of tissue hemorrhage about their wounds and no swelling. Lack of any type of "shock" reaction was striking. In contrast, however:

Clostridial Myositis: "J.H." tagged 3rd Bn. Aid. August 7 at 1414 hours. Shell fragment wound right thigh and leg. Sulfanilamide. Bandage. Plasma 250 cc. Admitted to 11th F.H. on August 8 at 2130 with B.P. 90/50 in definite shock. Operation August 9 at 0100; B.P. 80/?. The leg was very swollen as tight circular bandages had acted as compressors. Black blood was coming from small wound. Some subcutaneous gas was palpable but not considered evidence of infection. Given 5 units of plasma. Wide débridement with removal of blood clots. Sulfanilamide—surgical gauze and plaster. Marked *observe for gas* (Haggerty).

Transferred to 93rd Evac. on Aug. 9 with this note: Circulation at 1330 definitely better than at time of admission. The tight constricting bandage was present below knee on admission. Watch for gas (Haggerty).

At 93rd Evac. August 9 2130 negative smear for malaria. August 10 at 0900 entire right leg purple. Foot extremely cold. Air in foot, calf and popliteal tissues. Patient very toxic, disoriented and dehydrated. At 1100, 100,000 units of antitoxin and 2,000 cc. saline given; 3 units of plasma. At 1200 midthigh guillotine amputation. All great vessels of thigh thrombosed. Given 500 cc. blood and 5 gm. sulfa.

(continued)

Comment: This case was of interest—first because of the shock in contrast to the other three—and the location of the lost blood volume was obvious in the swollen leg. I do not believe he had gas infection at the time of débridement; the crepitation was very superficial and remote from the wound. The gas bacillus infection—if it was really that—developed as a result of circulatory complications. In battle casualties clostridium contamination is ubiquitous and *circulatory disturbance* the essential factor in development of infection.

ON THE ROAD AGAIN

The next day—August 9—I went with Pugsley, the 3rd Divisional Surgeon, to the 3rd Division Command Post to meet General Trescott and General Eagles. We then went on to an abandoned German field hospital at Acquedolci into which a collecting company was moving. The place was in disorder. Straw on the floor had evidently served for the wounded. The building had previously been an elementary school and some Italian posters instructing civilians in protective measures against chemical warfare and air raids, were "rescued" by Long and me from the walls. San Agata was still under shellfire but we rounded the corner just to the west of it and drove up the mountain to San Fratello. This mountainside was studded with strong points and pill boxes and had formed a defensive position commanding the valley to the west as well as the coast road. The battlefield was fresh: a panorama of scattered materials—dead horses—engineers with mine detectors sweeping the road—isolated squads of soldiers wandering around searching for their outfits. And there was the "odor of death," which seemed to be originating in the horses. These were beginning to swell up like barrage balloons.

The children of the little village of San Fratello were not yet "educated" to run out begging for "caramelli." When a piece of candy was tossed to them, they were not sure it could be picked up with safety.

Beyond San Fratello we stopped to eat some K-rations and then went along a bit farther to find a battalion aid post. An advanced group of soldiers had just struggled up the mountain and were eating their rations when we found them. The battalion surgeon was a very discouraged young man who in civilian life had specialized in treating psychoneuroses and now felt his Army effort was utterly fruitless—that any medical corps officer could perform his duties. I found myself thinking: These boys center their attention on the *technics* of their profession, medical as well as surgical, and do not realize that the *sense of responsibility* toward the sick and wounded is only developed in the doctor. The Oath of Hippocrates, even if written today, would not include "I shall scrub my hands for ten minutes by the clock and carefully clean my fingernails before undertaking an operation."

When we got back to the collecting station, it was beginning to swarm with Sicilian natives. One old man had picked up an incendiary bomb and had second-degree burns of both hands and face—not unlike the Cocoanut Grove pattern—but somehow he managed to maintain a smile.

Near the station was a small German cemetery, neatly laid out, as they all were, and marked with crosses, oftentimes with a helmet on the cross. The graves were covered with palm leaves and flowers. Down the road a short distance to the west, a barbed wire prisoner of war enclosure had filled up noticeably while we were in the mountains. Most of the prisoners were Italians; the few Germans seemed to keep to themselves.

Suddenly, every gun in the neighborhood began to fire and someone yelled: "Here he comes!" Everyone rushed into the building and snuggled down against the walls—myself included. The firing continued and then it was all over. It was said that a German plane had come in over the prisoner of war enclosure, machine guns blazing, headed down toward the hospital and then turned out to sea. Perhaps so—but I didn't see much. The prisoners were milling around in an excited manner and there was still lots of shooting. Perhaps I heard the plane but I am not sure. I didn't see it—I can't conceive of any likelihood of being hit—*yet* to make the story good "we were strafed."

After returning to 3rd Battalion headquarters, I went on to Palermo, stopping at the 10th Field Hospital for a talk with the commanding officer. He was rather puzzled at suddenly being assigned as a combat unit, having had the concept of field hospitals acting as small station hospital units.

On August 10 I arrived at the 91st Evacuation Hospital, now set up in the University Policlinic. I made rounds with Major Knapp, an extremely able young man from Cornell who was carrying the weight of the administration and surgical services on his shoulders. He had had only two years as assistant resident with George Heuer.

After supper, I drove over to the adjacent buildings of the University Policlinic where the 59th Evacuation Hospital had moved in. This outfit, professionally one of the best in the theater, had had a tough break. After a stalemate in Casablanca, acting as a holding and station hospital, they had been brought up to Bizerte for the Sicilian campaign. Here are my notes on some of the difficulties they ran into:

E.D.C. Comments: August 3 they left Bizerte on two LST's and one LCI at 1600. The equipment, headquarters, vehicles and 170 enlisted men loaded on one LST; 181 enlisted men and 28 officers on the second LST; 2 M.O.'s, 53 nurses and the Red Cross workers loaded on the LCI. The first LST with C.O., headquarters and equipment had engine trouble and turned back. The others arrived August 4 at 1500 hours and debarked at 1900.

(continued)

The surgeon's office of Seventh Army had no information of their arrival. The nurses were billeted at 91st Evac. The detachment at midnight marched to a staging area where they were eaten up by ants even though they stood up the rest of the night. The next morning Matheson went with Franklin to look at proposed sites and was assigned the Policlinic buildings, although they requested to set up in tents. At 1600 hours they moved into the dirty, bombed buildings, some still with civilian patients. At 1500 hours came an order for all personnel to be attached to 91st Evac.; at 1805 an order from the 91st Evac. for 6 M.O.'s, 10 nurses and 10 enlisted men to be attached to 91st Evac.; at 1810 they were notified to be ready to receive 150 patients. The 91st helped with cots and blankets—200 cots and blankets for 75; Ordnance supplied other cots and blankets. By working all night, began to receive patients at 1900 and had 139 by midnight. This was a swell job by Matheson, Riley, Roy Cohn and their professional staff. Two days later the C.O., headquarters and equipment arrived.

I walked around the Policlinic with Matheson and Roy Cohn. It was pathetic to see a university in ruins (**Figure 19.3**). The surgical operating room had received a direct hit and was a pile of concrete rubble. Large blocks of wall were hanging in midair by the reinforcing steel rods. Departmental libraries were in confusion. We looked through the surgical library—nothing of real value but many rows of bound periodicals, reports, reprints, and so forth. Instruments and apparatus were being salvaged by nuns.

E.D.C. Comments: "Back to Acquedolci on August 11 along the coast road," my notes read, "stopping at 128th Evac. near Cefalis. Wylie has this unit well polished up. Haynes as neurosurgeon has done a good job during this campaign. Also stopped at 56th Med. Bn. set up as holding hospital at Termini, West. Supper at 3rd Med. Bn. and later Perry achieved a haircut on the edge of the sea while the rest of us sat around enjoying the view. Pugsley gave us account of the tactical situation recorded on map.

"After dark Snyder and I went over to adjacent 10th F.H. and saw Higginbotham and talked with him about organization of F.H. for this combat function. This will be made the basis of a report as I am extremely anxious to use these platoons as surgical hospitals for first priority cases.

"On August 12 I went with 3rd Division veterinarian to inspect his newly acquired captured horses and mules. It has been difficult to round up these Italian army mules as the natives catch them and hide them. Several hundred have been secured however. An officer from New York City who had never seen a horse before is in charge and delighted with his assignment. We loaded up a pack mule with plasma and took some pictures for Red

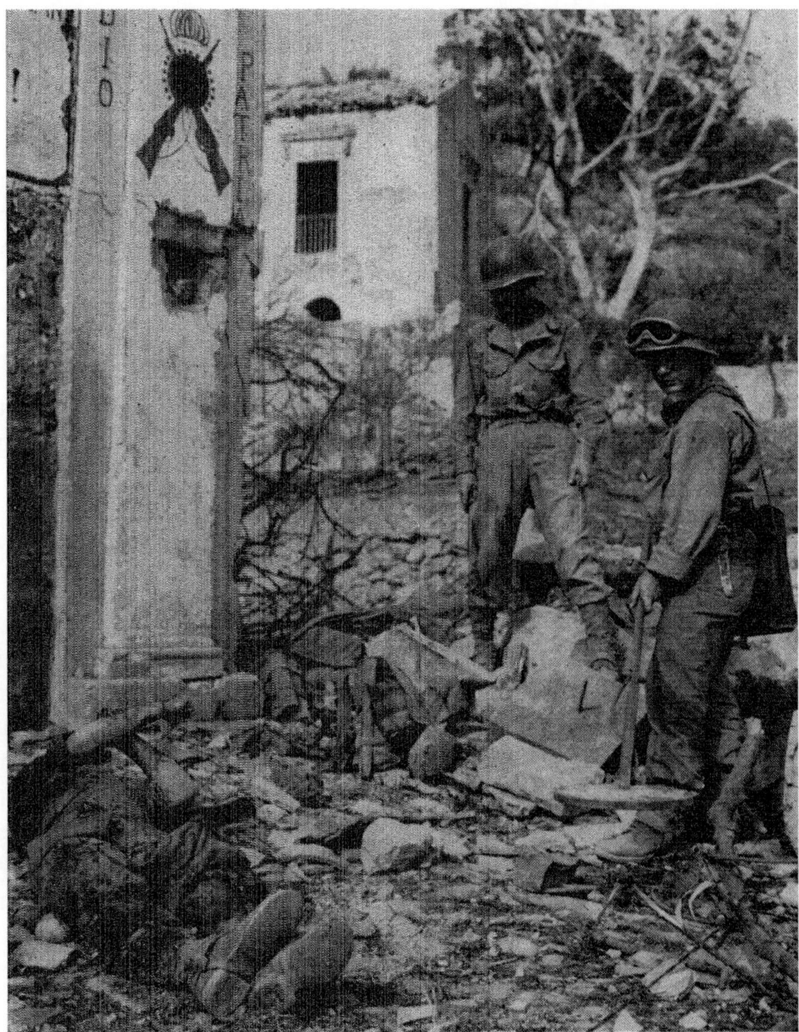

Figure 19.3. US soldiers, in Sicily, sweeping for mines near body of soldier killed by a booby trap.

Cross use. A horse with leeches under his tongue was presented, but even though twitched, it was impossible to get them out. This is reminiscent of Larrey's difficulty in Egypt with leeches in the noses of Napoleon's soldiers. A great pile of captured Italian pack saddles and saddlebags.

"After returning to 3rd Med. Bn. started for II Corps. Stopped at 93rd Evac. for Perry to collect some notes; meanwhile Currier, Eddie Harding, Rafe Hatt, Snyder and I went for a swim. Then back over the Mistretta road to find II Corps had moved forward today. Finally we reached headquarters just at dusk. This is a beautiful part of Sicily but

(continued)

the roads are extremely slow and the dust thick—fine volcanic ash. Mt. Etna was in full view most of the time. A pick-up ration supper.

"On August 13 back over the Cesaro road, reaching a ruined chapel just east of Troina for lunch. The cemetery behind had been badly machine-gunned and shelled. The marble slabs had fallen from the tombs, leaving gaping holes with skeletons and mummified bodies on display. Back through Troina still with the 'odor of death' about it; here was where the Germans left dead on the field contrary to their usual custom."

THOUGHTS ABOUT THE CAMPAIGN

On the journey back to Algiers, I had time to reflect on the strengths and weaknesses of the Sicilian campaign. What follows, here, are some thoughts I jotted down:

E.D.C. Comments: The characteristics of the Sicilian campaign (I wrote) have been described as:

(a) Continuous and unrelenting attack.
(b) Maneuver under cover of fire. No frontal attack by a large unit. This was made possible by superiority of fire power and air support which allowed troops to maneuver around the flanks of the enemy.
(c) Sweat has taken the place of blood. Men of Seventh Army marched tremendous distances over roughest possible terrain. This taxed to limits of physical exhaustion. Incredible marches allowed attacks to be launched from directions that would give the maximum of success with the minimum loss of life. And the military intensity of this campaign in part accounts for some of the weakness in the evacuation procedures; however, revision of some policies would have helped resolve some problems.

Field hospitals and 400-bed evacs. should be under control of Corps—not Army. Corps will try to maintain the evacuation policy established by Army but with changing tactical situations with which Corps alone is conversant; no policy in terms of days can be maintained over any period of time in combat.

Frozen surgical staffs in forward hospitals are a menace from professional aspect. The principle of surgical teams as in field hospitals might well be extended to 400-bed evacs. As it is now, the 400-bed evacs. are not staffed with the best qualified surgeons; these stay in 750-bed and G.H. units. The whole outfit moves into line inexperienced. Great difficulty is encountered in an overseas theater in making personnel shifts because of loyalty of group—inability of C.O. to pass judgment on professional qualifications—promises of C.O. to the group that "their day would come."

Consultants by echelon rather than by divisions of regional surgery. Procedures in military surgery are more dependent on *time* and *place* where certain operations should be done than on regional anatomy. A consultant must be an expert in principles of evacuation and field service to advise intelligently on problem of forward surgery. Professional services should be represented in Corps and Army. Possibly also periodically in divisions.

Social and organizational intricacies of the Army transcend in interest and importance the professional aspects. Wars within wars. The regular Army engages the enemy but at the same time carries on an internecine conflict that calls forth even greater strategic and tactical efforts.

Certainly the Seventh Army conducted this campaign totally unbalanced as far as hospital facilities are concerned. By deliberately refusing to accept reasonable responsibilities for care of their own sick and wounded, they seriously depleted divisional strength. In many tactical situations—and probably in all tactical situations now to be faced on the Continent—such a policy will be exceedingly dangerous. By transferring responsibility for hospitalization that is normally Army function, to base sections, the manpower of the Army is now scattered from Palermo to Oran.

In many ways it resembles a maniac driving a machine at high speed without pausing to oil or service the machine—only to put in more gasoline. One hates to see a fine machine with intricate specialized parts, built by years of training, permanently damaged by irresponsible staff work in 39 days. Misuse of a fine tool!

The number of beds (3,350) established was entirely inadequate for the force in Sicily; 5,760 beds in field and evacuation hospitals were allotted to Seventh Army, and 6,250 beds in station and general hospitals were available on call. This has resulted in several unfortunate situations. An excessive number of slight cases were transferred to North Africa and completely filled the beds in Eastern Base Section. More serious cases are rapidly transferred from one hospital to another without adequate rest during transit. The number of replacements required to maintain the strength on the island is excessive.

More beds in evacuation and station hospitals would have permitted retention of cases until the optimum time for evacuation by the several echelons of medical service.

A convalescent hospital is a very economical unit as far as personnel and equipment is concerned to hold a large number of mild cases awaiting return to duty. None was present in Sicily.

Air evacuation became the primary means of evacuating casualties from the combat zone. In spite of warning that this service could not be expected before D+14, it was established on D+3 and except on D+5 functioned daily.

July 10 to August 17, 11,157 sick and wounded were evacuated from Sicily to North Africa, 5,257 by water (combat loaders, LST's and hospital ships and carriers) and 5,900 by aircraft.

Mary F. Stuever, Paul K. Carlton, Jr, and Jay A. Johannigman

The Sicilian Campaign represented a brief but intense waypoint in the movement of Allied forces from the North African campaign toward southern Italy. The chapter is notable for several dramatic case reports, references to twitching a horse and using mules for transport, and visits to numerous medical facilities staffed by academic colleagues and associates of Colonel Churchill. Through all these interactions one appreciates the value of a surgical leader like Churchill, constantly observing, learning, and serving.

The author's travel through his area of responsibility (AOR)—from North Africa up to Sicily, back to North Africa, and then all around Sicily—allowed him to grasp the vast spread of the troops and the logistical challenges of moving personnel and equipment along bombed-out roads and through barely passable terrain. Taking almost an entire month to move supplies a short distance is hard to grasp in today's rapidly moving world, particularly given the air superiority characteristic of our recent campaigns in Iraq and Afghanistan. The recent COVID-19 pandemic did create delays and challenges similar to World War II by disrupting the global supply chain. Forward bases and medical facilities often had to make do with less than the people who were in those same locations just a few months prior to the global shutdown in response to the pandemic.

While damage control surgery per se was not known during Churchill's time, he appreciated that evacuation of patients with abdominal wounds to surgical teams was essential for survival. Examples of combat wounded evacuation by mules is quite telling of the extreme difficulties faced by combat medics at the point of injury. The discussion of the optimal location for surgical teams on the battlefield is very instructive. Churchill's visit to the 48th Surgical Hospital in southern Tunisia impresses the essential principle of positioning well-trained mobile hospitals near the point of injury. This chapter also highlights the need for medical teams to move as the front lines move and to flex to accept vast numbers of casualties. Modern readers should note the casualty flow reported by Churchill exceeds that of Korea, Vietnam, Desert Storm, Operation Iraqi Freedom (OIF), and Operation Enduring Freedom (OEF) by an order of magnitude. Agility is key.

Despite numerous medical advances in the 20th and 21st centuries, injury patterns during wartime have changed very little. Hemorrhagic shock remains the primary cause of unrecognized death. One reads between the lines of Churchill's description of the death of a casualty assumed to have a traumatic brain injury who ultimately died from an unrecognized massive hemothorax—the patient's altered mental status was a result of hemorrhagic shock. This is a haunting case as there were no external signs of chest trauma, yet the casualty bled to death in a field hospital. What is also notable is that the field hospitals performed their own autopsies on patients who expired under their care. This emphasizes the humbling necessity of closing the loop through performance improvement activities like the weekly Joint Trauma System Video Teleconference today. Finally, the discussion of clostridial myositis management is comparable to the invasive fungal infections experienced in OEF. Both situations require a high index of suspicion and resources to enable early surgical and antimicrobial intervention.

SUGGESTED READINGS

Ingalls N, Zonies D, Bailey JA, et al. A review of the first 10 years of critical care aeromedical transport during operation Iraqi freedom and operation enduring freedom: the importance of evacuation timing. *JAMA Surg*. 2014;149(8):807–813.

Rodriguez RCJ, Ganesan A, Shaikh F, et al. Combat-related invasive fungal wound infections. *Mil Med*. 2022 May 4;187(Suppl 2):34–41.

20

Penicillin in Tripoli

PENICILLIN WAS AVAILABLE by 1941 but in such small quantity that it could only be used for experimental purposes. And during the months following 1941, Sir Harold Florey, E. B. Chain and others were purifying penicillin to find a preparation that would be effective against infectious organisms and would be well tolerated by human tissues.

During my early months in North Africa I had made several visits to one of the British hospitals on the outskirts of Algiers where Sir Harold Florey and a small team, including Lieutenant Colonel Ian Fraser, were studying penicillin. The only penicillin available was a calcium solution which could not be administered intramuscularly but had to be applied directly to the wound. Florey was the scientist who had developed penicillin in England and he had come to North Africa to test it. They were seeking to find what this new agent could do.

Several times I examined the patients who were being treated in the British hospital. Florey was not a surgeon and it soon became obvious to me that he was tackling problems and expecting results from penicillin that could not be achieved under any circumstances, no matter how bactericidal his new preparation might be. The case that brought this most forcibly to my attention was a soldier who had been wounded in the chest about the level of the third rib anteriorly. The lung was totally collapsed. The entrance wound of the missile had been converted into a draining sinus. Once or twice a day they would turn the man head down and empty the pus out of the chest through this wound sinus. They would then fill the chest cavity with calcium penicillin solution, put a cork into the wound, expecting the action of the penicillin to sterilize the pleural cavity. This procedure to anyone who knew the rudiments of thoracic surgery, was about as silly as one could imagine. The pleural space was never going to be obliterated until the lung reexpanded. It was an ill-designed experiment. What was needed was a dependent opening in the chest to establish free drainage, followed by efforts directed toward expansion of the lung. Infection was not playing an important part in the disability of the patient.

There were many wounds that duplicated the descriptions of the wounds of World War I: enormous wound cavitation, compound fractures of the femur with rigid-walled cavities in the thigh muscles. Here again, the calcium penicillinase was being applied locally much as Dakin's solution had been applied during the First World War. They were culturing these wounds but not approaching the biologic problems from a broad standpoint. One day we all went out on the balcony for a breath of fresh air. The wards were quite unpleasant and the flies were thick. I talked with Florey and Fraser and urged that they go forward to try the effects of penicillin in wounds that were fresh. That was their ultimate procedure.

By the middle of 1943, the pharmaceutical industry had begun the manufacture of penicillin. On July 3, of that year I had returned to Algiers from Sicily to pick up a box of penicillin, brought by hand to the theater by Hugh Morgan, Consultant in Medicine, Surgeon General's Office. The campaign in Sicily was to mark the transition to the "penicillin era."

Therefore, when a conference of surgeons assembled in Tripoli on August 23 to smooth out imagined differences in surgical procedure between the British Eighth Army surgeons and the First Army surgeons—who had just come together in the Sicilian campaign—it is not surprising that penicillin would be one of the major topics. The following describes some of the events that took place before and during the meeting.

DIARY NOTES OF CONFERENCE

August 22

I invited Howard Naffziger, who had just arrived in Algiers, to join me on the trip to Tripoli. We had the plane to ourselves from Tunis to Tripoli. Landing at Castel Benito field we rode on a truck to British 48th General Hospital and were very well housed in an Italian sanitorium. There we met up with Brigadier Hugh Cairns and Florey who had come in from Cairo this afternoon, and with Ian Fraser and Scott Thompson. Ogilvie is here from Cairo so we hope for a round-up of surgical experience with particular emphasis on penicillin during the next day or two.

In Sicily, Fraser had worked up the Bronte road behind the Eighth Army. Wounds were trimmed by regular medical officers, but he watched them and made notes. Then, in his cases, a mixture of penicillin powder and sulfonamide was put in and a loose filling of petrolatum gauze. They were casted and marked "do not open until arrival at General Hospital No. 48." Here they were inspected, cultured, and sutured. Bacteriologic controls made at both ends. This working of two teams, one at the

(continued)

front and one to receive cases at the base, is an excellent idea. They say gram-negative infection, particularly pyocyaneus, results but does not materially impede wound healing with secondary suture. Florey finds about 5 per cent of staphylococci—morphologically indistinguishable from the rest—which are penicillin-resistant. The bad knee infection seen at 95th General Hospital with Fraser responded well to intramuscular penicillin; infection cleared. We both agreed that this was a real test case quite likely to end in amputation or death from chronic sepsis.

August 23

Florey and MacLennan see no theoretic or practical reason to withhold gas gangrene antitoxin when using penicillin. The two measures are complemental and not alternative methods of treatment. Florey believes that clostridia may continue to multiply with penicillin. I agree absolutely and was only persuaded away from this point of view by Long. Florey also believes that dead muscle should be surgically excised with penicillin treatment—obvious. Question how to apply penicillin practically with maximum economy of material.

The day was spent in the detailed discussion of wound management and the relation of the fragmentary experience with penicillin. Ian Fraser, Scott Thompson, MacLennan, Jolly, D'Abreu, Jeffrey, Ogilvie and others joined in debate about the merits of combining penicillin with sulfonamide. Conversation centered on the variable inherent in the surgery of war. My final comment was: Just what is being accomplished by flooding wound with penicillin during healing? Personally I should use penicillin for 2-3 days and then suture it and let it alone. In a dirty wound excise, pack with penicillin for 2-3 days, then suture. Strange mixture of Carrel-Dakin technic and modern bacteriology. Only effective method of suturing wound is systemic administration.

August 24

Naffziger and I up early on the balcony working over some neurosurgical reports loaned by Hugh Cairns. After breakfast to the 48th G.H. at 9:30. A parade of cases treated in various ways by penicillin and secondary or delayed primary suture. Examination of wounds and battle fractures by Florey, Col. Jeffrey, Cairns, Ogilvie, Fraser, Boyd, MacLennan, Major Thompson, Colonel Jolly, Col. Stout and Lt. Col. Button.

After lunch a long discussion was held following which we went to the beach for a swim, returning for tea and more discussion about how to best use penicillin. Naffziger and I left at 6:30 to have dinner at the

American mess with Major Crozier. After a drink on the roof of his villa we returned to the Grand Hotel where Naffziger disappeared for a bath to take the salt off his hide.

Florey has, I fear, stepped off his plane of research and is working at applied clinical level in an affair full of empiricism, surgical technics and innumerable variables. He is fully aware of the level at which he is working—that of applied technics—but I wonder if he knows the pitfalls into which he may be led. It is exactly what happened in the last war when physiologists undertook to solve shock, and some are still laboring at the misconceptions that clouded the issue then.

This afternoon on the beach Florey mentioned the fact that he was not doing research, that the problem was purely one of applied technics—but no one got the point. They think he is doing research at his accustomed level. He questioned Ogilvie about the M.E. system of giving sulfonamide at 8 and 12 hours and asked for water-tight proof that it was effective. The answer was that the wounds all looked better and after all it was the only way it could be given, and that the Australians or someone had shown that the blood levels were effectively maintained.

On the whole, the show today was disappointing. With so many variables I cannot see that they have "shown" anything. I don't believe their percentage of successful sutures is any greater with penicillin than without, from what I have seen of secondary sutures in our base sections. It should be of help in this problem, but we are far from proving it and even from finding the best method of application. If it must be given locally—then clean up the wound with it and suture it. Application in the forward area may be advantageous unless the surface infection hastens separation of the necrotic tissue due to injury that carries the bacterial growth as a surface rather than invasive infection. This concept, developed in my report to the Surgeon General, is fundamental, I believe.

August 25

Many British soldiers with large wounds and battle fractures were shown, contrasting the results in those given penicillin in the forward area with those who did not receive penicillin. Discussion was led by Jeffrey, Florey, Ogilvie and Jolly. Here are some of their remarks and some of my thoughts:

Jeffrey: Twenty out of 26 fractures shown. All others failures, mostly femurs, sutured and broken down with pus. One with denuded area of femur exposed will be amputated.

(continued)

E.D.C. Comment: In these deep compound fractures with shattered bones it is inconceivable that there can be adequate initial wound trimming. Therefore time must be taken for wound to separate slough. Early secondary suture not feasible. Careful aseptic dressings or saline dressings. Oral sulfonamide to prevent invasive infection presuture intramuscular penicillin—postoperative penicillin.

Florey: Do not suture completely—leave drainage.
Ogilvie: Fractures into joints most important problem for penicillin.

E.D.C. Comment: Can get rid of gram organisms but cannot get rid of dead putrefying tissues. Two barriers to secondary suture: (1) Invasive infection stirred up by it. (2) Delayed healing produced by inclosing dead tissues permeated with bacteria—produces moist purulent "low-grade" dissolution of wound.

Also incidence of area of invasive infection due to incomplete drainage of crevices and ramifications of wound. Must be high in compound fractures. Should be controlled preoperatively.
Jeffrey: If gram-pus discharge, you have created dead space.

E.D.C. Comment: I doubt necessity of applying penicillin locally to fresh wounds at time of débridement. If excision has been complete—don't need it; if incomplete, will do no good as organisms will propagate on slough until slough separates.

Jolly: Deep dry cavity does not exist in compound fracture in forward area. Blood would wash out powder.
Jeffrey: Medium-sized soft tissue wounds average 12 weeks before return to unit.
Jolly: The large soft tissue wound gets lost in base hospitals—neither Zone of Interior nor quick return to duty. Increased return to duty time. Gets passed back—loses benefits of continuity of treatment.
Jeffrey: Estimates with suture return to unit in six weeks.

E.D.C. Comment: Difficulties in base hospital giving q. 3 hours. Intramuscular injection painful varying with batch. Wasteful—needs special man.

Intravenous—100,000 units a day with 4 pints saline given with drip. Vein lasts two days. Thrombosis. Two of three samples pyogenic, to alarming degree. Temperature 105° but patients not very ill. When taken off intravenous and on intramuscular, no trouble. In dilute form must be continuous. 15,000 q. 4 hours intramuscular dosage.

SOME DIARY JOTTINGS OF STUDY

After returning to Algiers to clear up some paperwork, notes from Ian Fraser arrived. His series with local application of penicillin powder diluted with sulfanilamide powder (not sulfathiazole) in Sicily showed on return to base 85 per cent negative swab cultures at first dressing.

The series of 200 cases referred to by Scott Thomson are not true controls as they were not handled with same care in respect to no dressings en route after passing through other hospitals. Also may have included some undébrided cases. Control on cases badly needed.

An ideal study would be:

1. Débridement—sulfanilamide frosting.
2. Débridement—penicillin frosting.
3. Débridement—no frosting of any type.

Initial field culture—no touch transport—initial base culture.

1. Will initial systemic injection at time of débridement aid in getting wound to base with less gram and contamination?
2. Will pre- and postoperative dosage at base permit greater freedom in closure and platings of compound fracture? Complications most likely to come from gram and changes with transport to Z.I.
   a. Secondary infection—polybacterial.
   b. General decline in nutritional state.
   c. Local tissue changes that take place with weeks of infection, splinting, etc.

Mary A. Decoteau, Rosemary A. Kozar, and Lewis J. Kaplan

Churchill's chapter exploring the use of penicillin in Tripoli defined key issues that resonate with modern surgical care including: 1) the need for source control, 2) the synergy among debridement, altered host defense, and adjunctive antibiotic therapy, and 3) the key role of focused inquiries to answer clinically relevant questions. Each of these topics represents a domain of practice or inquiry of great relevance to patient care today. Mention of Tripoli in the title refers to a conference held in Tripoli shortly after the invasion of Sicily rather than the use of antibiotic therapy in Tripoli, per se. Refreshingly, Churchill's writing reflects a candid recounting of his observations and impressions unconstrained by any specific style required by peer-reviewed journals.

Source control of infected or devitalized tissue in wounds benefits from antibiotics to aid in reduction of bacterial bioburden that cannot be accomplished with surgery alone. Churchill's notions of limited antibiotic exposure falls just short of the current STOP-IT trial with 4 days of therapy after source control for intra-abdominal sepsis, but hews to the principles of antibiotic stewardship that had yet to be articulated in the early 1940s. An algorithmic approach to topical application of penicillin is logically presented as is the well-preserved technique of secondary closure of contaminated wounds.

The notion that scientific inquiry should be a carefully considered process is rendered in high relief during Churchill's musings about Florey and the potential pitfalls of his planned investigations into the appropriate use of penicillin. At that time, penicillin was available as a topical powder, an intramuscular injectable, and in intravenous (IV) form, albeit the latter appeared to induce fevers. The difficulties of obtaining effective antibiotic concentration at the site of fractures, including intra-articular fractures, marked a point of embarkation in local and systemic therapy. Modern approaches include antibiotic beads, antibiotic spacers, and antibiotic nails that help truncate the duration of IV antibiotic therapy but provide high local concentrations in areas that are difficult to debride.

Finally, that intervention efficacy must be measured against a control population is readily articulated as Churchill discusses combination therapy of penicillin and sulfanilamide. Appropriately, he outlines each "arm" of a suitably designed study. We continue to struggle with therapeutic interventions judged against historic controls instead of a concomitantly accrued control group. In characteristic fashion, at the end of the chapter, Churchill outlines a series of inquiries designed to improve combatant care in the particular while advancing the science of surgery and medicine in general. That the new knowledge discovery garnered from battlefield injured soldiers will translate to civilian care undoubtedly underpins Churchill's thoughts. We continue to leverage military discovery in caring for injured civilians using databases like the Department of Defense Trauma Registry to inform key aspects of care including hemorrhage control, resuscitation, wound management, and aeromedical evacuation.

SUGGESTED READINGS

Lax E. *The Mold in Dr. Florey's Coat: The Story of the Penicillin Miracle*. Henry Holt and Company; 2005.

Sawyer RG, Claridge JA, Nathens AB, et al. Trial of short-course antimicrobial therapy for intraabdominal infection. *N Engl J Med*. 2015 May 21;372(21):1996–2005.

Tarchini G, Liau KH, Solomkin JS. Antimicrobial stewardship in surgery: challenges and opportunities. *Clin Infect Dis*. 2017 May 15;64(suppl_2):S112–S114.

Van Vugt TA, Arts JJ, Geurts JA. Antibiotic-loaded polymethylmethacrylate beads and spacers in treatment of orthopedic infections and the role of biofilm formation. *Front Microbiol*. 2019 Jul 25;10:1626.

21

To Cairo

On August 26, 1943, Howard Naffziger and I left Castel Benito for Cairo at 7:30 A.M. and arrived at 2:15 at Heliopolis airport. The flight was monotonous, with desert extending to the level horizon on our right and usually the sea a pale blue horizon on the left. At times when we were out over the water, the desert appeared as a layer of cloud above the blue of the sea. The sharp edge of the green and cultivated Nile valley was a welcome sight and, with a glimpse of the pyramids in the distance, we crossed the Nile to the airport.

We went to pay our respects to the British Director of Medical Services in the Middle East, Major General Hartgill. Formerly Deputy Surgeon at the War Office, he had arrived in Cairo in May and had hardly caught up with problems of 10,000 beds over a wide area. While at his office I arranged a visit to the Scottish 15th General Hospital the following morning.

After our respects were duly paid, we went to our hotel for a very good dinner and had the best piece of steak since leaving the States. Then we did some window-shopping. The stores were a strange contrast to North Africa. All shop windows were full of things and bibelots like Atlantic City. Of course, we ended at the famed Shepheard's Hotel for a lime juice, it being quite too hot for anything stronger.

Cairo was, indeed, hot and humid. We were too far from the sea to get the breeze that made the balcony of the Grand Hotel in Tripoli so pleasant.

In the evening, we went to the Base Transfusion Unit No. 1. Everyone spoke of the admirable work of Lieutenant Colonel Buttle as contributing more to excellence of surgery in the Middle East (M.E.) than any other single individual. The unit had been built up with very little help from England. Reclaimed beer bottles were converted to containers for plasma, blood and saline. Simple, insulated boxes with ice were used for two day transportation of blood. There were two electric stills.

We then went to the 38th General Hospital (the Jefferson Unit). It was located eight miles out in the desert and was free of flies and mosquitoes.

Some visitors criticized placing this 5,000-bed hospital that far from communications, but the wisdom of this was obvious after seeing Cairo. Personnel rarely went to the city. They were content with the amusements and life where they were. Consequently, they had low diarrhea and venereal disease rates.

We were impressed by the good spirit of the group and excellent mess. Both Naffziger and I gave short talks. Then we were asked to go to the wards and see cases. One swelling of the thigh I considered neoplastic rather than vascular. Naffziger examined neurosurgical problems.

On August 29, I went to the Red Cross and found a Red Cross worker I knew—Charlotte Rantoul (Mrs. Charlotte Bonner). She had arrived there several weeks ago. I also met Mr. Banes, Director of the Red Cross in the Middle East, and then Charlotte took us shopping at E. Hatoun's, said to be the only one-price store in the Middle East. There were many interesting things, particularly old jewelry, reproductions of early Egyptian jewelry and Persian miniatures. I finally bought two brocaded capes and a few Egyptian cloth hangings to send home. I also bought some things for my sons—an ivory elephant for Fred, a very decorative, wooden camel for Pete, and a whole caravan of camels for Jerry. Mother and daughter, I thought, can don the capes if they don't appear at the same time.

Then I visited the M.E. Surgeon's office and looked over their vital statistics. A rate per 1,000 per annum still fails to register graphically in my mind. The Persian Gulf seemed to be the sore spot in everything.

CHEST CASES

After the M.E. Surgeon's office, I went to the British 9th General Hospital to see Major Logan's group of chest cases. Apparently there was another type of pneumatocele—traumatic, as some of these wounds left a large defect unassociated with the separation of sepsis. "They cross fissures indiscriminately," my notes read, "and present a nice problem in local resection." Logan had tried muscle implantation and thoracoplasty without success. There was an interesting case with fracture of costochondral junctures on left side and depression of sternum in which the F.S.U. surgeon did an open reduction after attempting traction—with excellent result. Strangely enough, the patient showed left lower lobe bronchiectasis of saccular variety that I felt must have been antecedent to the injury.

I then went on to the British 63rd General Hospital with Colonel Boyd, who had been collecting cases of peripheral vascular injury. "He has done," my notes read, "11 popliteal ligations (not acute injuries but for aneurysm) without gangrene. He does not believe in vein ligation concomitant, even with acute occlusion—always precedes when feasible with surgical interruption sympathetic chain or stellate ganglion." Some case histories follow:

Case 1: Aneurysm 2nd portion left axillary with stellate ganglionectomy 2 weeks before.

Still finds surgeons applying electric lamp cradles to limbs; believes in novocain block, keeping limb lower than the heart and at room temperature. In R.A.M.C. doubts ability of forward surgeons to do surgical interruption of sympathetics. Possibly surgery of the lumbar and novocain of the stellate is the answer for us.

Case 2: Common femoral aneurysm treated by lumbar resection and ligation of external iliac in one stage.

Has had 6 true causalgias—4 median, 2 sciatic treated successfully by sympathectomy.

Naffziger reports English work for painful amputation stumps of fingers; dissect digital nerve to level of carpal ligament, also liberal resection of digital arteries.

Causalgia relieved by cold; burning pain; shiny skin.

Case 3: First portion of left axillary aneurysm in Italian P.O.W. Stellate— div. clavicle, temporary ligature of subclavian, excision of artery.

Ligation of brachial artery while not productive of gangrene may in a few weeks be followed by mild Volkmann-like paralysis of arm. Precedes by sympathectomy. Segregation of cases in M.E. hospitals is surprising considering Ogilvie's writings on specialization in war surgery.

On August 29, Naffziger and I started driving across the desert to Suez, the desert through which Joseph came to Egypt, and which was later traversed by his many brothers. This is also the area in which Larrey followed Napoleon in his unsuccessful Egyptian campaign—recording in his memoirs a great many interesting observations.

The Gulf of Suez tapers into the canal, perhaps the most important ribbon of water in the world. We followed its left bank upwards through Ismailia to Port Said. On a Sunday afternoon this city was very quiet and there was no iniquity to be seen.

A large part of our drive back from Port Said to Cairo was along the bank of an irrigation canal. This was teeming with life: the large barges with triangular sails and unbelievably long booms and masts—camels—irrigation pumps—crude wooden wheels turned by cows to pump water into lateral canals—date palms with fruit just beginning to turn a purple bronze—and everywhere George the Wog busy with his affairs.

In the evening Naffziger and I were called to meet the Commanding General of the New Zealand forces in the Middle East. There we also met Wilder Penfield and went back to Shepheard's with him. We picked his brains about what he had seen during a trip to Moscow and the Far East, but there was seemingly nothing that could be translated into surgical procedure on our front. We were interested in the advanced echelon surgical specialization described in Russia and the separation of the lightly wounded from the seriously wounded, but I was not clear just how significant this was. Wilder described the work of Lena Stern, injecting potassium and calcium into the cisterna for shock—"traumatic shock." He also commented on the poor quality of certain nerve grafting procedures.

A TOURIST

The following day, August 30, the Red Cross arranged a trip for us, starting in El Mosky. I had lunch at El Mena House with Donald MacKenzie, of the Scottish 15th General Hospital, and Charlotte Rantoul and Naffziger. We then "reviewed" the pyramids and Sphinx in authentic tourist style—on camel back (**Figure 21.1**). In Cairo I saw the large mosque of Mohammed Ali in the Citadel. The view of Cairo from there was wide both in time and space, embracing ancient Egypt and the modern city.

Driving down from the Citadel through the so-called "Tombs of Khalifes" or "Dead City," I stopped at the tombs of the Royal Family, elaborately laid out in true Islamic style, which means leaving no surface without intricate ornamentation. The simplicity of the Greek—fortunately perpetuated in our taste, except for aberrations—as those that took place during the Victorian period—has much to recommend it.

I had dinner at Shepheard's with Naffziger, Penfield, MacKenzie and Cowdry, and discussed specialization in war surgery.

E.D.C. Comment: "MacKenzie, who ran F.S.C. for some months," I recorded later, "is all for having only the broadly trained surgeon with sound judgment in the forward area. Problems are those of resuscitation and general management rather than specialized technics. This is true, but where do these men exist?"

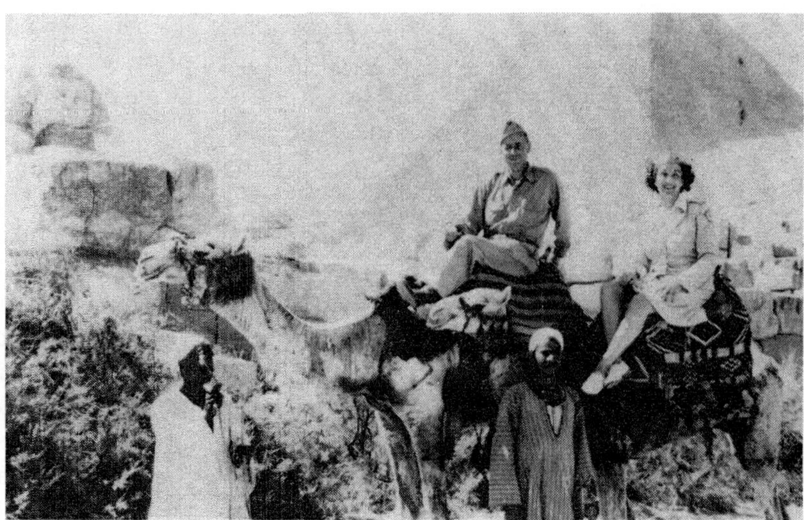

Figure 21.1 Mrs Charlotte Rantoul Bonner and the author as "tourists."

It is much easier to lay hands on five specialists than on one individual who can soundly practice the fundamentals of five specialties.

Douglas H. Anderson, John C. Mayberry, and Kenji Inaba

In the last chapter of "Part 3," Dr Churchill travels from the conference in Tripoli, as described in the previous chapter, to Cairo, along with reputed neurosurgeon Howard Naffziger. Notably, this trip occurred on the same day as the publication of the now infamous *New York Times* article calling for whole blood. Their fast-paced tour takes them across five different military hospitals in the region, where Churchill seamlessly weaves their personal and professional encounters. Almost as an aside, he briefly touches upon the challenges of blood procurement and distribution in the forward environment, illustrating innovative adaptations such as the use of "reclaimed beer bottles" for storing "plasma, blood, and saline."

The main focus of this chapter is on clinical cases relating to the injuries of the chest and extremities. The first case discusses a large traumatic pneumatocele (pulmonary pseudocyst), a recently defined phenomenon at the time. Although the cause of pneumatocele—whether penetrating or blunt trauma—is not mentioned, Dr Churchill later states in Appendix B, Wounds of the Thorax (page 442), that these pneumatoceles "develop in the course of the missile tract." The surgeon encountered difficulties in attempting to manage the large pleural space defect after resection, which appeared to be complicated by empyema or a bronchopleural fistula, subsequently requiring muscle implantation and thoracoplasty. With plain radiographs alone, pneumatoceles would have been difficult to diagnose, potentially leading to confusion with more common problems such as pneumothorax or lung abscess. The current management of pneumatocele is primarily observation, since most resolve on their own. One should exercise caution when placing a thoracostomy tube or attempt surgical resection, as these actions can cause infection into an otherwise sterile space or lead to the formation of a bronchopleural fistula, as likely occurred in the described case.

Churchill also describes the case of a patient with a depressed sternal fracture and costochondral junction fractures that failed "traction" but were successfully treated with open reduction—an interesting consideration for both modern military and civilian surgeons. He then describes cases involving both upper and lower extremity "vascular injuries," primarily nonacute peripheral arterial aneurysms, as well as cases of "causalgia," better known today as complex regional pain syndrome. The aneurysms were all managed with arterial ligation without reconstruction, preceded by sympathectomy.

These all had acceptable results without "gangrene" or the need for amputation, although universal ligation of arterial injuries was later challenged in Korea and Vietnam. The causalgia cases were treated successfully with sympathectomy alone. Before the development of contemporary arterial reconstruction, sympathectomy was the primary treatment for non-revascularizable arterial occlusive disease and vasospastic disorders. By disrupting sympathetic tone, sympathectomy promotes subsequent vasodilation and arteriovenous shunting in cutaneous capillary beds. Sympathectomy is still performed today for a variety of indications in a minimally invasive fashion, through either an anesthetic block or alcohol and radiofrequency ablation.

The chapter concludes with a discussion on "specialization in war surgery," a topic previously introduced in **Chapter 18: Preparation for Sicily—Operation Husky**. One surgeon advocates "for having only the broadly trained surgeon with sound judgement in the forward area." Churchill agrees but remarks that, "It is much easier to lay hands on five specialists than on one individual who can soundly practice the fundamentals of five specialties." This challenging paradox persists nearly 80 years later, a paradox mitigated by ensuring a solid foundation of comprehensive, broad-based training for modern military surgeons.

SUGGESTED READINGS

Barr J, Cherry KJ, Rich NM. Vascular surgery in World War II: the shift to repairing arteries. *Ann Surg.* 2016;263(3):615–620.

Karanth VK, Karanth TK, Karanth L. Lumbar sympathectomy techniques for critical lower limb ischaemia due to non-reconstructable peripheral arterial disease. *Cochrane Database Syst Rev.* 2016 Dec 13;12(12):CD011519.

Kuckelman J, Cuadrado D, Martin M. Thoracic trauma: a combat and military perspective. *Curr Trauma Rep.* 2018;4:77–87.

Phillips B, Shaw J, Turco L, et al. Traumatic pulmonary pseudocyst: an underreported entity. *Injury.* 2017 Feb;48(2):214-220.

Santos GH, Mahendra T. Traumatic pulmonary pseudocysts. *Ann Thorac Surg.* 1979 Apr;27(4): 359-362.

PART FOUR

Italy

22

My First Visit to Naples

THE LANDING in Salerno Bay (Operation Avalanche) took place on September 9, 1943. Naples was taken on October 1 and the Volturno crossed at Capua the same day. I remained in North Africa through September and most of October. Toward the end of October I visited the Fifth Army in Italy. Before leaving A.F.H.Q. in Algiers I made the following check list:

1. Selective hospitalization.
2. Blood Transfusion. Make delivery truck.
3. Placement of specialized surgical teams.
4. Movement of 2nd Auxiliary Group Headquarters.
5. Early closure of wounds.
6. Put penicillin under control of Gas Gangrene Committee—Jergeson and Simeone.
7. Serum albumin.
8. Anesthesia and shock.
9. Nutrition.
10. Requisition medical arts and photography unit from Washington.

Italy was the promised land after the deserts of North Africa and the scorching summer weeks in Sicily. The grapes were hanging in clusters in the vineyards and apples were plentiful in the orchards.

ITALY BY DIARY

These are excerpts from my notes of the trip:

October 21, 1943
I was up early with Fred Hanson but we did not get off until 0940 and did not put down at Tunis until 1210 hrs. Having had no breakfast, I found a quick C-ration lunch, taking off from Elowina at 1330 hrs. In Catania at 1525, I found no plane to Naples until the next day and stayed at the Transient Officers Hotel. On the flight over I met Major William

(continued)

Scully of Cambridge, Mass. Back in Gafsa when he was a patient in the 48th Surgical, Norman Wylie had me award the Purple Heart to Scully. He has recovered from his chest wall wound but still has two bits of mortar shell in him.

Catania was badly shot up. I visited the cathedral that was rebuilt after the eruption of Etna in 1916. There are still traces of the old arches in lava blocks. The inhabitants seem to be pulling themselves together with a bad hangover. These bourgeoise are not as friendly and joyful as the Sicilian peasants during the campaign. They seem surly and distinctly unfriendly. The Cathedral San Agata has fine old choir stalls carved with her life history; fortunately this cathedral was not damaged although other churches were.

For supper we went to a small restaurant where we had a morsel of steak and two plates of sardines—pickled and then fried. After the sardine supper, Fred Hanson and I persuaded an M.P. to drive out to the 5th Canadian General Hospital. At the officer's mess we dropped in on a game of penny ante. The C.O. was not particularly cordial, but unburdened a bit about having no liaison with the U.S.A. medical service about the treatment and disposition of U.S.A. patients. With a rather cool reception all around, Fred and I cleared out. At the hotel we made inquiries about the Air Force Surgeon in Catania and happened to meet the C.O. of the detachment. We told him about the feelings of the Canadian group, and he said he would try to correct the situation. Obviously, the A.F. Dispensary has not been cooperative in setting up friendly relations—it just dumps its patients there for Kahn tests and dark fields.

October 22

I had a scanty breakfast at a mess. The seasoning of sausages for Army rations is of interest. Both the Vienna sausage and the plump skin sausage that are always served boiled have peculiar and unpleasant seasoning. Very few like it. It is hard to see why frankfurters or country sausage have not been supplied. Both have stood the test of time as palatable to Americans.

There was a long argument in the next room last night touching upon fundamental interallied relations. How should a drunken British Tommy be treated when he called Americans sons of bitches? Why has AMGOT been so lenient with the civilian population? Did U.S.A. bombs or British naval shells wreck the city?

This morning I stopped at a bookshop. An old man and a girl were sorting books and putting them on the empty shelves. The man explained how ruinous American bombing had been. I picked up an Italian book entitled *Skies of Ethiopia* and showed him a picture of an Italian bomber over Addis Ababa, trying to explain that at that time America had no bombers, and that the Italians appeared to have had a good many. Then he started to berate the Germans.

Leaving Catania at 1100 hrs., we landed in Naples at about 1300 hrs. and went to Fifth Army Headquarters, then to the 95th Evacuation Hospital. I found the C.O., Lt. Col. Sauer, Howard Patterson and Larry Poole who were here on a trip.

Howard Patterson's notes of the 95th's landing at Naples provide a clear picture of the difficulties of a hospital accompanying an amphibious assault.

Red Beach was the only possible landing place; on other beaches the chance of survival was slim. Equipment was landed rapidly and mixed with other types in a "Miscellaneous Dump." The equipment of the 95th was assembled so far as possible, but surgical instruments did not arrive, or could not be found for several days. A platoon of the 162nd Medical Battalion joined with the 95th, setting up five tents which were used as a surgery for less serious cases. The 95th admitted 495 casualties on the first day. Many were kept in the open air.

Surgical teams were used a great deal. They were picked up from a Clearing Platoon supposed to be set up on the beach. Palmer had told them not to be fancy— to bring a first-aid kit, extra dressings, a pocketknife and two curved clamps. They landed at Yellow Beach and went to the Clearing Station which soon became a Graves Registration Depot. Bodies were gathered and brought there so they wouldn't be run over by jeeps and trucks. The beaches were under fire and in all ways a shambles— no surgery possible. The 95th had been working two days when some Auxiliary Group surgeons blew in and said they had been assigned to help. Shorbe, Poole, Capt. Lowry and Sydoriac, all were able and needed. (See **Figure 22.1**.)

On D + 6 the 95th borrowed six nurses from the 93rd. The faces of the patients had not been washed; their shoes not taken off. The enlisted men had not slept for several days. Poole feels that the thing that they did worst was keeping records, and that this was because of lack of time.

J——— was responsible for making the arrangements to set up the 95th in the hospital it occupied. The British were already here and wouldn't let them in. Apparently a lot of argument went on and J——— would do nothing about it. The 95th equipment was dumped on the ground in the rain. Some was ruined. The executive officer was sick; the detachment commander and the transport officer were laid up with injuries so Baxter and Larry Poole took over, Sydoriac being an excellent contact man. Poole hired 36 civilians to clean up, arrange the supplies, allocated space, and set up the equipment.

Surgery was handicapped by the lack of positive pressure anesthesia apparatus. They had tried desperately to get a machine in Oran where there were several in the Supply Depot but they were turned down by 5th Army and are now borrowing from the British.

(continued)

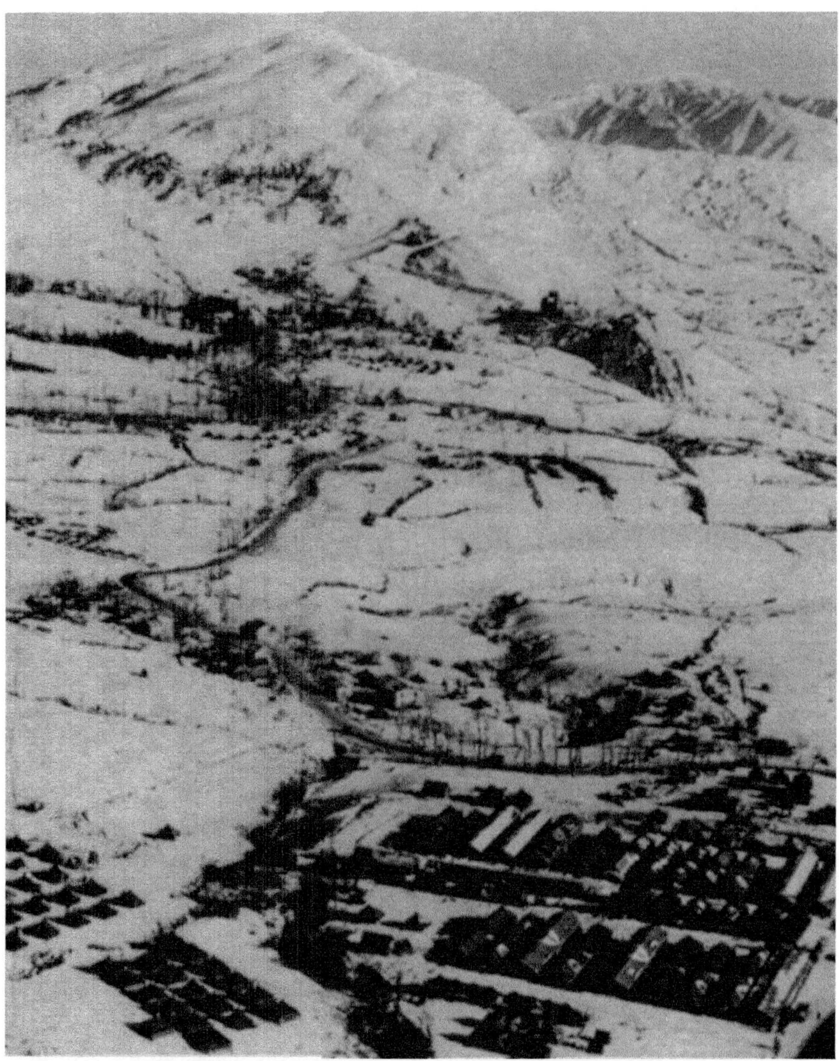

Figure 22.1 The 8th Evacuation Hospital at Pietramala, Italy.

Later I discussed wounds of cecum and right colon with Howard Patterson with reference to a patient seen by Poole at the 3rd General Hospital. Poole also recalls the case of R.Z. Pfc. on 17 April evacuated by plane from the 9th Evac. 10 days after operation. Also a patient now in 95th in whom a Lahey type exteriorization was done. A rifle bullet deformed by passing through the seat of a jeep entered the right flank, badly damaging cecum so as to require its resection. In these cases would it not be better to separate the ileostomy from the stump of the colon, forming the ileostomy through a stab incision near the midline? The difficulty seems to lie in infection from inoculating the belly wall with feces at the time of operation. This is further augmented by the ileostomy.[1]

October 23

It is taking 6,800 tons daily to supply Army. The port of Naples is difficult to recondition because underwater demolition is being held up by unloading ships. The reserve of essential supplies—ammunition, food, etc.—is sufficient for three to seven days. Still landing over beaches. This information was passed along to surgeons who were frustrated and at times resentful because they lacked some special piece of equipment for the care of the wounded.

At Fifth Army Headquarters, Col. Martin (Fifth Army Surgeon) was concerned about gas gangrene and Howard Snyder is looking into the subject. Army is trying to maintain a 30 day holding policy for sick and wounded. It is thought that if Army can maintain this policy in mobile hospitals then a base of 15,000 fixed beds would be sufficient to maintain 120 day policy in Italy and evacuate directly to the Z.I.

Returning to the 95th Evac, watched a brisk air raid with many bombs dropped in the harbor and dock area. There was an extensive use of flares, a technique rarely used in Algiers. After the raid a few casualties were brought into the surgical service. One with a wound of the left costal margin that tore the colon in two places. Resection of the splenic flexure was required and the colostomy openings were placed some distance apart. Nephrectomy was required for a shattered left kidney. Another interesting flak wound entered the left deltoid region and coursing down along the spine produced a physiologic transection of the spinal cord. Profound shock—a good deal of blood loss into deep structures of the back. There was complete loss of superficial and deep sensation as well as muscular action. Absent reflexes except normal plantar reflex on the right. Muscle tremors—a great deal like a pithed frog.

(continued)

---

[1] The following extract from a letter written by Howard Patterson on December 13, 1943, refers to the outcome of our conversation: "For the past twelve days we have had plenty of work with a large proportion of 'big' cases, including many abdominal cases. I had one right hemicolectomy in which I followed your advice and brought the ileum and transverse colon stumps out through separate incisions. This is his ninth postoperative day, he is eating well, his condition is highly satisfactory, and his main wound has remained clean thus far."

Here's another interesting case:

R.E.P. 101st Tank Destroyer. 3rd Division. Age 24. G.S.W. left thigh accidentally incurred when he discharged his pistol at 0030 hrs. October 5, 1943, injuring his left femoral artery. The severed artery and vein were ligated and a foreign body removed at 2000 hrs. at 93rd Evac. The leg was pulseless, cold and remained so. A lumbar sympathetic block was done on two occasions, 5 October. When admitted here on 12 October he was seriously ill, dehydrated and confused. There was a 3 inch infected wound over the femoral artery just below the inguinal ligament. The entire left leg and foot were swollen. The thigh was warm but the leg and foot were hard and cold. He was given I.V. fluids and a 500 cc. blood transfusion on 13, 15 and 18 October. Following this treatment he was no longer confused. The discoloration of leg and foot became more pronounced. Amputation was delayed to allow the infection in the thigh to subside but finally had to be performed because of gas in the tissues over the calf. Low thigh amputation was done under sodium pentothal anesthesia. Skin traction was applied immediately and has been maintained. Postoperative course was uneventful. The granulation tissue is clean. Sulfadiazine therapy. Organism: *Clostridium fallax.*

October 24

The man with the cord injury recovered from his shock but is still paralyzed. The Lt. Col. shot a few nights ago with bad wounds of cecum near ileocecal valve and ascending colon on whom Patterson did a Lahey type of placement after resection of right colon looks better. A badly infected shoulder wound in a P.O.W. probably has intermittent leakage from the right subclavian artery. Talked to surgical staff.

At Fifth Army headquarters after dinner, I talked with Bruce about professional organization and suggested bringing II Auxiliary Group Headquarters over to Italy. At British 92nd on invitation of Col. C. J. Callan-Jones, I outlined our policies on management of chest injuries. Col. C-J. has had two years' experience on Malta and a period on Suez Canal before coming to Italy. There was no gas gangrene on Malta. Casualties there were from bomb fragments and flak. Bomb fragments caused extensive pulping of muscles but all were treated within six hours. He prefers to wait nine days before aspirating blood from the chest because of the danger of reactivating hemorrhage and has found air replacement ineffective. Possibility that plasma exudation into pleura following aspiration increases the deposition of fibrin. Snyder believes blood acts as foreign body and after three days in itself produces exudation.

Back to 95th Evac., I chatted with Patterson about the following case:
J.C.A. Private. 468th Q.M. Shot through upper part of left thigh. Extensive hemorrhage chiefly external. Exploration under ether showed complete division of femoral artery just at point of origin of the profunda femoris. Also laceration of veins. Very badly bled out and was pulseless and without obtainable blood pressure. Plasma replenishment was vigorous but blood replacement slow. This man died during the night. Here is another instance of death from slow and inadequate blood replacement. The man was conscious and shock was not "irreversible" when he was admitted. The bleeding was controlled surgically. 2,500 cc. of whole blood administered rapidly might not have saved his life but would have been the best and only safeguard against the loss of his leg had he survived.

October 25

I rode to 38th Evac. with Capt. Ashworth of 1st Armored Division and had a long bull session in evening on cast splitting, débridement, and exteriorization of large bowel.

October 26

I took a time-lag census on 50 wounded to compare with series of gas gangrene cases. Lever and Wasden blew in after dinner. The 15th Evac has just come up from Sicily in a convoy of "ducks." Cato Drash and Blackford (Chiefs of Surgery and Medicine of 8th Evac.) came over to see me about some bad news (trouble with their C.O.). Drash is tense about the situation. He must have relief. The C.O. asked to meet all surgical captains and lieutenants. Drash was not informed of the meeting and did not go. The C.O. asked for 5 volunteers for *temporary* detached duty at clearing stations. As the 8th Evac. was not functioning, *ALL* volunteered. The 5 were selected by the C.O. without consulting his chief surgeon and turned in to Fifth Army. They were not called for temporary duty and a week ago 4 of the 5 were *assigned* to forward areas. Four replacements were sent but without surgical training.

Joe Martin plans to assign one Medical Battalion and a Field Hospital to Corps. Everything else will be under Fifth Army.

(continued)

October 27

At 94th Evac. I made rounds. Slightly wounded cases have been nearly all evacuated. I was particularly interested in a series of abdominal incisions—many were transverse, about one inch above the umbilicus. Nearly all abdominal incisions show infection, caused in part by meticulous closure of the skin. The pulley stitch used by Howard Patterson has been adopted by many in the 94th Evac. I believe it produces too much tissue strangulation to be advisable in heavily contaminated abdominal incisions for large bowel perforations. One answer to the infected laparotomy incisions is certainly to be found in avoiding suture of the skin. I talked at length about gas gangrene which is being found with increasing frequency and spent the night at the 94th.

October 28

Quite a crowd gathered for a conference on gas gangrene. Jergeson presented the material from the 94th. Lyman Brewer then presented his chest cases—an excellent record, and Charlie Dowman gave a synopsis of head wounds—the results were not so good. McClennan dropped by for a short talk. He is now with Eighth Army.

Back to Fifth Army Headquarters I had a talk with Martin. He was very receptive with what we want to do with a surgical program; *viz.*, use Jergeson and Simeone for survey of gas gangrene and vascular injuries; Beecher and Lalich for evaluation of shock and anesthesia, and in a short time, John Stewart for nutritional and metabolic studies. Also, Martin wants Howard Snyder for Army Consultant.

October 29

I picked up Jergy at the 94th Evac. to start him collecting data on gas gangrene and went into Naples to the 2nd Medical Laboratory to show them the meat broth bottle used by McClellan for cultures of anaerobes. Then I looked about for Fifth Army Base Headquarters and ran into Shefts and some of his team down from the front where they are attached to the 33rd Field Hospital. This is a new outfit and Snyder is now up there looking it over. Shefts wants an anesthesia machine badly. It is hard to understand why we should have had so much difficulty with the supply of anesthesia machines. They have been at a premium during the whole North African campaign.

I stopped at the 118th Station Hospital in an Italian military hospital where Col. Huntington commands. It was a rambling, dirty old building but now appears satisfactory. In the operating room an inguinal hernia was being repaired. I couldn't help thinking of the GI who appeared for prophylaxis 15 minutes after the landing at Oran. Here we are in Naples a couple of weeks after evacuation by the Germans and already repairing inguinal hernias!

Up at the 95th Evac. I had a bull session with Shorbe, Lowry, Jr. and Poole. They seem optimistic about the end of the war and say that German P.O.W.'s have a greatly different attitude than they showed in Tunisia. Now all admit they are licked and want to end the war quickly. This hardly checks with the fact that four fresh German divisions are being moved into line. Speculation on the end of the war is something indulged in rarely. I should reckon as follows: By early spring (March 1944) the Allied Force in Italy will be at the line dividing the peninsula from northern Italy—approximately Pisa-Rimini. In the interval we shall have assembled a large force in England with a great deal of publicity and propaganda. The Russians will start a spring offensive in the south. This theater will start either toward southern France or the Balkans or both and then the *coup de grace* will be delivered across channel. Germany should fold up about the middle of July.[2]

October 30
At Fifth Army Base Section I met Lt. Col. Jeffers at the fairground which is being taken over as a hospital center. This is an amazing place, a rundown and badly bombed "world of tomorrow" without the trylon and perisphere (New York City 1938-9). The fairgrounds in Pozzuoli were approached from Naples through a long tunnel used as an air raid shelter by the local inhabitants. Posillipo is a long promontory separating the Bay of Pozzuoli from the Bay of Naples. A road through a long tunnel beneath the ridge of Posillipo runs from Mergellina to Posillipo and the fairgrounds were located shortly after the end of the tunnel.

This entire region is of volcanic origin and sulphur-charged steam emerges from apertures in the ground. Close to Pozzuoli is the ancient doorway to Hell pictured in old prints as a water-filled crater—Lago d'Averno—which emitted such poisonous gases that birds flying over it

(*continued*)

______

[2]As an amateur strategist I missed by a year.

were overcome and fell into its depths. Other prints show visitors tying a dog to the end of a stick and exposing it to poisonous gas, then pulling the dog out and resuscitating it by dunking in the lake. The river Styx emerges from the ground as a spring where Aeneas made his descent into Hades guided by the Cumaean Sibyl.

The 182nd Station Hospital has set up in two buildings; Major Harry Jenkins in command and doing a swell job. The mess hall is a terraced restaurant overlooking a swimming pool. Two bombs came through the roof in a recent air raid but both were duds. One could be pulled out for demolition but the engineers thought the other had best be detonated *in situ*. Jenkins objected so strenuously that they tried a trick I have never heard of—set off dynamite around the bomb to split the casing, then spooned out the nitroglycerine and removed the cap. Apparently it worked!

Major Kenwall of Buffalo is Chief Surgeon. Making rounds with him we discussed a few problems, particularly delayed closure of wounds which I want to get started actively in this new base. One of the medical officers running to get to his ward during the air raid a few nights ago received a small bit of H.E. in his abdomen that perforated the cecum. Operated on within an hour and closed primarily. With pea-sized fragment and early operation this appears correct policy; not with large fragments and long time-lag, however.

Major Harwell Wilson, one of Phemister's former residents, is now Chief Surgeon of 225th Station Hospital that is moving into the fairgrounds. He was with us on rounds. This (225th S.H.) is an unusually good outfit with the Hughes twins from Memphis as C.O. and Executive Officer. They want to take on some special work rather than routine and this obviously is the hospital for special problems if we can set it up. Their interest is in burns and plastic surgery problems. If we can get penicillin and start plating and closing compound fractures, the cases could be segregated here at least for a time.

I spent the evening with the C.O. and the Chief Surgeon of the 11th General Hospital, the Harper Hospital Unit moving into the building now occupied by the 95th Evac. Their equipment has not yet arrived. When the 23rd General Hospital came in a couple of days ago, they lined up their detachment on the beach on a land mine. Several casualties resulted. The shrapnel balls of these mines penetrate rather deeply but do not cause much muscle damage because of their low velocity. I saw several of these wounds today.

October 31

The rotor was gone from Jergy's jeep this morning but after a short delay he got a replacement. At Caserta I met with Snyder and Hanson and had another talk with Col. Joe Martin about the problems posed by rotating officers between hospitals and field. I pointed out the danger of selection by C.O.'s who ignored needs of their professional staffs and was able to cite examples from two evacs. where officers with specialized surgical training had been moved to a battalion and replaced by officers with but one year of rotating internship. Martin urges NATOUSA Headquarters advanced echelon or U.S. representation in Medical Section of Allied Force advanced echelon. He feels that our cousins (British) are taking up what they want in the usual way. This recurring difficulty is by no means one-sided. We seem to remain isolationists and "inferiorists" sullenly wanting our own show. If we had brisk, capable officers to work alongside of the British we could hold our own. This is no affair for amateur diplomacy!

I finished my report on gas gangrene and turned it in to Fifth Army Headquarters. (See Chapter 23, Gas Gangrene.) Harry Beecher has been sent for. Jergy has been replaced by Shorbe and Lyman Brewer will take over Jergy's team. Remainder of teams and 11 Auxiliary Group Headquarters have been requested. I hope they will leave Paul Sampson at the 24th General Hospital to carry on the chest center as I requested.

On the top floor of the palace at Caserta is a large Italian aviation school. Many plane motors, wind tunnels, even a large bomber fuselage with wing tips removed are set up for demonstration. Some neat little pressure tanks. I picked up a few students' drawings to send home.

I went to 38th Evac. Halloween celebration. Paul Sanger had arranged a concert troupe—baritone with violin, accordion and guitar. They delivered the genuine article here a few miles from Naples. O Sole Mio from Rigoletto with full lyrical quality. George Wood told the story of his southern Baptist chaplain who asked permission to baptize a patient. On questioning, George found the plan was that of a real Baptist dunking in the Volturno which was still under shellfire! If the preacher was sincere and not seeking publicity, this provided an interesting parallelism with a surgeon's undertaking an elective operation in a forward evacuation hospital—which has been done. The urge for technical expression and carrying out the ritual is irrepressible. Is baptism under these circumstances an elective or emergency procedure—granted the patient was not in extremis? Perhaps it was an

(continued)

essential step in rehabilitation. At any rate, if the patient was spiritually transportable and not subject to relapse, the baptism should be carried out at the base.

An article by Fine *et al.* in the August issue of *The Annals* announced that there is no generalized increase in capillary permeability in shock! What grounds (other than the response to amputation) ever existed for assuming there was? The great shock hoax goes marching on despite the bodies that molder in their graves.

Fred Hanson and a Britisher argue about how flies make a landing on the ceiling; simple loop or side loop. Our observation is imperfect in the dim lighting.

> "The time has come," the Walrus said,
> "To talk of many things:
> Of shoes—and ships—and sealing-wax—
> Of cabbages—and kings—
> And why the sea is boiling hot—
> And whether pigs have wings."

Do pigs have wings? No, they have flies—was my contribution to the discussion. In *vino veritas*.

November 1

I went to Naples with Fred, Snyder and Nancy Wright. Naples was being evacuated of all inhabitants so the electric current could be turned on at noon. This was a precaution against the possibility that Hitler had ordered demolition charges fired by electric current. Thousands of civilians were streaming out of the city into parks or farther into the country. The city near the waterfront was already deserted except for military police and a few squads of GI's and Tommies. We met the stream of evacuees coming up the hill as we were driving down. Raggle-taggle gypsies poured from the narrow streets of the Neapolitan slums. Some hobbling with canes, some with a crutch, blind being led. Poverty-stricken humanity en masse is not a pretty sight.

I picked up air transport tickets for tomorrow and headed out to II Corps Headquarters for dinner. Pleasant sunny afternoon in a walnut orchard. Later I went to a "smoker" at II Corps rear and primed the Chief of Staff, Col. Williams, about dry socks for combat troops. (This was a warning based on the "trench foot" cold injury of World War I.)

Excellent view of an air raid over Naples. A cheering section broke loose when a Jerry plane was caught in a searchlight beam. Night at II Corps. Heavy artillery fire at the front about 18 miles away.

November 2

I was up early to drive into the Pomegliano airport for the courier plane back to Algiers. Took off at 1005 hrs. laying a course over Naples harbor passing close to the active cone of Vesuvius on our left. Then directly over Capri which we have just now left behind. Landed at Elewina 1230 and took off at 1345 hrs. I reached Maison Blanche at 1620 hrs. in a hard rainstorm.

TWO NEW PROBLEMS

It is obvious that the long and weary months of the Italian campaign cannot be reproduced by the transcription of detailed diary notations. The entries during my first tour in Italy—October 21 to November 2—show the advance in the treatment of the wounded as a result of the experience in North Africa and Sicily. The delayed or reparative suture of wounds was well in hand although we were waiting for penicillin to be in ample supply before undertaking the plating and closure of compound battle fractures. Whole blood for transfusion was the responsibility of hospital units equipped with vacuum bottles for bleeding service troop donors and refrigerators for storage. X-ray equipment was available, and foreign bodies that might delay healing were being removed at the initial débridement. The treatment of thermal burns had been simplified and early grafting was routine. The field hospital for the wounded requiring urgent surgery, and sited at the rear boundary of the division adjacent to the clearing station, had been used in Sicily and the auxiliary group surgeons had gained valuable, if sobering, experience.

In this brief first visit to Italy, two new problems were identified, one of which was already confronting us—gas gangrene. The other was to appear with the cold and wet winter months that lay ahead. Both gas gangrene and cold injury to the extremities were destined to become major problems in a few more weeks.

23

Gas Gangrene

Edward Archibald (1872-1945), Professor of Surgery at McGill University, was a pioneer in the development of thoracic surgery. During World War II the annual meetings of the American Association for Thoracic Surgery were discontinued. At the last meeting before the United States entered the war, there were only 124 members present in Montreal. Those present were deeply stirred at the dinner by the singing of a young Canadian medical officer, particularly when he sang "There'll Always be an England."

Shortly after this meeting, Professor Archibald called on me at the M.G.H. "Churchill," he said, "lobectomy and the surgery of tuberculosis have disappeared beyond the horizon. Take me to see what you are doing for wounds and fractures." He was writing a book on military surgery. After his death in 1945 I was sent the typescript that he had compiled, and asked if I thought it should be published. My advice, based on there having been so many developments in surgery during the war, was that the typescript be placed in the archives of the Osler Library.

Professor Archibald's section on gas gangrene included the reports by MacLennan from the Middle East and set forth our knowledge concerning clostridial infections of war wounds at the outset of World War II. I would like to pay tribute to this scholarly endeavor of Professor Archibald to do "his bit" for the Allied cause when over seventy years of age and shortly before his death. An extract from his manuscript follows:

REPORT FROM

Edward Archibald (1872-1945),

on Gas Gangrene

When one surveys the history of our gradually acquired knowledge of gas gangrene one is struck with the fact that this type of infection was but little known to the general surgeon before the war of 1914-1918, and that that war, in which it was at first almost endemic in severe wounds, afforded for the first time the opportunity of intensive study both of the causal organisms and of the clinical course. The military surgeons on both sides during the fall of 1914 and most of 1915 were confronted with an avalanche of gas gangrene that astonished them and against which, as they slowly realized, the standard antiseptics of the time were helpless.

Why did they not know and expect it? Welch and Nuttall had discovered the *B. aerogenes capsulatus* in 1892. But there were good reasons. To begin with, anaerobic infection rarely complicates the injuries of civil life, and few were acquainted with it. But there were many wars even during the generation preceding 1914. But there were also, in respect to gas gangrene, great differences between the last war and previous ones. And although an occasional surgeon was doubtless acquainted with this new type of infection the military surgeons of the Balkan, the Boer, the Spanish-American, and the Russo-Japanese wars remained ignorant of it. Yet that was excusable, for gas gangrene was rare in these wars. The difference lay, first, in the predominance of clean bullet wounds over high-explosive shell wounds until 1914 reversed that proportion; and, second, in the absence of conditions of trench warfare at close quarters. Moreover the soil of the intensively manured land of France and Belgium swarming with the organisms contrasted strongly with the relative sterility of the uncultivated ground and sandy soil in South Africa, Russia, and the Balkans. All these factors in former wars tended to keep low the incidence of gas gangrene in wounds. Thus the landslide of infection in 1914-15 constituted a new experience for the surgeons of the time.

The Medical Corps, French as well as English, were not organized in August, 1914, to take care of the unexpectedly large number of casualties. The field ambulances and the casualty clearing stations had but small staffs, and were not expected to do more than apply antiseptic dressings and evacuate all wounded to general hospitals in the rear. It is not surprising, therefore, that, in August and September of 1914, in their retreat from Mons, and also during that extraordinary recovery and the advance into Flanders, both causing great difficulties in the collection and the evacuation of the wounded, the incidence of gas gangrene rose to an estimated 12 per cent of the wounded, and among the French considerably higher. Overcrowding, delay and ignorance of the dangers of delay, combined to give the anaerobes the best of opportunities to multiply and produce their fatal toxins. In a total ration strength of 220,572 in the British Expeditionary Force engaged in France and

(continued)

Flanders during the five months of 1914, there were 59,346 battle casualties treated by the medical services. The task of doing any surgery in the field ambulance or in the few casualty clearing stations, with their small staffs and equipment, was an almost impossible one, even if they had known at the time the value of early wound excision. Nevertheless in late 1914 surgeons of the casualty clearing stations, governed by surgical common sense rather than by Listerian tradition, began to lay open freely these lacerated wounds in swollen limbs which obviously needed release from tension; and the surgeons at the base soon reported that these wounds that had been given free drainage were in much better condition than the others not so treated. This confirmation of front line surgical judgment led to a more general use of early incisions and drainage. In spite of a gratifying reduction in the incidence of gas gangrene, this remained a serious problem.

So matters continued during the winter of 1914-15. But to the north of the line on our left there was the Belgian front, and at La Panne there was a Belgian "Ambulance du Front" of which the surgical chief was Depage. The French word "Ambulance" designates a hospital unit situated well forward, just outside enemy gunfire, and equipped for emergency surgery and for the holding of casualties for a reasonable period after operation. In January 1915 Depage, convinced of the necessity of doing more than the mere débridement, or laying open, of shell wounds, began to do a more extensive operation, which at the time, being quite atypical, received no formal name, but which consisted essentially in proceeding, after free incision, to the superficial excision of the whole wound interior, in the manner since recognized as the standard wound excision.

Many visitors in the spring and summer of 1915 came to LaPanne from the Medical Corps of other armies, and Depage's doctrine began to spread. Through 1915 individual surgeons in the Royal Army Medical Corps and the Canadian Army Medical Corps, that is those acting in casualty clearing stations adopted this operation of wound excision, with the approval of the Chief Consultant Surgeon to the British Expeditionary Force. By early 1916, the method was officially sanctioned and widely adopted. Arrangements were made to provide a special motor ambulance service direct from field ambulances for all severe cases requiring early treatment at a casualty clearing station. Such cases, to use Bowlby's words, "should not be kept waiting for the regular convoys." Meanwhile many of the forward area surgeons of the French Army had already in early 1915 adopted independently the same surgical rules, and Carrel was urging it as a means of securing complete access for his hypochlorite solution to all parts of the wound.

By early 1916, it became obvious that the surgical staff of the casualty clearing station was insufficient to carry out the largely increased numbers of these operations which were considered emergency in nature. While that increase occurred chiefly in the field of extremity wounds it was also due to the decision that abdominal wounds, open chest wounds and to some extent cranial wounds, should also be treated in casualty clearing stations. Consequently, not only was the number of clearing stations augmented, their equipment and bed capacity much increased, but there was also formed a large pool of mobile surgical teams to be sent to the casualty clearing stations wherever the need for help was anticipated. The offensive on the Somme in July 1916, in the words of the Official History, "gave the first opportunity of arranging for surgery on a large scale in heavy fighting." The attack was launched on the first of July and that night several of the fourteen casualty clearing stations in the Fourth Army accommodated twelve to thirteen hundred casualties each. There were on that day 14,400 men admitted into thirteen clearing stations; on the second day 13,806; and on the third day 8,793. Many hundreds of operations were performed, even when the stress was greatest, and in the four and a half months during which the Somme offensive lasted, more than 30,000 operations were carried out in the forward area of the Fourth and Fifth Armies alone. The great majority of these were débridements and excisions.

One of the immediate and striking results was a great decrease in gas gangrene infections. In fact, the incidence of gas gangrene was generally taken as the one reliable yardstick by which to measure these and other improvements in field evacuation and in forward area surgery. It is well to realize the extraordinary results that were attained by the third year of that war through early wound excision alone, not only as regards the prevention of gas gangrene but also its cure. When one reflects that at the start of the war knowledge of gas gangrene was extremely limited, forward area surgery was confined to dressings and antiseptics on the surface, and operative surgery was limited to hospitals far in the rear, it is amazing to realize that within three years the gas gangrene problem, both in its scientific and its surgical aspects, was practically resolved. The additions to our knowledge in the intervening years have been chiefly those of detail in what was already known rather than in the discovery of new knowledge.

WORLD WAR II: GAS GANGRENE APPEARS

IN ITALY

The following is the report I wrote on gas gangrene which I mentioned in my diary in the preceding chapter:

HEADQUARTERS FIFTH ARMY
Office of the Surgeon
A.P.O. #464, U.S. ARMY

31 October 1943

700-M

Subject: Gas Gangrene.

To: Surgeon, Fifth Army.

1. Incidence.
   a. 19 cases of gas gangrene have been recorded in the 94th, 95th, 8th and 16th Evacuation Hospitals during the Italian campaign. 2 cases were observed in Bizerte area in casualties evacuated from the Salerno beach. Complete clinical records of these cases are being assembled for critical appraisal.
   b. Instances of anaerobic wound infection including gas gangrene have been carefully tabulated by Major McClennan, R.A.M.C. He provides the information that the incidence of gas gangrene has definitely increased in the Eighth Army in Italy. Figures given (verbal report) are:

Desert campaign	3 per 1,000
Tripoli—Tunisia	7–8 per 1,000
Sicily	10 per 1,000
Italy	20 per 1,000

   c. Gas gangrene infection has been observed in the Fifth Army and also the Eighth Army arising in simple wounds of a type that has not hitherto been attended by complications.
2. Causative Factors.
   a. In Tunisia the recorded cases of gas gangrene were in the majority of instances associated with a demonstrable and obvious cause, usually delayed evacuation from the field, error in surgical judgment, such as suture of wound, tight packing or incomplete débridement, impaired vascular supply to an extremity.

b. A survey of 50 battle casualties at the 38th Evacuation Hospital showed the following facts.

Average Time Lag Wounding to Tagging	5.4 hrs.
Average Time Lag Wounding to Arrival 38th Evac.	12.7 hrs.

Excluding 6 patients in whom the wounding-tagging lag was 8 hours or over (these were isolated incidences of soldiers far in advance on patrol, reconnaissance, or attacking company missions):

Average Time Lag Wounding to Tagging	1.4 hrs.
Average Time Lag Wounding to Arrival 38th Evac.	8.8 hrs.

c. The same 50 casualties were questioned as to the missile causing their wounds.

Bullet wounds (machine gun, rifle or pistol)	17–34%
Artillery or mortar	31–62%
Mines	2–4%
Rifle grenade	1–2%

d. Of these 50 wounded, 8% had not had sulfonamide applied to the wound before arrival at hospital; 22% had not had oral dosage of sulfonamide.

e. 32 of the 50 casualties were from 3rd Division. 18 of the 50 casualties were from the 34th Division.

f. Standards of surgical management of battle casualties, as observed, have been satisfactory. Cases of gas gangrene have not been due to errors of surgical judgment.

g. From this random sampling it would appear that conditions governing wounding, evacuation, and management of wounds are not essentially different from those prevailing in Tunisia and Sicily.

3. Changed Factors That May Be Significant.

a. Terrain. It appears that the coastal plain of Italy is more intensively fertilized and cultivated than the terrain of Tunisia or Sicily. This provides a commonly recognized source of infection.

b. Weather conditions. Mud and surface water is more prevalent than has been encountered since the first phase of the Tunisian campaign. Colder weather may also be significant. Both of these factors have been recognized as important in gas gangrene.

(*continued*)

c. The incidence of infection with the Welch bacillus as contrasted with B. oedematiens has been greater than previously encountered in the Eighth Army. This further suggests a difference in underlying conditions.

4. Summary.

a. Basic management of battle casualties in the field does not appear to be responsible for the increase in the incidence of gas gangrene.

b. Changes in uncontrollable conditions may provide an adequate explanation.

5. Action Taken and Recommendations.

a. Medical Circular Number 4, issued on 20 October by Headquarters Fifth Army, provides sound and adequate information on the subject for the guidance of medical officers. Minor changes in the instructions regarding the combined use of penicillin and anti-toxin will be made when penicillin is available.

b. Captain F. Jergesen has been designated to collect and consolidate pertinent data regarding cases. He will work in association with Major F. Simeone when this officer is secured from North Africa.

c. Active cooperation of the 2nd Medical Laboratory has been assured by Lt. Col. Ernst. The problem has been discussed with the bacteriologic division and the preparation of proper culture media for preservation of specimens instituted.

d. Conferences with surgical staffs of hospitals have been held.

e. Action will be taken to secure a supply of penicillin at the earliest possible date.

f. Major Hansen will submit facts and recommendations regarding the condition of the feet of combat troops with reference to contamination of wounds and also circulatory disturbances (trench foot) that may be anticipated with colder weather.

g. It is recommended that Supply Officer take steps to insure adequate stocks of polyvalent anti-toxin for prophylactic use in selected cases and therapeutic use in established cases.

h. A form of Case Reports is submitted for mimeographing and distribution to hospitals.

EDWARD D. CHURCHILL
Colonel, Medical Corps
Consulting Surgeon, NATOUSA

CONFERENCE ON CLOSTRIDIAL INFECTIONS

The cold, wet weather of the late autumn in the Naples region was accompanied by a significant increase in clostridial infections. A conference was held on the subject at the 15th Medical Laboratory with the following in attendance: Virgil Cornell, the Commanding Officer of the Laboratory; Joseph Martin, Surgeon, Fifth Army; Elliott Cutler, visiting from E.T.O.; Tracy Mallory, Head of Pathology; Floyd Jergesen, 2nd Auxiliary Surgical Group on detached service collecting data on cases in the field; Howard Snyder, Surgical Consultant, Fifth Army; Fiorindo Simeone and John Stewart, Surgical Consultants, A.F.H.Q.; and Lieutenant Colonel Ernst and Major Stock of the 2nd Medical Laboratory. Cornell asked Martin to speak and then turned the meeting over to me as chairman.

Joe Martin spoke briefly on the need for a combined clinical and laboratory approach to the subject. I outlined the problem and the reason for undertaking it. These reasons were the preparation of a polyvalent antitoxin; the preparation of toxoids other than that available for *cl. perfringens*; the evaluation of treatment by antitoxin, sulfonamides and penicillin.

Jergesen had found between 60 and 70 per cent of cases associated with injured blood vessels. The infections endangering life were those that developed gas myositis early after wounding. He had assembled records on some 60 cases that fell into three groups: clostridial myositis; clostridial cellulitis; clostridial infection in dead limbs (deprived of blood supply).

Jergesen had become an expert on the diagnosis and management of gas gangrene. At the meeting I questioned one of his statements which he, in turn, said was valid "north of Caserta." This was a gentle dig at those from the base who presumed to know about affairs in the forward area. When the following item appeared in *The Saturday Evening Post*[1] on January 1, 1944, I could not resist sending it to "Jergy" with an appropriate title.

> *DIAGNOSIS OF GAS GANGRENE NORTH OF CASERTA*
> *(As recorded by War Correspondent from a Field Hospital)*
> *At the end of an hour and a half, the surgeon working on his leg looked up with a muttered exclamation of wrath and dismay. "Smell it?" he said. "Gas," whispered a nurse. There was no question about it. Gas gangrene had set in.*

Not much was accomplished at the meeting beyond getting this group thinking about the subject and stimulating Cornell to send a small laboratory group forward to begin work. Tracy Mallory did not believe that the solution was as difficult as MacLennan had described it.

---

[1] Reprinted with permission from *The Saturday Evening Post* © 1944, The Curtis Publishing Company.

In the "Report of the Fifth Army Medical Service for 1944," the subject of gas gangrene is covered as follows (p. 124, par. VII):

> The study of gas gangrene, completed in 1944 by Captain Floyd H. Jergesen, Lt. Col. Simeone and the 15th Med. Lab. is one of the outstanding contributions of the year. The improved surgical management of those wounds in which gas gangrene is likely to develop and the improved treatment of those in which clostridial myositis did develop has resulted in a lower incidence and mortality in clostridial myositis. Good surgery has accounted for much of this improvement. The availability and use of penicillin, blood transfusion and serum therapy have all played a part in the results obtained. Before the routine use of penicillin in all severely wounded battle casualties, the incidence of clostridial myositis had been reduced to five or six cases per 1,000. With routine penicillin therapy there were only nine cases of clostridial myositis in the last four months of 1944, during which time 15,553 battle casualties were admitted to Fifth Army hospitals.

The mortality rate of gas bacillus infection in World War I had been calculated as 44.6 per cent.

Speaking before the American College of Surgeons in Boston in May 1946, Simeone gave the following account of the experience in Italy:

> Early in the Italian Campaign of World War II, the incidence of clostridial myositis was 6.6 per thousand battle casualties; the mortality was 65 per cent. By the end of the campaign the incidence had dropped to less than 0.5 per thousand and the mortality to less than 25 per cent. This improvement resulted from studying the disease and disseminating the knowledge gained from the study.
>
> Early adequate débridement was the most important preventive measure. While penicillin given to control the activity of contaminating organisms may have been helpful, the administration of sulfonamides did not prevent the infection. Prophylactic administration of antitoxin was of no demonstrable benefit.
>
> Ignorance of the responsible organisms handicapped the therapeutic use of antitoxin. An attempt to diagnose the predominant organism by associating it with certain clinical types of the infection failed. Large doses of polyvalent antitoxin produced demonstrable clinical improvement in some cases, but there was no effect upon the mortality.
>
> Penicillin improved the results of treatment, probably by converting the invasive form of gas gangrene, "clostridial myositis," to the noninvasive "anaerobic cellulitis." It helped save both life and limb by making local incision of infected tissue possible, a procedure which previously had been invariably fatal.

ARTERIAL BLOOD SUPPLY

An important predisposing cause of clostridial myositis is interruption of the arterial blood supply of a limb. This may be by direct arterial injury or by the displacement of bone in a battle fracture.

In a letter dated September 2, 1950, addressed to the N.R.C., DeBakey wrote as follows:

Analysis of World War II experience with acute injuries of major arteries revealed the following significant facts:

1. The incidence is relatively low—about 1 per 100 battle casualties. Approximately 2 of every 5 major arterial injuries result in amputation. Thus, the incidence of arterial injuries sufficiently serious to cause amputation of the limb is about 4 per 1,000 wounded.

2. The time elapsing between wounding and institution of therapy is of such vital significance that it may seal the fate of the limb regardless of any form of therapy. Under the best conditions during World War II this time-lag averaged over 12 hours and it is doubtful that this can be greatly reduced. Clinical and experimental evidence would indicate that the survival rate following restoration of the circulation after such a time-lag is less than 50 per cent.

3. Methods to preserve the circulation, including the use of anti-coagulants, during this time-lag are simply not practical under military conditions.

4. Vascular surgery and blood vessel banks require special equipment and facilities and a surgeon with specialized experience. It would be necessary to make such facilities and personnel available in every forward installation where initial wound surgery is done since it would be difficult, if not impossible, to handle the wounded with vascular injuries as a special category by a special routine in the forward links of the chain of evacuation.

In the light of these facts, particularly the low incidence of major arterial injuries among the total wounded and the relatively small yield even under the best conditions, the establishment of blood vessel banks and vascular surgery centers in forward installations is considered of dubious value. The imposition of such a costly procedure in terms of specialized personnel and equipment on the military organization, already greatly burdened at this level, would seem scarcely justified.

(continued)

This does not mean, however, that no efforts should be directed toward restoration of vascular function in these cases. Consideration should be given to the achievements of this objective at two points in the phasing of wound management: (1) at the time of initial wound surgery and (2) during the time of reparative surgery. The former must be concerned with the pressing need to save the limb. This can be done by the use of venous autografts with suture anastomosis. The special equipment required for this purpose may be easily provided at forward installations and the technical ability should be readily acquired by an adequately trained surgeon. It would seem possible that this much could be done and encouraged with relatively little effort without imposing much of a burden upon the military organization. Moreover, the main purpose, survival of the limb within the limits of practicability, could be accomplished just as effectively by this means as by the establishment of blood vessel banks.

During the period of reparative wound surgery, most of which will take place in the Z. of I., blood vessel banks may have real usefulness. The problem here is not concerned with survival of the limb but with normal functional activity. Viability of the part has already been assured by this time but frequently there is present varying degrees of chronic circulatory deficiency. The objective here is restitution of vascular function with the purpose of restoring ultimate normal functional activity of the extremity. This is best done by restoring continuity of circulation through the original channels. Preserved arterial homografts may be especially useful for this purpose and the establishment of a blood vessel bank in a vascular surgery center should be considered at this level in the care of the wounded.

Jane J. Keating, Alexander L. Eastman, and Juan C. Duchesne

This early chapter of "Part Four" consists of documents compiled by Churchill on the subject of gas gangrene since the discovery of *Bacillus aerogenes capsulatus* in 1892. This topic gained much attention early in the Italian campaign due to the apparent increase in this wound complication. Although not described in the text, no story better portrays the danger of infection more so than that of Union General Charles F. Smith during the American Civil War. After leading a Union victory resulting in promotion, he sustained a minor leg injury while exiting a gunboat in Pittsburgh and succumbed to infection and death nine days later.

Churchill's chapter begins with Dr. Archibald's description of gas gangrene during World War I. In previous conflict, there was poor recording of tetanus infection during the American Civil War. Archibald attributes the emergence of infections to high-velocity wounds, close-quarter warfare, and the manure covering Flanders and eastern France. He estimated that at one point during World War I approximately 12% of the wounded might have been affected by gas gangrene. However, Archibald introduces the Depage Doctrine, describing the Belgian surgeon's practice of extensive debridement beyond limited incisions, which became widely adopted during wartime and reduced infection.

Between World Wars I and II, important advancements included the availability of sulfa drugs, penicillin, and polyvalent tetanus antitoxin. These improvements are reflected in Churchill's second report describing decreasing incidence of gas gangrene in World War II. Churchill acknowledges that while a conference discussing clostridial infections took place, little was accomplished; however, this served as a commitment to study the problem in the forward environment.

A significant study came out of work by Jergesen and Simeone in 1944 outlining the importance of adequate debridement for the initial wounds and subsequent management of high-risk wounds. Even in the presence of improved resuscitation and availability of both topical and intravenous penicillin, adequate debridement was likely to be the cause of improved outcomes.

Toward the end of the war, surgeons recognized that arterial insufficiency contributed to infection. In the final section of this chapter, Churchill cites a 1950 letter from Dr DeBakey to the National Research Council on the topic of arterial injuries. DeBakey recognized the benefit of reestablishment of circulation but prolonged evacuation times, need for anticoagulation, and specialized surgical expertise made routine vascular reconstruction impractical. Indeed, of the 2,471 arterial injuries reported by Simeone and DeBakey, only 81 were repaired. The pioneering work of Carl Hughes and Frank Spencer during the Korean War shifted the primary management paradigm from ligation to repair or reconstruction. Then, in Vietnam the majority of arterial injuries were repaired while a small minority were ligated.

With the use of chronologic documents, this chapter describes advancements in gas gangrene prevention and treatment, including widespread and timely debridement, early antibiotics, and resuscitation with minimization of ischemia. While much has changed in the current understanding of this infectious complication, including a name change to the more all-encompassing term necrotizing soft tissue infection (NSTI), a system of classification, and the introduction of the laboratory risk indicator for necrotizing fasciitis (LRINEC) score, these initial strategies remain the cornerstones of prevention and treatment today.

SUGGESTED READINGS

Debakey ME, Simeone FA. Battle injuries of the arteries in World War II: an analysis of 2,471 cases. *Ann Surg.* 1946 Apr;123(4):534–579.

Foote S. *The Civil War: A Narrative.* Vol 1. Random House; 1958, p.323.

Hughes CW. Arterial repair during the Korean war. *Ann Surg.* 1958 Apr;147(4):555–561.

Rich NM, Baugh JH, Hughes CW. Acute arterial injuries in Vietnam: 1,000 cases. *J Trauma.* 1970 May;10(5):359–369.

Stevens DL, Bryant AE. Necrotizing soft-tissue infections. *N Engl J Med.* 2017;377(23):2253–2265.

24

Cold Injury

THE FEET of the combat soldier have been one of the prime concerns of his commander from the most remote times. It was not by chance that the infantryman, marching and fighting on foot, was *known* as a "foot" soldier. Fifteen miles per day was considered a fair average for infantry in short marches; ten miles, including necessary delays, was considered good traveling in long marches.

Some of the longest marches of infantry were made by American troops. During the first year of the Mexican war, the "Army of the West" set forth to conquer New Mexico and California. General Kearney with his army left Fort Leavenworth, Kansas, in June, and after a journey of 900 miles over the great plains and mountain ranges, arrived at Santa Fe on the eighteenth of August. In 1860, the 7th Regiment spent 140 days on the road, traveling 1,000 miles to reach Fort Buchanan in New Mexico. Another regiment in 1859 marched from Fort Leavenworth to California, a distance of 1,800 miles, spending 190 days on the road. One hundred and sixty-two of those days were actually passed in marching at the rate of about eleven miles a day.

The infantryman of World War II was more "on wheels" than the infantryman of the past. Jeeps and command cars carried the officers, and trucks conveyed the GI's. In contact with the enemy, however, the infantryman again became a foot soldier; his feet were soaked by rain and mud, by crossing streams, or simply by his own sweat. As the winter approached in Italy, the ankle-high boots of the foot soldier offered little protection against cold injury intensified by the other factors of immobility and dependent position of the lower extremities.

It is accepted generally that protection of the soldier from cold injury is the responsibility of command. The military surgeon may advise the combat commanders but they alone determine the cost in manpower that a military objective may exact. Casualties from cold injury are to be reckoned with those from bullets, land mines and other more direct forms of enemy action.

As I related in Chapter 22 (My First Visit to Naples), my diary records that, on my first trip to Italy, I "primed" Colonel Williams, the Chief of Staff II Corps, "about dry socks for combat troops."

COLD INJURY HAS BEEN DESCRIBED UNDER MANY DIFFERENT NAMES:

Chilblains are usually on the hands, most frequently on the dorsal surface of the phalanges between the joints. On the leg they occur most frequently over the anterior surface of the tibia. The lesion appears first as a red, swollen and itching area which subsides in a few days or continues in a chronic or recurrent form. Blister formation or ulceration may develop, and in chronic cases tenderness and pain may become manifest.

Shelter leg was described during the London bombing of 1940. All ages and both sexes were affected among the civilians who spent the nights in the subways in a sitting posture. The subways were crowded and people brought their own chairs. The subways were cold and damp, but dependency of the legs and pressure on the popliteal space seemed to be the chief etiologic factors. Civilians seeking shelter in the tunnel leading from Naples to Pozzuoli were affected likewise by "shelter leg."

Immersion foot came into prominence during World War II as a condition affecting passengers and crews of ships. Not only complete immersion in water, but sitting in lifeboats or afloat on life rafts caused this cold injury.

Trench foot was the name for cold injury sustained in the wet and muddy trenches of World War I. This term was used frequently in World War II although trenches were replaced by foxholes or slit trenches. Trench foot is said to occur in the temperature range of 32° and 50°F.

Frostbite. Actual freezing of the skin and subcutaneous tissues results from exposure to freezing and subfreezing temperatures. The lower the temperature, the shorter the exposure. In World War II this was encountered chiefly in fliers exposed to the slipstream of aircraft. It was known as high-altitude frostbite and affected fingers, ears, chin, nose and feet. The penis may be frostbitten if exposed for urination; it also may be affected by a wind quartering into the trouser fly. A local burning sensation is followed by numbness. The skin assumes a waxen pallor.

Frostbite is well known to skiers, bobsled runners, mountaineers and, of course, polar explorers. The saga of Scott's expedition to the South Pole only to find that Amundsen had reached the goal a few weeks before him is a tragic record of cold injury and death by freezing. In military history it is paralleled by Napoleon's retreat from Moscow (**Figure 24.1**).

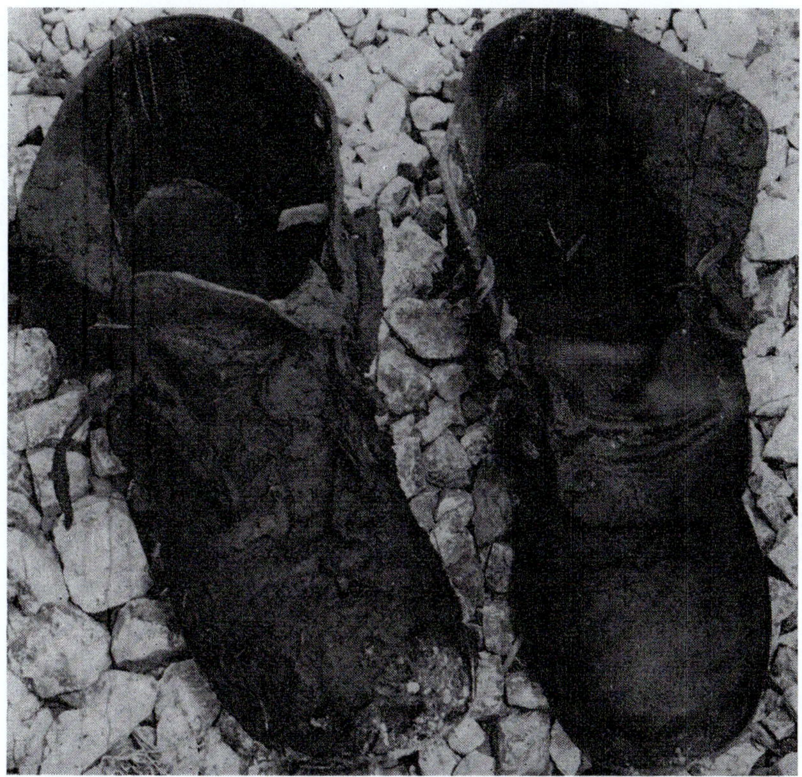

Figure 24.1 Soaked by rain and mud, by crossing streams. . . .

FIRST KNOWN COLD INJURIES IN THE WAR

In North Africa during the winter of 1942-43, and in Sicily during the summer of 1943, if cold injury occurred we were unaware of it. The Fifth Army in Italy was first subjected to the environmental conditions that produce cold injury in appreciable numbers. The volume of the Surgeon General's *History of World War II* devoted to cold injury contains the following (p. 101):

> Colonel Edward D. Churchill, M.C. Consultant in Surgery, Office of the Surgeon, NATOUSA, was, however, sufficiently aware of the possibilities of trouble to write the Surgeon on 31 October, 1943, that, with the approach of cold weather during the forthcoming fighting in the Apennines, circulatory disturbances (trench foot) were to be anticipated. Even before this date, informal consultations had been held with a number of medical officers with combat units concerning the possible occurrence of cold injury and its dangerous potentialities.

(continued)

It was only a week after Colonel Churchill had alerted the Surgeon to the possibility of cold injuries that the first patients with trench foot to be observed in Italy passed through a clearing station south of Cassino. By 12 November, 6 cases are known to have occurred. Not all had been recognized immediately as instances of cold injury. One or two of the first casualties were thought to have suffered sprains and were treated with hot applications.

After trench foot once began to appear, the incidence increased rapidly, and, over the 6-month period ending on April 30, 1944, there were more than 5,700 casualties from this cause in the Fifth U.S. Army.

For the full story of cold injury in World War II in the Mediterranean Theater and again in the European Theater, the reader must consult the official statistics, photographs and descriptions contained in the volume referred to earlier.

Cold Injury
COMMENTARY

Julie A. Rizzo, Jay A. Yelon, Rob L. Sheridan

In this monograph, Dr Churchill provides a relatively concise description of the topic of cold injury—a condition of significant importance in combat casualty care. He uses a variety of descriptive circumstances leading to cold injury as a resource to help untangle a surfeit of confusing nomenclature. The ubiquitous and crippling implications to military operations when troops are not adequately trained to perform in cold environments are highlighted. Over the ensuing eight decades, our understanding of cold injury has expanded significantly.

The concept of systemic hypothermia and its anticipation, prevention, and management have come to the forefront since Churchill's anticipatory memo to the theater surgeon in October 1943, during the early phases of the Italian campaign of World War II. Training and equipping troops to recognize the early symptoms of hypothermia has become an essential part of military and winter adventure preparation. An understanding that hypothermia (as well as other environmental injuries) are frequent secondary complications in soldiers suffering from non-cold trauma is now understood and anticipated by health care teams.

The terminology has become less confusing regarding frostbite, the local freezing tissue injury. Indeed, several classification systems have been developed to predict tissue viability. Prevention remains the most effective way to managing systemic and local cold injuries. This is accomplished by the modern military through focused training to avoid exposure, moisture and submersion and well designed equipment for protection and monitoring. Training emphasizes increased caloric intake, appropriate layering of clothes for insulation, ventilation, and protection from the wind, as well as observing fellow service members for signs of hypothermia. Early recognition of cognitive symptoms of hypothermia in oneself and fellow warfighters dramatically reduces the occurrence of overt hypothermia and frostbite.

Timely treatment of hypothermia and frostbite at the point of injury can reduce morbidity and mortality in military operations, wilderness adventures, and urban settings alike. When prevention fails and hypothermia or frostbite occur, immediate circumstances, available equipment, transport distance to medical treatment, and pharmacologic agents on hand will define the immediate treatment plan. In most cases, treatment at the point of injury consists of supportive care, including rewarming and hydration.

Although iloprost as an intravenous infusion is available in some parts of the world, complications, logistical challenges, and available data have limited its widespread adoption internationally. If long-distance transport in cold conditions is anticipated, avoiding freeze-thaw-refreeze injuries is vital to limiting injury severity.

Once transportation to a warm health care environment is accomplished, definitive treatment ensues. Supportive care should be continued, and the grade of the injury should be defined. Tissue that demarcates as nonviable is removed in a delayed fashion, and the resulting wounds are closed with a creative combination of skin grafts and flaps. Rehabilitation commences early after rewarming to provide the best chance of regaining full mobility.

In recent years, there has been a growing experience with early thrombolytic therapy for frostbite cases associated with absent perfusion after tissue thawing. Currently, such therapies are limited to centers with available vascular radiology services and expertise. Going forward, preventative measures should remain the top training priority to minimize the need for such invasive therapies. Nevertheless, research and innovation aimed at making effective frostbit treatment more accessible, without the need for sophisticated interventions or monitoring, will serve as a safety net. This is particularly crucial in potential future conflicts with contested battlefields and airspace, where prolonged prehospital phases of combat casualty care may become more common.

SUGGESTED READINGS

Cancio LC, Lundy JB, Sheridan RL. Evolving changes in the management of burns and environmental injuries. *Surg Clin North Am.* 2012 Aug;92(4):959-986.

Gauthier J, Morris-Janzen D, Poole A. Iloprost for the treatment of frostbite: a scoping review. *Int J Circumpolar Health.* 2023 Dec;82(1):2189552.

Handford C, Thomas O, Imray CHE. Frostbite. *Emerg Med Clin North Am.* 2017 May;35(2):281-299.

Sheridan RL, Goverman JM, Walker TG. Diagnosis and treatment of frostbite. *N Engl J Med.* 2022 Jun 9;386(23):2213-2220.

25

From Capri to Typhus

I Returned to Italy from North Africa early in December, 1943, and stayed in the Parco Hotel, which was set aside for the billeting of transient officers in Naples. It was far enough back from the docks to be off the target in air raids. This was a period of great confusion in Naples. Rest camps for troops were established in the city by the Fifth Army, and soldiers were sent down on five-day leaves. The venereal disease rate was at an unprecedented height and bad liquor was plentiful as local plants bottled and labeled many kinds of decoctions. One enterprising scoundrel sold liquor fortified with methyl alcohol, which was responsible for several American soldiers going blind. When tracked down, I heard, he was made to drink his own brew!

When a disciplinary barracks was established, in order to man it a one per cent assessment was made on all organizations in the Peninsular Base Section (P.B.S.). Taken from medical sources were four noncommissioned officers, two cooks and twenty-eight enlisted men of various grades and skills—typists, chauffeurs and others. Actually the hospitals were the only medical source of supply used. The personnel taken from hospitals were used as guards at the stockade.

Prophylactic stations also caused a heavy drain on hospital personnel. A sergeant and two privates, under medical officer supervision, were required for each station. By December 4, nine prophylactic stations had been set up and three more were to open. One station, for instance, opened at 3:00 P.M. and gave 115 treatments before the next morning.

TO CAPRI

Shortly after I arrived in Naples, Bruce Hopper, Major Sherry and I drove to the docks for a brief trip to Capri. My companions were "retreads" of the World War I Air Force. Boarding a decrepit Italian excursion steamer of narrow beam and a list to starboard, we put out to sea in the Golfo di Napoli. A strong wind was blowing and the sea was rough, so the little boat hugged the lee shore of Sorrento. The small harbor on the Island of Capri was protected by a breakwater. A funicular hoisted us to the village square where Lieutenant Bond, of the Troop Carrier Command, arranged billets at La Palma. This was a small hotel just opened as part of the project to turn Capri into an Air Force rest camp.

In the dusk a walk about the square and its side streets ended at Luigi's for a cognac and then the Quiziano for dinner. At Luigi's I found a bottle of Orvieto wine after prolonged search. It fitted snugly into my musette bag.

At the Quiziano we had dinner with Don Beachcomber, a restaurateur of Hollywood, assigned by the Air Force to provide meals for the rest camp.

The next morning we moved to the Villa Vismarro, which was to be set up as a "General's Villa." By providing one luxurious villa it was hoped to reduce the number of establishments that would be demanded by general officers on the island. The General's Villa was staffed with servants and supplies but occupied only sporadically.

The Villa Vismarro had been built by a fascist who made a fortune in the hydroelectric development of Sicily under Mussolini. It was large, modernistic in design and occupied one of the picture postcard sites on Capri.

Our first call was on Baronessa Uxhäll, a disciple of Axel Munthe. The Baroness took us to San Michele, then to the far end of Anacapri, where by descending through the fields to Torre di Materita we reached the home of Munthe. San Michele had been converted into a museum some years previously. Torre di Materita looks off toward Ischia.

After other excursions to the historic sites of the island we had tea with the Baroness and her husband, formerly Professor of Physiology at Hamburg. His sole interest in old age was American detective stories. They had left their books and all other possessions behind in their hurried flight from Esthonia.

At the Villa Vismarro, Bruce, Major Sherry and I sat in the garden in the late afternoon, watching the sun slowly sink into the sea. The first dinner party at the villa was served at the round marble table with a water garden sunken in its center and lighted from below. Red camellias drifted on the surface of the water. An exotic setting and a strange mixture of guests: Don Beachcomber; Lieutenant Colonel Woodward, New Orleans sportsman; an Italian contessa of decadent nobility; Major Sherry, banker from Syracuse, New York; Bruce Hopper, Professor of History, Harvard University; Lieutenant Commander Roberts, manager of the Mayflower Hotel, Washington, D.C.; and the Surgical Consultant, A.F.H.Q.

It was a short walk to the Quiziano to see a show staged for the rest camp. On return to our villa we took with us the itinerant Neapolitan floor show singers and dancers and went up to the so-called music room on the top floor.

Having no knowledge of the copulatory rituals of the fascists at the time of Benito Mussolini, it took a moment for the significance of the "Music Room" to be grasped. The only pieces of furniture in the room were a grand piano and an ancient, gilded, four-posted, canopied bed.

The bed was huge. I christened it "The Great Bed of Ware." Shakespeare, in *Twelfth Night*, gave the line to Sir Toby Belch:—"and as many lies as will lie in thy sheet of paper, although the sheet were big enough for the bed of Ware in England." Ware is a town of Hertfordshire on the Lea. The Great Bed formerly was at the Saracen's Head and was removed to Rye House two miles distant.

The setting, designed by Mussolini in the back room of the Palazzo Venezia for assignations with Clara Petucci, has been described in a footnote by Tompkins.[1]

> It was a large room with tinted-glass windows and a ceiling decorated with the signs of the Zodiac; its antique Venetian furniture had been supplemented by a king-sized bed, a phonograph (for Chopin and Beethoven), a solitary framed photograph of the Duce, and a wardrobe full of negligees, mostly pink and blue, with goosefeather boas personally selected by Mussolini. Arriving shortly after 2 P.M., Clara would undress, put on a nightgown and negligee, and dutifully wait for the appearance of her lover.

Sprawled on the great bed, we were entertained by the Neapolitan singers until our glowing sunburns and Orvieto wine made us so sleepy that we welcomed a return to the safety of our rooms below.

In the morning Bruce Hopper wakened me at seven o'clock for the return trip to Naples. We sailed about an hour later and docked at Naples at about half-past ten.

CUTLER VISITS ITALY

It was at this time that Elliott Cutler arrived from London and he joined me in a visit to the Medical School of the University of Naples. The rooms used for instruction in microscopic anatomy were in shambles. Glass microscope slides littered the floor and the microscopes despoiled of all lenses. Allied troops had been quartered in the Medical School, and stories had spread that microscope lenses were valuable. I had seen this type of destructive looting in the post office of Palermo. It was not always a search for something of value, but something small enough to carry away in a pocket. Something to mail home as a souvenir or swap for a pack of cigarettes. Many things taken were discarded on the road. Officers could, and did, carry more weighty objects—collections of postal stamps, Oriental rugs, oil paintings ripped from their frames.

The following morning Howard Snyder, Elliott Cutler and I drove north from Caserta through Capua, the oldest Greek colony in Italy. The Volturno River was in full flood from the recent rains. The 11th Field Hospital was

---

[1]Tompkins P. *Italy Betrayed*, Simon & Schuster; 1966.

receiving the seriously wounded from the 36th Division and was sited near a Long Tom battery that was firing intermittently. A shell from the counter-battery fire had hit the mess tent shortly before our arrival. The surgical operations in progress were demonstrations which I was proud to have Cutler witness.

Jim Mason and Phil Giddings were at the 33rd Field Hospital. Both platoons of the 33rd Field Hospital were adjacent to the divisional clearing station. They had been moved up for an advance that had been postponed. Because of the scarcity of sites in the mountains and heavy use of the road it was thought best not to move them back. The artillery was close by. The patients were so exhausted that the firing seemed to make little difference to them. The doctors and nurses slept in foxholes dug in their tents.

At the 94th Evacuation Hospital, which was badly bogged down in the mud, Colonel Pierce, "Sig" Sanzene, Charlie Rife, Charlie Dowman and Lyman Brewer were working hard. Pierce, the Commanding Officer, had designed a new operating tent made by stretching tarpaulin over a light wooden frame. A note in my diary records that, "We entered this war with the tentage designed for the Spanish-American War. Here again is reflected the failure of the Army to keep abreast of changes in civilian surgery during peacetime, and failure to realize that the overall pattern of surgery changes. The use of plasma to save lives will yield a group of living patients that will require many other adjuvants to treatment."

At the medical battalion headquarters of the 3rd Division, McCarthy was looking tired. I had last seen "Mac" on the northern coast of Sicily. His division had been taking a beating and was no longer the cocky, trim outfit that was in Palermo last summer. He showed us his report on the health of the division. Venereal disease, especially syphilis, had risen rapidly as the division rested and was given the freedom of Naples. The ancient Neapolitan Disease! He also showed me a new litter he had designed for mountain work. The front poles were carried on the saddle of a mule and bearers carried the rear.

A long drive brought us to the 56th Evacuation Hospital near Dragoni. Howard Snyder and Elliott Cutler shared a tent; I shared another with Harry Blesse, the Commanding Officer. Back on August 17, I had written in my diary:

> *E.D.C. Comments:* Today Long submitted a report on the state of affairs in Sicily that now cannot "be put on paper." The episode which could not "be put on paper" at that time was the "slapping" incident involving General Patton.[2] Now, in our tent, Harry Blesse and I talked about the episode, which had since been publicized. He told me that his brother Fred had carried a reprimand from Eisenhower to Patton on his second trip to Sicily.

---

[2] The original edition contained an Appendix F on the "Patton Slapping Episode."

Chris Carter, who was in charge of the surgical staff, told me about a patient who had been evacuated from the 56th Evacuation Hospital with a diagnosis of "ileus." The surgeon in charge of the patient had been told that the soldier had peritonitis, but remained unconvinced. It was a well-proven instance of survival following a penetrating wound of the descending colon untreated by operation. I eventually saw the patient several times at the 300th General Hospital in Naples where he had been sent from the 56th Evacuation Hospital. Several metallic fragments in the left upper abdomen showed clearly on x-ray films. An enema came out through the unhealed wound and demonstrated the fecal fistula. For further management I advised dependent drainage in the left flank with a subsequent transverse colostomy.

The next day we visited the 15th Evacuation Hospital, which had crossed the Volturno on a pontoon bridge and had become bogged down in one of the worst seas of mud I had seen. It was impossible to get in or about the hospital without wading through thick "custard." The Commanding Officer, Frank Lever, was just out of bed after an attack of grippe and looked pale and thin. A French battalion on its way forward was moving across the pontoon bridge and delayed our departure. The delay gave us an opportunity to talk with an officer of the 100th Battalion of Japanese infantry from Hawaii. This Nisei battalion became famous in Italy and took severe punishment in combat. The officer told us that there was no "trench foot" in his outfit because his men were careful to wash and dry their feet, and always carried an extra pair of socks sewn into their shirts. During subsequent days, however, I saw many patients with cold injury from the 100th Battalion. I recall talking with a Nisei captain who had been wounded by a machine gun bullet. He was anxious to get back to his men because their morale might deteriorate with him away. From his account and from many others, both enlisted men and officers, there was no opportunity for men in the advanced assault companies to take care of their feet. Conditions were different from warfare in trenches where a man could find shelter or at least unlace his boots.

"A man will become a casualty," I noted, "if he fights under these conditions for longer than five days at a stretch. Some of the soldiers I have seen as patients have not had their shoes off for nine to twelve days—cold, rain and mud. The answer lies in more frequent relief. This is a command responsibility."

During our return toward Naples, I spent a night in Caserta. Part of the royal palace—La Reggia di Caserta—was the headquarters of the Fifth Army Rear. "Dinner in the Colonel's Mess" I noted. "A stuffy, swank private dining room full of elderly colonels dining on broiled steak and other luxuries. Then to the palace opera house where La Boheme was given by the San Carlo Opera Company. General Clark and staff were in the royal box. 'Looking Glass' world of contrasts, mud to opera" (**Figure 25.1**).

In the morning we toured the royal suite of the palace with a guide. The colors of the ceiling paintings were gorgeous; this was, in every way, a regal palace, even to the queen's tub, which was plated with gold, and the bas-reliefs on the walls with closed eyes so not to "see" the queen at her bath. The chapel had been badly damaged by a bomb hit. Gilt veneer, column capitals and other debris were mixed into the crumbled masonry on the floor. The pipes of the organ were bent and twisted by the blast. The altar itself was not destroyed.

We then went to the hospital train loading near the bombed station and yards at Caserta. The train company was commanded by Major Fisk. Officers from the 300th General Hospital were sorting the patients. The train ran every day between Caserta and Naples, saving by its capacity 2,500 miles of ambulance lift.

The Chief of Staff, Major General Gruenther, asked to see Elliott Cutler regarding a trip Elliot had made to Russia. He wanted to know how the American GI could be made to hate the Germans. We told him certainly not by running such soft spots as the "Colonel's Mess" at the palace! "This whole palace headquarters, in my opinion," my diary notes say, "is bad for the morale of an army in the field. They should be up in the mud with their men, doing a little hating themselves! One doesn't hate on a full stomach and a hot bath."

Our next stop was the 36th General Hospital, set up in an Italian military hospital which was well adapted to our purposes except for the plumbing. I talked with Jim Winfield about some problems he brought to my attention.

Later, writing of my tour, I noted, "All want confirmation of decisions relative to the disposition of patients. Few discuss the problems of surgery or postoperative care unless on actual ward rounds."

We were back in Naples the second week of December. I checked with the 15th Medical Laboratory about gas gangrene and the blood bank. Arnest—then the Surgeon of the Peninsular Base Section—had asked the blood bank to keep a backlog of 140 units for emergency use in the Naples area. This interlock with the Fifth Army's needs seemed important. The Fifth Army Surgeon had told me that he was requesting a British Base Transfusion Unit from Tunis. From my point of view I saw that "things were getting mixed up because of lack of definitive policy and supplies."

The 52nd Station Hospital, with Guy Wells of Providence as Commanding Officer, and Lang Parsons as Chief of Surgery, had just arrived to set up in Naples. Hospitals in Naples were very crowded. The plan at that time was to have six general hospitals and eight 500-bed station hospitals. I was again deploring the use of station hospitals for battle casualties in an expanding base section behind an army in combat. We needed more flexible units with less

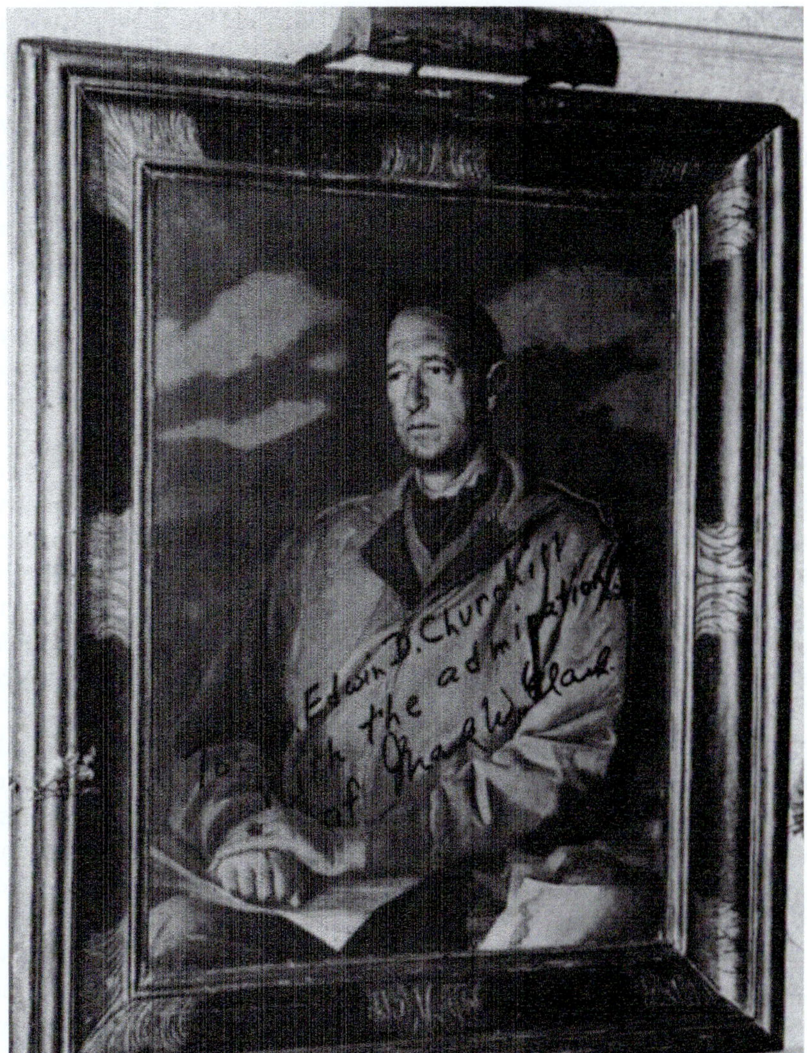

Figure 25.1 Portrait of General Mark Clark at the time of the Anzio landing.

elaborate equipment and more competent staffs. I advised Arnest to delay the establishment of special centers for the present and to get battle casualties out of station hospitals and into general hospitals as soon as feasible.

TYPHUS

In the winter of 1943-44 there was a small epidemic of typhus in Naples. A.F.H.Q. had been alerted to the dangers of insect-borne disease during the North African campaign. The Committee on Hygiene and Epidemiology, Technical Section for Public Health, French High Commissioner of North

Africa, had met in Algiers on March 24 to 26, 1943. A full report of this meeting had been made to the Surgeon, NATOUSA, on March 27 by Perrin Long. At this meeting Dr. Gaud, Director General of Public Health, Morocco, had discussed the situation in Morocco, where typhus and plague were then causing alarm. Morocco was having an epidemic of typhus, and from October, 1942, to the time of the conference 7,879 cases of this disease had been reported. In contrast to the epidemic of 1941-42, the area of Oudjda was relatively free from typhus while the Casablanca area suffered heavily. Case fatality rate among Europeans was 26.5 per cent while that among natives was 14.5 per cent. Vaccination with the living murine vaccine of Blane and the dead vaccine of Algeria was carried out extensively and considered to be of value. Dr. Gaud also discussed plague on the basis of 201 cases reported during the same period.

In the Naples epidemic, 2,250 cases of typhus were reported between October, 1943, and March, 1944. The introduction of typhus to Naples was thought to have come from Italian soldiers returning from Yugoslavia and Russia. In my own notes I refer to its appearance in a Serbian prisoner and its spread to other inmates. The prison was bombed and many of the prisoners escaped. Some were rounded up but many cases of typhus appeared scattered widely over Naples. The disease was a virulent type, running 25 per cent mortality rate.

Infectious and insect-borne diseases were not in my field of responsibility, so, as with venereal disease, I was merely a bystander. Bill Stone was our expert at A.F.H.Q. at the time of the Naples epidemic. My interest lies in picturing the conditions in Naples that were conducive to its spread. There was widespread destruction of dwellings, and families were crowded together in hovels or lice-infested air raid shelters. Hot water for bathing was nonexistent and soap was not available. The streets were littered with rubbish and fallen masonry. Yet every combat soldier relieved from combat duty for a rest period was eager to go to Naples and perhaps "shack up" with an obliging girl or queue up in a house of prostitution.

Beginning in November, 1943, the Fifth Army Surgeon, Joe Martin, began issuing systematic instructions to the troops in methods of controlling body louse infestation. (These were the "cooties" of World War I.) Starting on January 1, the rest camps in Naples received particular attention. A special detail, made up of an officer and seven enlisted men, was assigned the task of applying insecticide powder to soldiers on their arrival and departure. All bunks were kept dusted. Finally, Naples was placed off limits and the rest camps were moved north to Caserta. Ambulances and litters used in transporting patients to and from the Naples hospitals were carefully dusted with DDT; airplanes and their passengers were sprayed with "bombs" and dusted.

Reported cases dropped from 219 in December to 35 in March, 1944. By March 27, the incidence of typhus had so diminished that the order placing Naples off-limits to troops was rescinded. Spending the night in Naples, however, was still forbidden, and troops were not allowed to enter restaurants, public transport or crowded buildings. With the coming of spring the danger of typhus disappeared.

On October 2, 1944, a new educational program in body louse control was started and the winter of 1944-45 passed without danger of typhus.

Timothy P. Plackett, Ronald I. Gross, and Karen J. Brasel

In **Chapter 25: From Capri to Typhus,** Churchill recalls his visit to the rest camps on Capri and his stay at the luxurious Villa Vismarro. After this brief sojourn, he returned to Naples and completed a battlefield rotation of the surrounding field hospitals accompanied by Dr Elliott Cutler, the chief consultant in surgery in the European Theater of Operations, US Army. The chapter concludes with a retelling of the typhus outbreak in Naples during the winter of 1943-1944. While Churchill acknowledges that the prevention and treatment of typhus were not under his purview, he once again highlights that disease and non-battle injuries are among the most frequently encountered medical problems during combat operations. This is further amplified through the chapter as he mentions a variety of other nonsurgical conditions such as venereal disease and trench foot.

Epidemic typhus was a significant problem throughout the North African and Eastern European theaters. Caused by an infection of *Rickettsia prowazekii* and spread from human to human by body lice, epidemic typhus has typically been associated with poor hygiene, unsanitary living conditions, and overcrowding. Acute infection can prove fatal if untreated; Churchill cites a 25% mortality rate. The mainstays of prevention focus on addressing the underlying conditions in which the vector thrives, namely the use of insecticides, washing clothes and bedding at high temperatures, preventing overcrowding, and avoiding high-risk areas. Modern infection control practices addressing infections transmitted by arthropods have changed little from the prevention measures described by Churchill. Military field hygiene teams continue to focus on the importance of applying *N,N*-diethyl-meta-toluamide (DEET)-based insect repellent, washing uniforms at least once a week, and using high water temperatures ($\geq$130 °F) to ensure any lice or other vectors are killed. The one significant advancement since Churchill's time is the addition of permethrin-impregnated uniforms and recommendation to repeat its application after 50 launderings. Treatment with doxycycline or chloramphenicol generally leads to rapid resolution.

Although epidemic typhus may seem a disease of the past, sporadic outbreaks still occur when conditions are ripe for the spread of body lice. Large outbreaks are seen when armed conflict results in a disruption of basic services and significant numbers of people are forced to live in displaced persons camps. This was seen during the recent Syrian conflicts and there is rising concern that it could occur during the current war in Ukraine. Heightening the potential risk in Ukraine is the observation that high levels of typhus were seen in this region during World War II. Indeed, Churchill alludes to Italian soldiers returning from the Russian front as a potential source for the Neapolitan outbreak. Untreated survivors are at risk for spontaneous recrudescence years or decades after the initial infection (Brill-Zinsser disease, akin to shingles after chickenpox). Such individuals can serve as reservoirs for future outbreaks.

This chapter reminds the modern military surgeon that while their primary focus is on the treatment of combat injuries, an understanding of public health principles and field sanitation must remain a part of training. The military surgeon is first and foremost a medical officer and needs to be prepared to address the full spectrum of medical issues when subspecialist expertise is not available. Whether it's venereal disease in **Chapter 17: Prostitution and Venereal Disease,** trench foot in **Chapter 24: Cold Injury,** or typhus in the present chapter, Churchill emphasizes this invaluable and time-honored truth throughout his writing.

SUGGESTED READINGS

Bechah Y, Capo C, Mege JL, Raoult D. Epidemic typhus. *Lancet Infect Dis*. 2008;8:417–426.
Field Hygiene and Sanitation. TC 4-02.3 Department of the Army, May 2015.
Newton PN, Fournier PE, Tapps D, Richards AL. Renewed risk for epidemic typhus related to war and massive population displacement, Ukraine. *Emerg Infect Dis*. 2022;28:2125–2126.

26

Mustard Gas in Bari Harbor

THE VESICANT type of gas made its appearance in the First World War later than the others, but soon became the most important in gas warfare. It first came into prominence at Ypres on July 12, 1917, dichlordiethylsulphide being the chemical used. It was called by the French soldiers "ypérite," by the Italians "yprite," and by the British "mustard gas." Gas mask discipline offered ample protection to the eyes and lungs, but very important—and horrendous—military results were obtained from skin burns which caused the evacuation of enormous numbers of casualties. The Central Powers considered dichlordiethylsulphide their most pernicious gas and the experience of the Allies certainly confirmed the opinion that it had won this place in military importance. This gas had many features which rendered it especially suitable. It was toxic in a concentration which could not be detected by the sense of smell; the person affected suffered no discomfort at the time of the exposure and symptoms were not evident until many hours later. Mustard gas penetrated all clothing and was remarkably persistent on the earth or on foliage over which it had been scattered. These factors tended to increase its effectiveness; in addition to the physical action of the gas on the men themselves, the morale of troops was impaired.

Truly speaking, dichlordiethylsulphide is not a gas, but a liquid, which slowly vaporizes, and is effective in either state. It volatilizes slowly at ordinary temperatures and dissociates only at high temperatures. This latter fact was taken advantage of in the treatment of contaminated clothing. Furthermore, it is readily oxidized by such substances as chlorine or bleaching powder, and these chemicals were used in purifying dugouts, trenches, and ground or foliage saturated with the gas.

GREATEST SINGLE LOSS

On December 2, 1943, the Luftwaffe staged an air raid on the shipping in the harbor of Bari, an important port on the Adriatic Sea just above the "Heel of the Boot" on the map of Italy. In the words of General Eisenhower it caused the greatest single loss "inflicted upon us during the entire period of Allied campaigning in the Mediterranean and in Europe."

The air raid began at 1930 hours and was over in twenty minutes. In the *History of U.S. Naval Operations* the estimate is given that the attacking aircraft numbered 105 JU-88 bombers and that radar detection of their approach was confused by the foremost planes creating a "window." High-explosive bombs were dropped and direct hits were scored on some three or four ships. Sixteen vessels in all were completely destroyed and, since a convoy had arrived recently, many were still loaded with valuable parts and instruments for the Air Force. The destroyed ships were carrying 38,000 tons of cargo.

The ship *John Harvey*, loaded with 100 tons of mustard in 100-pound bombs, as well as a large quantity of munitions, was tied up at berth 29 on the mole. Other ships were berthed side to side against the *John Harvey*. Another ship closeby was loaded with ammunition and explosives. The *John Harvey* was not hit during the air raid. Shortly after the raid, an oil tanker exploded and started to burn. There were two big explosions, the second of which blew up the *John Harvey* and sank her at 2210 hours. An order had been issued to scuttle the *John Harvey* after the fire began but it is not known whether the message was received. There were no survivors from the *John Harvey*.

The harbor was covered with flaming oil and gasoline. In this maelstrom of fire and explosion, sixteen ships were sunk and four partly destroyed. Survivors were blown into the water or forced to jump in and swim for their lives. In parts of the harbor heavy oil covered the surface of the water.

Most of the mustard released from the *John Harvey* was destroyed by the fire. Empty bomb casings on the mole accounted for the release of at least 2,000 to 3,000 pounds of mustard just above the mole. The wind was offshore and carried this out to sea. Had it been in the opposite direction a far greater disaster could have resulted.

It seems remarkable that no general alarm of gas was spread that evening, but few survivors identified the characteristic odor. On direct questioning, some of the survivors spoke of having commented on a "garlicky" odor. Some had joked about the odor and attributed it to the quantities of garlic eaten by the Italians. The *Lyman Abbott* was lying in the harbor and someone aboard yelled "Gas!" Many of the crew put on their gas masks and wore them for about a half hour. No one could be found who personally had recognized gas.

No official information concerning the possibility of mustard exposure was communicated to the hospitals. A rumor reached one hospital but it was denied by an unidentified Naval officer.

The mustard that was not burned either sank to the bottom of the harbor or was mixed and dissolved in the oil. Exposure to the mixture of mustard and oil caused most of the casualties and deaths. The amount of mustard in the oil varied in different parts of the harbor. Some casualties were caused by vapor alone, but the greater number and the serious casualties were those who had been covered with oil. This occurred from swimming or being splashed with oil. A few were contaminated while sitting or standing in lifeboats or clinging to life rafts.

More than 1,000 men were killed or missing following the disaster. More than 800 reached hospitals and, of these, 628 were suffering from exposure to mustard. Sixty-nine deaths, wholly or partly caused by mustard, had occurred by December 17.

Rescue squads at the port and hospital staffs had no inkling that the injured men were contaminated with mustard. They were covered with crude oil and suffering from immersion and exposure. They were wrapped in blankets and given hot tea to sip. Those with injuries requiring surgical attention were cared for first and those merely covered with oil were left wrapped in blankets for twelve to twenty-four hours. The mustard-oil mixture was not washed off and contaminated clothing was not removed. A few uninjured men, on their own initiative, cleaned all of the oil off themselves that night and as a result suffered only slight burns. No specific anti-gas treatment was thought of. Many men who appeared in good condition after several hours were sent to a Seaman's Home still wearing their contaminated clothing.

Few of the medical attendants sustained burns, although several had irritation of the eyes. This suggests that the solution of mustard-in-oil was quite dilute. Patients were taken to three British General Hospitals—the 98th, 70th, and 84th—and to the 14th Combined General Hospital (Indian), and the 3rd New Zealand Hospital.

The main explosion in the harbor was of tremendous violence. Window glass seven miles away was shattered. It was anticipated that many cases of blast injury would be observed, and patients initially were considered as such or as suffering from immersion and exposure. The first suggestion of anything unusual came from the resuscitation wards. Men were brought in supposedly in shock. The pulse was either imperceptible or barely palpable and the blood pressure in the range of 40 to 60 mm. of mercury. Notwithstanding these observations, the appearance of the patients did not conform with shock from hemorrhage. There was no restlessness or anxiety, no rapid shallow respirations, and the pulse rate was only moderately rapid, 110 to 120. In contrast to the effects of blast injury, these patients did not have chest pain, altered respiration, injured eardrums or blood-tinged sputum. They were somewhat apathetic. When spoken to they could sit up in bed and would say that they felt well at a time when their pulse was barely perceptible and their systolic blood pressure as low as 50 mm. of mercury.

A striking feature was the lack of response of the hypotension to the usual resuscitation measures. Plasma infusion gave only a small and transient rise of blood pressure, and most patients showed no rise in pressure in response to plasma, warmth, stimulants and morphia. Adrenalin gave no rise in pressure even when given as intravenous infusion. Coramine gave a transient but not significant effect.

About six hours after the disaster, patients began to have eye symptoms. Patients in the hospitals, and those not yet admitted, noticed a burning of the eyes and a flow of tears. Lacrimation increased and was associated with squinting and spasm of the eyelids and sensitivity to light. Within twenty-four hours, eyes became swollen and the men feared that they were blind. There was no actual loss of vision but the spasm of the eyelids was so severe that the eyes could not be opened.

Redness of the skin became apparent early the next morning with daylight. Blisters appeared at about this time, some twelve hours after the first exposure. It was at this time that the hospitals first were notified of the possibility of "blister gas" exposure among the injured. Nearly all patients were nauseated and vomiting when they reached hospitals, but only scant information could be gathered about the appearance of the vomitus.

The first death occurred eighteen hours after exposure to mustard. Several others took place within the first twenty-four hours. The early deaths deserve special mention because they were both dramatic and unpredicted. Men who appeared in good condition save for low blood pressure, redness of the skin and eyes, became moribund within minutes. Their deaths were not associated with respiratory distress, cyanosis or restlessness. Patients who were able to talk and say they felt well would be dead within a few minutes. One patient, for example, was pulseless but warm and able to talk sensibly— he then turned cold and soon his heart stopped. Examination of their hearts, lungs, abdomens and nervous systems showed no abnormal findings or but minimal ones at such times.

In 54 carefully studied cases (not selected) the times of death were as follows:

DAY	DEATHS	DAY	DEATHS
1st	5	8th	8
2nd	8	9th	6
3rd	6	10th	3
4th	4	11th	3
5th	4	12th	0
6th	3	13th	1
7th	2	14th	1

Two peaks are apparent in the incidence of deaths: the first on the second and third days, and the second on the eighth and ninth.

Symptoms and signs of upper respiratory tract irritation appeared by the second or third day. These took the form of hoarseness and soreness of the throat, especially on swallowing. At first, cough was "brassy" and only later was productive of purulent sputum. Irritation of the lower respiratory tract was not noteworthy until well toward the end of the first week. Signs of lung involvement in the patients who were to die early were chiefly tracheal rhonchi.

The general apathy of the patients was universal and impressive. They could be roused but quickly resumed a listless and somnolent state. The injured included men of at least twelve nationalities or races, and the apathy was equally striking in all.

The clinical observations and response to treatment were taken up sequentially according to the part or organ injured.

EYE LESIONS

The eyes were involved to some degree in every patient who sustained any other lesion from mustard. The immediate involvement of the eyes by vapor or mustard-in-oil solution produced severe and distressing symptoms, but it was believed that the eye lesions would not produce permanent damage. Burning and soreness of the eyes were first noted by the men four to six hours after exposure but were not intense until several hours later. The eyes at first felt "gritty," or "as though sand particles had gotten in the eyes." This soon was associated with lacrimation, pain and burning, photophobia and blepharospasm. By twenty-four to thirty hours these symptoms became maximal and many were kept in hospital only because of their eyes. Corneal lesions were few and there was no denudation or ulceration.

The acute features of eye involvement subsided rapidly after three to four days, and after the first week eyes were rarely causing difficulty. Secondary infections were mild. This is in contrast to the eye lesions caused by liquid mustard splash or saturated vapor. The military significance of acute eye lesions should not be underestimated. This was shown by the experience on the destroyer *Bistera*.

The *Bistera* was in the Bari harbor the night of the raid and, after picking up some thirty injured men from the water, put to sea for Taranto. Six hours out of port, eye symptoms appeared in the ship's officers and most of the crew. These became so severe that it was only with great difficulty that the ship was brought into Taranto harbor eighteen hours later. The crew practically was blinded by eye lesions.

The more severe eye lesions were associated with the more severe face burns, and after the first week the burns of the skin surface of the eyelids accounted for much of the remaining eye trouble.

In the treatment of the eyes no first aid was given to any of the disaster victims. The two men who wore gas masks that evening did not experience eye or respiratory tract irritation. All eyes were irrigated one to three times a day. Atropine solution drops were used three times daily. Albucid solution in varying strengths was without detectable effect on a controlled group of patients. In the more severe cases and in those with secondary infection, 10 per cent albucid solution was used in one group and penicillin in a comparable group. An attending ophthalmologist planned a detailed report.

The use of "eye teams" was initiated in one hospital, centering the responsibility on the ophthalmologic service. After examination the treatment was done by this service. The "eye team"—one or more nurses with corps men—moved from ward to ward, caring only for eyes. Treatments were thus standardized and the eyes not overlooked in a busy ward.

INJURY TO THE SKIN

The first evidence of reddening of the skin was apparent on the morning of December 3. The redness became more obvious in the eighteen to thirty-six hour period and blisters appeared. These were quite superficial but widely spread. Over the span of the first four days the skin involvement became more and more extensive as wider areas of redness and blistering developed. Edema of the skin was noted from the first. The skin was brawny, thickened and its texture was altered. It was tender on pressure and did not pit. As subcutaneous edema developed, this did pit on pressure. Large areas of skin later were to strip off their superficial layers; in some instances up to 80 to 90 per cent of the body surface was lost.

The coloration of the skin that developed was striking—bronze, reddish brown or tan in some, and very red in others. There was resemblance to sunburn and suntan. Part of the coloration was attributable to erythema, as it could be faded out with pressure; part was a change in the skin itself and disappeared when the desquamation took place.

The nature of the exposure determined the pattern and distribution of the burns—wherever mustard-in-oil had been in contact. Men who had been immersed were burned in all areas. Others had a more limited distribution. Vapor burns were in the exposed areas, the axillae and groins. The soles of the feet and palms of the hands were quite free of injury.

Subcutaneous edema of the genitals was extensive and paraphimosis common. These lesions were painful and, as usual, caused the patient apprehension.

The simplest treatments of the skin were the most satisfactory. Surgical gauze or bland ointments were satisfactory. The blisters and skin loss were quite superficial and many were healed in a fortnight. A few patients were cleaned with liquid petrolatum and then with warm water and soap. They developed only a diffuse and mild erythema and showed no toxic effects. It is probable that early cleansing saved their lives. A few doctors and nurses showed injury to their hands or mild irritation of their eyes. With the dilute mustard-in-oil solution, a long period of exposure was necessary to produce significant effects.

Systemic effects of mustard have usually been considered insignificant. In this group of patients, however, the victims were immersed in a solution of mustard-in-oil, wrapped in blankets, given warm tea and then allowed a prolonged period for absorption. The blood showed mild concentration. The white cells were normal in number until the third day. In the fatal cases both granulocytes and lymphocytes fell as low as 50 or 100/cu. mm.

In autopsied patients, some but not all showed evidence of blast injury to the lungs. When exposure to vapor had been intense, edema, congestion, ulceration and denudation extended from the larynx to the smaller bronchi. Gross liver changes were described.

Tissue was sent to centers in Porton and Edgewood for microscopic examination.

In concluding a report he made on the disaster, Lieutenant Stewart Alexander, the Consultant in Chemical Warfare Medicine at A.F.H.Q., gave the following summary:

1. Of 628 mustard casualties, 69 died within the first two weeks. Some of these casualties had associated injuries, primarily blast effects.
2. Casualties were due to mustard vapor and to a mustard-in-oil solution being in contact with the skin for prolonged periods of time.
3. The systemic effects were very severe and of far greater significance than has been associated with mustard burns in the past. This is attributed to prolonged absorption over an enormous body surface exposure.

VIOLATION OF DISASTER MANAGEMENT

In studying the Bari disaster I noted that the lack of any warning that mustard gas was loose, and the failure of decontamination precautions before rushing the injured to hospitals, violated one of the principles of disaster management pointed out by the experience of the Cocoanut Grove fire. *The pattern and nature of the trauma must be ascertained by observers who are not responsible for rescue work and first aid efforts.*

In retrospect the question may be asked, "Why in World War II did the United States have a ship in Italy loaded with mustard gas?"

Eisenhower explained that "we were always forced to carry [it] with us because of uncertainty of German intentions in the use of this weapon . . . we manufactured and carried this material only for reprisal purposes in case of surprise action on the part of the enemy . . . war is always conducted in the realm of the possible and of the estimated rather than of the certainly known." President Franklin D. Roosevelt had declared in 1943 that the United States in accordance with the Geneva Convention would renounce the use of gas warfare unless first used by an enemy.

"On the afternoon preceding the attack on Bari, Air Marshal Sir Arthur Coningham, commanding the British air forces supporting the Eighth Army, held a press conference. The German air forces had been so thoroughly defeated—almost eliminated from the immediate front— that Coningham estimated they had no power to intervene further in the operation. To the assembled press he stated flatly: 'I would regard it as a personal affront and insult if the *Luftwaffe* should attempt any significant action in this area.' The next morning he was definitely more than embarrassed. His newspaper friends did not, by any means, allow him to forget his arbitrary and unqualified statement of the day before." General Eisenhower probably enjoyed the mischief of passing along this story about the Air Marshal, for the Air Force was striving to attain complete independence from the Army. A customary viewpoint of the Army was to accuse the Air Force of having no interest in anything beyond the airstrip.

Dale F. Butler, Travis M. Polk, and Joseph F. Rappold

This chapter highlights the complex machinations of world leaders, international intrigue, and ethical concerns during an often-overlooked historical incident. Dichlorodiethyl sulfide, or mustard gas as it is commonly known, was deployed throughout World War I, but was deemed unlawful in World War II. Despite this, both the Allies and Axis powers regarded it as a necessary countermeasure should the other side deploy it first. This fatal and ultimately preventable disaster was a direct result of these decisions.

Despite chemical weapon use representing a clear violation of international law, today's combat surgeon requires familiarity with all weaponizable caustic agents. Mustard gas was used during the Iraq-Iran War of the 1980s with exposed patients still requiring treatment today. Other chemical weapons such as chlorine and nerve agents have been used during more recent conflicts and terrorist events. Therefore, all deployed surgeons should heed the education on the symptoms and signs of gaseous attacks. Furthermore, physicians in combat must prepare to isolate and decontaminate patients prior to operating on their traumatic injuries.

The Joint Trauma System (JTS) provides education for chemical, biologic, radiologic, and nuclear (CBRN) injuries within its repository of clinical practice guidelines. Perhaps the single most important point is recognizing that a CBRN attack has occurred. During the fog of war, clinicians may miss the manifestations of such an attack in real time, especially while under fire. Thus, it is important for all team members to commit such symptoms to memory and operate under a heightened level of concern in any conflict. If any concern is noted, all personnel must don the appropriate personal protective equipment (PPE) immediately. Failure to apply adequate PPE can quickly convert military medical personnel into additional casualties. In Bari Harbor, due to the clandestine nature of the mustard gas storage, medical personnel were at a significant disadvantage in containing exposure.

Unfortunately, confirmatory testing for mustard gas exposure does not exist; so the physician is left to interpret symptoms under the umbrella of heightened suspicion. Most vesicant agents impact the skin first, causing blistering and wounds appearing as burns. These agents have similar effects on the eyes and respiratory tract during inhalation. Once recognized, time to decontamination is the greatest predictor of ultimate severity for the patient. For ongoing treatment, patients will likely require topical ocular medications to protect the eyes. Cutaneous wounds benefit from local wound care, like thermal burns. Pulmonary symptoms are treated as a chemical pneumonitis and require the appropriate supportive care. British anti-lewisite (BAL) is a chelating agent for use in patients with severe respiratory compromise exposed to a specific form of mustard gas known as lewisite. Due to their mechanism of action via nonspecific DNA alkylation, mustard agents cause significant leukopenia after the third postexposure day, contributing to lethality. Ironically, evaluation of the bone marrow during autopsies conducted by the US Army on Bari Harbor casualties contributed to the early understanding that nitrogen mustard compounds could be used as chemotherapy for cancer treatments.

Experiences from prior engagements—both positive and negative—continuously propel military medicine into the future. The mustard gas exposure in Bari Harbor illustrates how potentially defunct weapons can resurface in any conflict. Military clinicians must maintain a high level of familiarity with all potential battlefield weaponry and their effects.

SUGGESTED READINGS

Amini H, Solaymani-Dodaran M, Mousavi B, et al. Long-term health outcomes among survivors exposed to sulfur mustard in Iran. *JAMA Netw Open*. 2020;3(12): 1–11.

Barbee G, Defeo D, Gonzalez C, et al. (2018). Chemical, radiological, and nuclear injury response part 1: initial response to CBRN agents. Joint Trauma System Clinical Practice Guidelines. Accessed September 17, 2023. https://jts.health.mil/index.cfm/PI_CPGs/cpgs.

Barbee G, Defeo D, Gonzalez C, et al. (2022). Chemical, radiological, and nuclear injury response part 2: medical management of chemical agent exposure. Joint Trauma System Clinical Practice Guidelines. Accessed September 17, 2023. https://jts.health.mil/index.cfm/PI_CPGs/cpgs.

Conant J. *The Great Secret: The Classified World War II Disaster that Launched the War on Cancer*. WW Norton and Company; 2020.

27

Conference—A Trip to Oran[1]

DOCTORS ARE ADDICTED to medical meetings where they can mingle with each other and talk shop to their hearts' content. Colonel Howard H. Hutter, the Surgeon of the Mediterranean Base Section (M.B.S.) was to leave on rotation for the Zone of the Interior and a big farewell party was planned for him in Oran. The program was laid out in an 83-page booklet, the cover of which carried the title: "The Medical Services of the French, British and American Armed Forces and the Physicians and Surgeons of the Department of Oran, Algeria, Present a Clinical Conference on Recent Advances of Medicine in War Time." The conference was scheduled for January 11, 1944. The raison d'être for such a pretentious program booklet was the printing of long abstracts of each presentation in two languages—English and French. The dedication on the third page was as follows:

This clinical conference given under the joint auspices of the medical services of the French, British, and American Armed Forces, and the civilian physicians and surgeons of North Africa, is an attempt to bring to all members of the Medical Profession the knowledge of the most recent advances in Medical Science. As an initial effort, there will be errors in organization, omissions of topics of interest to some, and justifiable complaints from many, on our selection of papiers (sic) for discussion. We ask your indulgence for these mistakes, for there was another purpose for this conference than the dissemination of medical knowledge . . . it endeavors to create a closer and better understanding among the physicians of the United Nations, not only in their relationship as members of the medical profession, but as citizens of a free and democratic world.

---

[1]National Academies of Sciences, Engineering, and Medicine. *A National Trauma Care System: Integrating Military and Civilian Trauma Systems to Achieve Zero Preventable Deaths After Injury* National Academies Press; 2016.

In that spirit, we welcome you. We beg of you to forget nationalistic prejudice, jealousies of civil versus military medicine. We urge you to be physicians first and foremost in an international world of science. We have visualized only one difficulty, that of language differences, and therefore you will find interpreters in every hall, who stand ready to diminish the difficulty of communication you may meet. With that obstacle to our closer friendship mitigated, meet your fellow members of medicine, listen to them, argue with them, talk to them, but out of this conference let us have one lasting benefit . . . a mutual understanding for all problems, not only those of medicine.

The conference boasted of Patrons, a Professional Committee, an Exhibition Committee and an Organization Committee. Listed as Patrons were: M. le Docteur Jules Gasser, Président de la Délégation Spéciale de la Ville d'Oran; Arthur R. Wilson, Brigadier General, U.S.A.; Howard J. Hutter, Colonel, U.S.A., President of the Committee; Xavier G. Cazalas, Colonel, Armée française.

On January 9, Fred Blesse, John Stewart and I flew to Oran so we could reach the municipal theater for the opening of the conference at 9:30 A.M. on the eleventh. It began with an invocation, four welcome addresses and two introductory addresses. Perrin Long and I gave the introductory addresses. I have forgotten what Perry said—perhaps he spoke in French; my address was designed to bring in Ambrose Paré and Baron Larrey as the prototypes of military surgeons, and end on the "miracle" drugs.

E.D.C. Comment: War offers to the military surgeon an opportunity and responsibility for the development of his science that is nonexistent during time of peace. It may be of interest to examine more closely into this opportunity—what it really is and what may be done about it. At first glance it might appear that the only opportunity offered to the military surgeon is the task of raising the surgery of the battlefield to the approximate level of prewar civilian surgery. Certainly many of us responsible for the care of the wounded soldier would find real satisfaction if even this humble goal could always be achieved.

After tracing the history of the evolution of surgery on the battlefields of medieval and renaissance Europe, Sir Clifford Allbutt exclaimed "How large and various was the experience of the battlefield, and how fertile the blood of warriors in rearing good surgeons." The history of surgery repeatedly confirms this statement.

(continued)

The story of Ambrose Paré is all too familiar to recount. One aspect, however, should not be forgotten. It was during a campaign and not in peace time that he perceived that the application of boiling oil to wounds was based on a false doctrine. It was under combat conditions that he set about to perfect methods of amputation because of the prevalence of wound fever. It was at the Siege of Damolliers in 1552 that a successful early amputation of a smashed leg established this operation as a life saving measure for compound fractures.

Baron Larrey, the great surgeon of the Armies of Napoleon, discovered the principle of immediate closure of open pneumothorax by being on the battlefield and actually closing a wound in order to spare the bystanders the spectacle of outpouring blood. To his amazement the desperate condition of the patient improved, and the man recovered. (The soundness of the principle was proved on subsequent cases.)

It is not so easy to point to single dramatic advances that occurred during the War of 1914-18. Surgery at that time was already well along in the era of elaboration of technics that exploited the advent of aseptic technics. As far as technical advances were concerned, Harvey Cushing, in a realistic frame of mind during the Passchendaele Battles of 1917, wrote, "It's an awful business, probably the worst possible training in surgery for a young man and ruinous for the carefully acquired technic of the oldster."

We may well ask what forces have combined against our craft to bring about the startling change from the viewpoint of Allbutt in 1905 to that of Cushing in 1917. Is our experience here and now in this war to be merely an "awful business" or can we make it "large and fertile"?

It is unlikely that great technical advances such as arose from the genius of Paré will be witnessed. The lay press is on the "red alert" for such happenings and fails to understand why accounts of "miracle" operations are not available for every press dispatch. We as surgeons know that there are what the lay consider "miracle" operations being performed daily. Also, as surgeons, we know that they represent only the established standards of our craft.

There are, however, real "miracles" awaiting to be done. Miracles that will further decrease the number of days lost from duty and increase the salvage of manpower for the theater. Miracles that will reduce the disability and invalidism of soldiers who cannot fight again.

To find these miracles one need only set his course by the direction in which peacetime surgery has progressed in recent years. Preoperative care, known now as "resuscitation," needs accurate appraisal and improvement. The methods of use of the sulfonamides call for review to give assurance that these valuable agents are put to the most effective use.

Methods of anesthesia need study as this subspecialty of surgery has not yet found the proper balance between what is convenient and what may be dangerous. The sphere of usefulness of penicillin must now be determined. Early closure of wounds by reparative suture and skin grafting is a matter of untold importance to the strength of the combat force; it is our duty to speed this program to the utmost, armed with the new concepts of infection and the assistance of chemo-therapeutic drugs. The effects of the nutritional state on wound healing, a subject about which a great deal is already known in civilian practice, must be studied and corrective measures instituted in our hospitals. I need not enumerate more.

Only by fostering this type of military surgery can the Medical Corps maintain the prestige set by the great military surgeons of the past. Only a balance between administrative service and professional functions can fulfill our responsibility to our commanders and our patients.

One criticism of these remarks can be answered before it is raised. Civilization does not stage a war to advance the science of surgery—that is obvious. Routine responsibilities of medical officers must be fulfilled and tactical plans for bringing the war to a rapid and victorious ending be relentlessly carried out.

All that is asked is that advantage be taken of the byproducts of our routine work—that surgeons be given the opportunity and facilities to work longer hours and with even more intense application. By simple and entirely practical measures we will be able to seize something constructive from what is otherwise an acme of destruction. As a result of this type of work the proud tradition of the Medical Corps will be carried down the pages of history to future generations of military surgeons; we will have made the most of our opportunity and will have fulfilled our responsibility.

GENERAL PROGRAM

The general program in the municipal theater started at 10:10 A.M. and continued through the remainder of the morning. J. Couniot, lieutenant, Armée francaise, led off with: "Des amputations en chirurgie de guerre." "Noting the silence of our learned societies on this question since 1919, it may seem useless to-day to speak of amputations in war." "Mais: 'si la chirurgie doit rester toujours le même, fût-elle pratiquée sous l'habit militaire' (Lećcne), les conditions stratégiques des guerres diffèrent."

Couniot then referred to the diversified geographic conditions, motorized warfare, new methods of warfare such as land mines and aircraft bombs, the development of sulfa drugs and anti-shock measures. These are the factors, he said, which permit us to look on war amputations in 1943 under a different light than in 1914-1918.

Major Tracy B. Mallory, U.S.A. reported that the files of the Army Medical Museum had already accumulated more than 100 cases of a fatal disease called "lower nephron nephrosis." Two main categories were recognized: those secondary to agents producing extensive hemolysis, and those which appear following sulfonamides.

Major James E. Flinn, Venereal Disease Control, M.B.S., spoke on the recent advances in venereal disease treatment by the use of mapharsen intravenously, in conjunction with intramuscular bismuth subsalicylate in early syphilis and the use of the sulfonamides, fever therapy and penicillin in gonorrhea. At another session in the afternoon, D. J. Djian-Wall of Paris spoke on hereditary syphilis in the city of Oran. In 1936 when the population of the city was 189,240, the known death of 372 newborns from hereditary syphilis occurred. Among the natives it was five times more prevalent than among Europeans. For the last nine months of 1943, these percentages, based on a population of 241,295, "are nearly the same for the mortality and are increased for the mortality in the first year of syphilitic debility; that may be in connection with the conditions of war. . . ."

A paper by Commander F. C. Greaves, U.S. Navy, was so interesting that I noted it at length in my diary. It was entitled: "Experimental Study of Underwater Concussion." He had demonstrated on laboratory animals that blast injury resulting in death was attributable to pulmonary damage. Intestinal lesions were inconstant and there were no injuries to the central nervous system. The determining factor in injury to the tissues is the presence of air or gas in the tissues; the more air or gas that is present, the greater the injury. Protection with kapok or rubber foam reduced injuries. Greaves gave an exposition of the zones of dangerous effects to a swimmer on the surface with varying depths of the explosion.

Two papers were given on the treatment of burns. The first was by Henri Laborit, a doctor of the French Navy. He had never heard of the Koch-Allen school or of the Cocoanut Grove fire, so recommended avoidance of greasy dressings and advocated tannic acid, mercurochrome or gentian violet as local applications. Harvey Allen expounded the gospel of aseptic care of the open burned surfaces and early closure of granulating areas. Plasma requirements, he said, may amount to several liters and secondary anemia and reduced plasma proteins must be corrected. "The burned surface," Allen continued, "should be cared for as any other open wound, with the same aseptic and gentle handling of tissues as are demanded in the operating theater. The wounds should be cleansed carefully and covered with a nonadherent dressing and this followed by a large resilient pressure dressing. Splinting is as necessary for a burned part as for a fracture."

Members of the Army Nurse Corps, directed by Captain Lucille Spaulding, then ended the morning program with a demonstration of the new wardrobe for nurses which was gradually replacing the old issue models.

In the afternoon, as in a state medical society meeting, the program was divided into sections: one in surgery, two in medicine, one in laboratory and diagnostic medicine, and one in dentistry, the latter including the management of wounds of the face. Exhibits in the Lycée Lamoricière included the mobile optical unit of the U.S. Army—a soldier might be helpless, and thereby doomed, if his glasses were broken during combat. It was equally impossible for a soldier to get along on the American or British field ration without proper chewing surfaces.

Major Henry G. Schwartz, U.S.A., and Captain George E. Rhoulhac had prepared a demonstration on neurosurgical technics. F. L. Soper, of the Rockefeller Foundation, demonstrated a method of delousing, a subject which was of great practical importance as a preventive measure to avoid typhus.

The section on surgery met at 2:00 P.M. in the municipal theater. Pelham Glasier led off with a paper on varicose veins. This was followed by Samuel P. Harbison on traumatic aneurysm; Major Roland R. Best, U.S.A., spoke on wounds of the intestine and Major John Martin, of the 12th General Hospital, spoke on the immediate treatment of craniocerebral injuries. Lieutenant Colonel Earl R. Crowder, who was of great assistance as Consultant in Radiology, read a contribution on spondylolisthesis. I was delighted to renew my acquaintance with Capitaine E. Curtillet, of the French Army, who read a paper on wounds of the thorax. He advocated immediate closure of an open pneumothorax at the earliest possible moment.

> . . .l'oxygenothérapie doit être continue et massive—aspiration et hémostase par coagulation sont de première utilité.
>
> L'intervention complète peut être remise de 24 à 48 heures dans certains cas.
>
> 2. Le problème des premiers jours est un problème d'évacuation. Intérêt de fixer le blessé dans une formation de l'arrière, difficultés de transport dues à la fragilité de son état s'y opposent. Le transport par avion, sous réserve de certaines précautions (pas dans le première semaine, a rendu de trés grande services en Tunisie.
>
> 3. Le problème des semaines suivantes est double:
>
>   a) Traitement des infections secondaires, bien classiques:
>
>   b) Traitement des corps étrangers inclus. Le procédé de la pince de Petit de la Villeon est parfois indiqué, d'autres fois on devra intervenir à ciel ouvert.

Colonel Lee Cady, of the 21st General Hospital, presided at one of the medical sections and Colonel Merritt G. Ringer at the other. Leprosy, amoebiasis, typhus, bacillary dysentery and malaria, as well as the prevalent epidemic hepatitis, were subjects discussed. The physicians of North Africa were excellent clinicians and had far greater experience with these tropical and subtropical diseases than the physicians of our Medical Corps. This was also true in the section on laboratory and diagnostic medicine.

John Devin B. Watson, Dawn M. Coleman, and Marc A. de Moya

This chapter ostensibly focuses on a 1944 clinical conference of the American, French, and Allied forces in the Mediterranean theater. The first half of the chapter quotes from Churchill's plenary address in which he examines the foundational contributions of "military surgeon prototypes" Ambrose Paré and Baron Larrey while pondering various "miracles." He cites, "War offers to the military surgeon an opportunity and responsibility for the development of his science that is nonexistent during time of peace." He qualifies that while many seek surgical "miracles" from the war, the real miracles come from the medical advances on the battlefield. He concludes his address with a simple request: that surgeons be permitted to "take advantage of the byproducts of (their) routine work . . . to seize something constructive from what is otherwise an acme of destruction," thus further advancing care.

The remainder of the chapter summarizes the general program and the various presentations given by the numerous Allied clinicians, nurses, and dentists, both in English and in French. While Churchill expresses enthusiasm for the intellectual stimulation from the academic topics addressed, war-weary clinicians derived perhaps even more benefit from the esprit de corps with colleagues and the *je ne sais quoi* from an in-person meeting many months into this brutal conflict.

Churchill submits that during World War II, surgery and medicine were unlikely to have the "great technical advances" that were observed during the times of Ambrose Paré and Baron Larrey. In hindsight, we now appreciate that the early 1940s began what many consider the sweet spot of medicine—a period spanning the widespread availability of penicillin through the era of managed care—in which surgical innovation exploded. Churchill cites various clinical entities such as lower nephron nephrosis post sulfonamide administration that would have taken years or perhaps decades to characterize without the continuous influx of relatively young, healthy wounded troops. Viewed within the context of contemporary war surgery, how many years would it have taken to advance the concepts of damage control surgery, temporary abdominal closure, tourniquets, and shunting for civilian trauma, if not for the surgical experiences in Iraq and Afghanistan? While Churchill suggests that the surgical miracles seen in the Paré/Larrey era are not readily visible, the actual data presented clearly suggest otherwise.

The trip's most important value to Churchill was the synthesis of unity and understanding among the Allied clinicians. In modern parlance, this would be framed as burnout prevention. Sadly, post-COVID, continuing medical education (CME), society meetings, and even oral board exams are conducted virtually or in hybrid configurations. While this virtual approach to medical education has some pragmatic benefits, it threatens the "unity and understanding" that Churchill describes. The salutary effects on surgeon wellness are degraded. Reflecting on our own experiences, these meetings offered innumerable opportunities for mentorship and sponsorship through networking in person at conferences. How many academic projects have stemmed from chance meetings with other surgeons? "A Trip to Oran" describes the truth that most of us already know: we attend conferences during deployments and in civilian life under the auspices of CME and academic presentations, but we benefit perhaps even more from reconnecting with old friends and colleagues, making new alliances, and recharging our batteries in a way that allows us to return refreshed to the trenches of clinical medicine.

SUGGESTED READINGS

Duchesne JC, McSwain NE, Cotton BA, et al. Damage control resuscitation: the new face of damage control. *J Trauma*. 2010:69(4):976-990.

Gifford SM, Aidinian G, Clouse WD, et al. Effect of temporary shunting on extremity vascular injury: an outcome analysis from the Global War on Terror vascular injury initiative. *J Vasc Surg*. 2009;50(3):549-555; discussion 555-556.

Meredith JW. Looking to the future on the shoulders of giants. *J Am Coll Surg*. 2012;214(4): 385-389.

Sibley JB. Meeting the future: how CME portfolios must change in the post-COVID era. *J Eur CME*. 2022; 11(1):2058452.

28

Italy After the Fall of Rome

ALLIED TROOPS arrived at Rome on June 4, 1944, Rome having been declared an "open city." General Martin was in the first party to enter Rome. As Fifth Army Surgeon, his first urgent task was to find structures for use by three Evacuation Hospitals—the 15th, the 56th and the 94th. The 38th Evacuation Hospital was set up in tents in a grove of the "Pines of Rome." Buildings were also selected to be used by station hospitals and general hospitals. In moving into buildings, the first thing that had to be done was eliminate booby traps; reconstruction of plumbing facilities and of the electrical wiring followed. Fifth Army engineers were well versed in this from their experience in Naples.

Between May 25 and June 4, during the so-called "battle of pursuit" with the retreating Germans, the wounded had been evacuated by plane and boats, thereby avoiding the overland journey to Naples. North of Rome the pursuit still continued for 150 miles—to the Arno River. Destruction of bridges and roads by the Germans delayed the Allied Armies so that it took six weeks to reach the Arno. The main axis of progress for the U.S. Army was Highway 1, the coastal road through Civitavecchia, Grosseto, Piombino, Livorno and Pisa. The French used Highway 2, the inland route through Viterbo, Siena and Poggibonsi to Firenze. The Arno was reached on the twenty-third of July and the advance was brought to a halt by General Clark to give the Army a well-earned rest.

The expression "The Fall of Rome" is used by many writers. Strictly speaking, an open city cannot "fall"; only armed bastions or defended cities "fall." I used the phrase in the title of an article sent to the Surgeon General at this time. The "Fall of Rome" was used deliberately in the title to establish priority for the surgeons of the North African-Mediterranean Theater for their many important contributions to military surgery (see Appendix E, The Surgical Management of the Wounded in the Mediterranean Theater at the Time of the Fall of Rome).

On the day the troops entered Rome, I was in Naples. From 800 to 900 casualties a day were being evacuated. A row of eight C-47's, with nurses busily working with the casualties as they were being loaded on, were standing on the dusty field. The Tyrrhenian Sea in the background cooled the breeze. Thunderbolt fighter planes were zooming about—landing, taking off, curving past as if standing on wing-tip. Ambulances with litter cases kept pulling in with passive casualties whose personal effects were in plasma boxes. Litter handlers passed leisure time with small talk reminiscent of a midwest railroad station. Dusty drivers with goggles sat in jeeps waiting. Occasional tanks or armored vehicles clanked down the road to Ordnance repair or from Ordnance to the front.

My mind goes back, now, to a flight I took that day with some of the wounded. Once again I am there—in a plane with nineteen litter cases, twelve of them with chest wounds. It is hot; the smell of sweat is heavy. I sit in the tail on a pile of parachutes and May Wests and watch the take off over flooded Pontine marshes and over the coast. I put on the ear-phones of the tail radio set and enter the world of the air—most of it is completely unintelligible. "Leader-over your landing gear—Roger—over—Ba-a—Ba-a—Ba-a—Ba-a—runway—over—One at a time—One at a time—coming in—Ba-a—Ba-a—Ba-a—runway—over. Remain clear of runway until further advice—over—Blue Three—There have been two trucks down there since 8:00. Shall we go down for them? Roger—B-Baker—D-Dog. Blue Four—the runway is clear for you—Ba-a—Ba-a—Ba-a. There seems to be some M.P.s on the road just south of where the smoke is coming from—pancake—over. Go ahead—until further advice—over—Roger."

I stopped at a number of hospitals that day, including the 225th Station Hospital. There I found quite a bit of excitement—a British bomb had been found behind the hospital and preparations were being made for opening it. Everyone was cleared from the nearby area but, fortunately, the detonator was unscrewed successfully and there was no explosion.

TRANSFUSION AND HEPATITIS

The next day, June 5, Bill Stone and Bill Munly called a meeting to discuss the meaning of the greatly increased usage of whole blood for transfusion in the base section hospitals. Bill Stone and General Stayer had the erroneous impression that blood transfusions were being used on patients with advanced sepsis merely to build them up. John Stewart, Frank Berry, Tracy Mallory, Gene Sullivan, Perrin Long, Virgil Cornell and I were at this meeting. I presented the surgical aspects of the program of reparative wound surgery and early delayed closure which had led to the increased usage of whole blood for transfusion—that we were preventing the deterioration and anemia of advanced sepsis by penicillin, blood and reparative surgery. With the use of a blackboard I explained that transfusion was used in the forward area for resuscitation and the preparation of the patient to withstand surgery. In certain instances it was used for the supportive treatment of patients held because of the nature of the wound, early infection or delay in evacuation. At the base, transfusion was used for the correction of secondary anemia to prepare the patient to withstand reparative surgery with its added loss of blood.

In the 21st General Hospital during April, 1944, United States Army battle casualties admitted numbered 283; accidental injuries, 125. In May, 789 battle casualties and 107 injuries were admitted. French admissions were 437. Blood transfusions numbered 545 in April and 579 in May. In April, with a backlog of septic cases being cleaned up, transfusions numbered 2 per battle casualty; in May, keeping abreast of current admissions, there were 0.5 transfusions per battle casualty.

At this time the medical staffs and consultants were busy with the growing incidence of infectious hepatitis. Some interesting observations were recorded for the first time, throwing light on such features as the incubation period. The following case was of particular interest:

A member of a hospital detachment played baseball and was strong enough to hit a home run. This was on a Saturday. He donated blood on Tuesday afternoon. This blood was given to a recipient on Wednesday morning. The donor felt poorly for the first time on Thursday, and on Saturday was admitted as a patient with jaundice. On Sunday he was delirious, then comatose and died that evening. An autopsy was performed. The recipient, on the seventh day after the transfusion, showed increase in lymphocytes. On the tenth day the cephalin test was positive. Headaches began on the seventeenth day. On the twenty-third day chemical tests showed the disease but patient denied all symptoms. On the night of the twenty-third day following the transfusion, he had a chill and fever and became jaundiced.

The physicians were beginning to recognize that variance in severity of hepatitis may not be attributable to increased virulence of the virus but to changes in the resistance of the host, one determinant being diet. I wrote in my notes, on June 5, 1944, that the same consideration holds for the treatment of wounds—and that it must be ascertained what can be carried out in any particular theater or group of troops.

On the evening of June 6, I was with Jack McKittrick, Red Burrage and Frank Berry listening to late radio reports of the Normandy invasion. There was a "sad" note in the broadcast from Berlin: "What is this you are doing to us and to yourselves?"

On June 7, Trygve Gundersen expressed his discouragement about getting the ophthalmic surgery organized and in competent hands. General Stayer told him that a Boston man had tried to set up special centers in World War I and it didn't work. He was referring to Harvey Cushing's attempt to centralize head wounds. Stayer insisted that a general hospital could handle everything. I agreed that they should be able to do so, but the fact remained that some could not. Also, battle casualties were still widely scattered in station hospitals.

MEDICAL HISTORY OF SALERNO

It was on the seventh of June that Frank Berry, Guy Wells and I made a pilgrimage to Salerno to see if any trace existed of the School of Salerno, famous in the history of medicine. We finally located a small Franciscan church with a plump, soft-eyed priest who claimed this was the site, or at least the area of, the original school. Later it was moved to the Dom which we then visited. It is also the burial place of St. Thomas Aquinas. The cathedral with its fancy marbled basilica enshrines the tomb of St. Matthew. To me, the most beautiful thing in the cathedral was a faded mural depicting the walled city of Salerno with a landing assault being made with ancient men-of-war and galleys.

Salerno had been a health resort in ancient times. The traditions of Greek medicine lingered for centuries in southern Italy and Sicily and some type of medical corporation existed in Salerno in the ninth century. Attacks by sea, such as pictured in the cathedral, had been made by the Saracens and by the Normans and helped make Salerno a clearing house of medical ideas and recipes. It reflected a grand mixture of barbarian, Latin, Greek, Jewish and Muslim influences. The so-called "School of Salerno" came into existence over a period of time although the activity centered in it was not tangible until the first half of the eleventh century. It was the earliest scientific school of Christian Europe.

Salerno was never a fountainhead of scientific and medical learning, such as were many cities of the Po Valley compared with which its literary contributions were very humble. It was, however, the earliest distributing center of medical ideas in Europe. The first step in a long evolution which was to culminate in the production of Pasteur. The earliest official document of the school was a charter granted in 1231 by the Emperor Frederick II, but as George Sarton remarks: "By that time the heyday of Salerno was over." The importance of the school had grown rapidly in the second half of the eleventh century and the heyday was the twelfth century.

AFTER SALERNO

That same day Frank Berry, Jim Thompson, Clarence Dunn and I visited the 1st Canadian General Hospital at Avellino. A few days earlier I had made an indiscreet remark to Cliff Thompson at the Orange Grove Allied Officers' Club overlooking the Bay of Naples. I had expressed a fear that there would be many Canadians with one short leg limping about after the war because of the method they were using to treat compound battle fractures of the femur. Thompson sent for Gardner and we had a long discussion on fractures of the femur. "The basic difference between Gardner and our fracture experts," I noted in my diary, "lies in his claim that he can reduce the fracture and maintain length and alignment by a single plaster spica during 'closed plaster' treatment of the compounding soft part wound. In the U.S. Army we admit that the closed plaster may be useful as an expedient during an overwhelming rush of casualties or in hospitals subject to unexpected evacuation, but beyond this usage we see no place for Truetta types of treatment." On the subject of the Spanish Civil War, the conversation turned to Jolley's "three-point-forward system," and I explained the improvement we had made in Sicily by having a hospital physical proximity to the triage point.

At the officers' mess another guest, in addition to our group, was Brigadier Hollenby in tartans. We were piped in and the formal toast to the piper followed. The 1st Canadian General Hospital had brought two pipers with them—two Scots from Saskatchewan piping in Avellino, Italy!

I spent the next day, June 8, with Lang Parsons in the 52nd Station Hospital in Naples. Patients with maxillofacial wounds were being concentrated in this hospital, designed as a special center.

I learned a great deal from him about the problems of this type of patient. The total admissions from April 9, 1944, to June 8, 1944, numbered 334; of these, 87 had been discharged to duty by the end of the period, 4 to the Zone of the Interior, and 1 had died. The census on May 31 was 220—compound fractures of the mandible or maxilla, 76; serious soft tissue wounds, 95; minor wounds, 49. It was believed that they were achieving a higher salvage for duty, a quicker turnover of patients and a more effective reduction in deformities.

Parsons was most perceptive about the needs of these patients, both physical and morale. He wrote an excellent and full report that was forwarded to the Surgeon General. My own notes on the basis of this visit were as follows:

E.D.C. Comments: These patients require constant supervision and treatment rather than an emphasis on operation and gadgeteering. Dietetics are a major consideration as a liquid diet and special feeding devices are needed for patients with wired jaws. The nursing load is heavy with irrigations, mouth washes and hot packs. Tracheostomy care is time-consuming.

At the time of admission the morale of patients is at a low ebb because of the emotional stress that accompanies facial wounds. A deep sense of personal integrity centers in the face and it is helpful to their morale for patients to be grouped when there is necessity for facial bandages, or an inability to speak because of jaw wiring or tracheostomy. Many of these patients walk about and must assemble in the mess for ambulatory patients. In a general hospital these men feel conspicuous and are stared at by other patients. In a special center they become inconspicuous in a group with similar defects. Also, they see the favorable results of corrective surgery and early rehabilitation. The sum of these considerations probably outweighs the expertness of technical management in the creation of a special center.

The large soft part defects are conspicuous by their absence. Certainly in the past many of these hideous deformities were caused by retraction of the superficial muscles of the face added to sepsis and fibrosis in the contracted position. Early splinting of bony parts— control of infection by proper drainage, hot dressings, pressure bandages and chemotherapy, careful approximation in the forward area, all tend to minimize these shocking mutilations. Here again, skin defects produced *by the missile itself* are rare and when they do occur are likely to be fatal immediately because of hemorrhage, asphyxia or the lethal nature of the wound.

Tracheostomy has not been stressed sufficiently in the early management, but is being done with increasing frequency. Efforts to create a special center in a base section are justified.

Both World War I and World War II have developed a generation of plastic surgeons and oral surgeons skilled and experienced in the management of maxillofacial wounds. Air evacuation, special centers, both overseas and in the Zone of Interior, have contributed to the better management in addition to technical advancements in prosthetic oral surgery.

By June 9, disquieting reports were pouring into Naples that the hospitals in Rome were choked with German wounded. The radio reported 8,000 wounded prisoners of war. An organizational change had set up an echelon known as Allied Armies in Italy (A.A.I.) responsible for correlation between the Fifth Army and P.B.S. "Of course" I recorded in my diary, "there is no U.S.A. Medical Corps representative in A.A.I.!"

At dinner with Frank Berry, Jack McKittrick and Claude Welch the conversation drifted to the surgical experience of war. "We are not," I noted, "training general surgeons in war, but giving an intensive, postgraduate course in the surgery of trauma from which experienced surgeons will profit but men without basic training will only acquire bad habits. The 'tendon-lengthening-scoliosis arthropods' are unhappy in wound surgery, just as the 'chest-wall-ribcutting thoracic surgeons' are unhappy. Broad experience in the surgery of trauma throws the short-comings of narrow regional specialties into the spotlight. Specialties may be built about diagnostic instruments such as the cystoscope or the bronchoscope. The art of looking down holes includes the otoscope and the proctoscope. The surgery of trauma is more comparable to the surgery of neoplastic disease or the 'surgery of infection.' Trauma also cuts across all regional specialties."

The following morning Eldridge Campbell came over and we talked about the quality of neurosurgery. He was working to clean up a heavy workload at the 66th Station Hospital, where many prisoners of war with head wounds were lodged. After lunch, Larry Poole, Eldridge and I paid a visit to a French Hospital to see Pierre Stricker. A nurse was wrestling with a huge cerebral fungus which had erupted through a fractured skull. (Herniation of the brain with sepsis is an interesting phenomenon and it also occurs in the eyeball.) There are other distressing cases in Stricker's neurosurgical ward—incontinent colonial troops—flies. The small staff was working under terrible handicaps.

On June 13, a cable came, requesting that Frank Berry return to the United States for assignment as Consultant to the Army Ground Forces. This obviously emanated from Fred Blesse, who had returned to the States in May for duty at the headquarters of the Army Ground Forces. General Stayer had been appointed Surgeon of NATOUSA to succeed him.

We had had little opportunity to become acquainted with General Stayer so Frank and I went to P.B.S. headquarters to discuss the matter with Arnest and Bill Munly. Munly said he thought that refusal was impossible. He also thought that the position could be a particularly important one in bringing a different professional point of view to the ground forces.

Frank and I planned a visit to Rome and to some of the Fifth Army medical installations before he left for the States. The Fifth Army was now strung out 100 miles beyond Rome with virtually no contact with the enemy. The tales of 8,000 wounded prisoners of war in Rome had not been confirmed. In fact, Arnest and Munly said there were only twelve in Rome and about 100 in some hospital north of Rome.

The next day, before we left, Charlotte Rantoul came for lunch. She was now a Red Cross worker with the 340th Bomb Group, an outfit that had lost eighty-eight bombers when Vesuvius had erupted recently. On moving to Corsica, the group had then lost both personnel and planes when twenty-four German planes raided their base a week after they arrived.

Frank and I intended spending the night at the 59th Evacuation Hospital on the former Anzio beachhead, so we drove along the shore road and across the Pontine marshes. We found Mathewson and Roy Cohn, who reported that the hospital was badly upset by "C.O.itis"—a new term that was coming into my diary notes meaning: Inflamed at or by the commanding officer.

On the morning of June 15, Berry and Churchill entered Rome. We found our way past the Coliseum, around St. Peter's, out the road toward Civitavecchia to the 59th Evacuation Hospital, which was in the House of the Good Shepherd on the northern outskirts of the city. We spent that afternoon seeing the sights with Jim Forsee, who was looking for a site for the 2nd Auxiliary Group.

Continuing north on Highway 1 the following morning, we arrived at the 93rd Evacuation Hospital, which was located in a wheat field. There we had lunch with Don Currier, Howard Patterson, Eddie Harding and Stamford. We then went on to the 94th Evacuation Hospital where we sat around in the x-ray room discussing clinical problems until late in the evening. A patient with a machine gun bullet in the mediastinum stirred up an argument about surgical exploration on the basis of possible injury to the esophagus.

The following day, June 17, we reached a platoon of the 33rd Field Hospital, located near Oribello. Tom Ballantine, Luther Wolf, Fred Jarvis and others of the 2nd Auxiliary Group made rounds, concentrating on a number of seriously wounded men. The triage had been selective and the surgery excellent. Returning to the 94th Evacuation Hospital, we had a session on chest wounds with Larry Shefts, Sig Sanzene, Charlie Rife and Howard Snyder. Howard "cross examined" Shefts to bring out how radical he was in the indications for operation—always a subject for argument in World War II. It seemed to me we were in agreement on all major points. After supper, on our way back, we stopped at Civitavecchia to see two railway guns captured from the Germans. Nearby was a bronze statue of St. Francis d'Assisi with arms outstretched, standing before his ruined church.

A TALK WITH GENERAL STAYER

My diary records that we were back in Rome on June 18 and that Champ Lyons, Oscar Hampton and Howard Snyder "were holding a 'session' on the usage of penicillin." Afterwards we paid a visit to the Vatican and the Sistine Chapel. His Holiness Pope Pius XII granted an audience to British and Americans, which we attended, and then we toured parts of the Vatican Museum. In the late afternoon we went to the 15th Evacuation Hospital where we had supper and sat on the roof in the warm evening with Frank Lever, Charlie Wasden and Dan Mulvihill.

My diary also notes that I had located "Rappaport's old book shop" at the top of the Spanish Steps that lead from the Palazzo di Spagna to the terrace in front of the S. Trinita de Monti and Hotel Hassler, and that "I bought a copy of Carsten Niebuhr's *Description de L'Arabie*—a book often referred to by Doughty" (**Figure 28.1**).

The drive back to Anzio was a long one, but on arrival one of the surgeons cooked us a late supper of shad roe and scallops. The following night a farewell party was given for Frank by the 9th Evacuation Hospital, replete with beefsteaks, speeches and toasts.

ALLIED FORCE HEADQUARTERS

2 May, 1945

SPECIAL ORDER OF THE DAY

Soldiers, Sailors and Airmen of the Allied Forces in the Mediterranean Theatre

After nearly two years of hard and continuous fighting which started in Sicily in the summer of 1943, you stand today as the victors of the Italian Campaign.

You have won a victory which has ended in the complete and utter rout of the German armed forces in the Mediterranean. By clearing Italy of the last Nazi aggressor, you have liberated a country of over 40,000,000 people.

Today the remnants of a once proud Army have laid down their arms to you—close on a million men with all their arms, equipment and impedimenta.

You may well be proud of this great and victorious campaign which will long live in history as one of the greatest and most successful ever waged.

No praise is high enough for you sailors, soldiers, airmen and workers of the United Forces in Italy for your magnificent triumph.

My gratitude to you and my admiration is unbounded and only equalled by the pride which is mine in being your Commander-in-Chief.

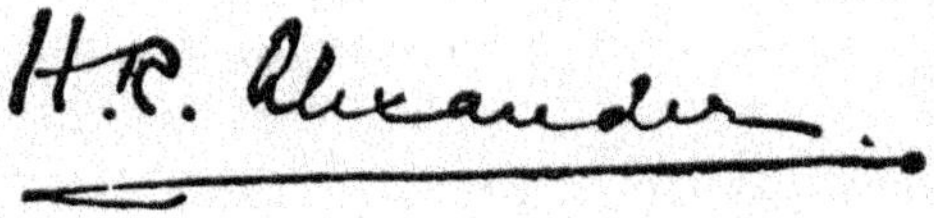

H. R. Alexander

Field-Marshal,
Supreme Allied Commander,
Mediterranean Theatre.

Figure 28.1 A special order of the day.

On June 20, Frank and I took a plane back to Algiers where he shared my billet. General Stayer was in his office, and this time I spoke to him. I told him about the cable requesting Frank as Consultant to the Ground Forces in Washington, that we could not afford to lose him and that, furthermore,

Frank did not want to leave. General Stayer was quite annoyed—he said that I should have brought the matter to him immediately.

"Are you afraid of me?" he asked.

"No, sir," I replied. "Should I be?"

General Stayer moved quickly to get Frank's orders cancelled and arranged that he be made Surgical Consultant to the Seventh Army in Colonel Myron Rudolph's office.

Reynold Henry, Robert B. Lim, and Scott B. Armen

In this chapter, Dr Churchill recounts his experiences upon arriving in Rome, where advanced care facilities were being positioned to care for the wounded returning from the front lines as Allied Forces pushed deep into Axis territory. Dr Churchill spent much of his time in Rome conferencing with colleagues, reviewing complications and treatment strategies, and discussing trauma systems issues. A casual reader might even suggest that he neatly assumed the role of a trauma system medical director. Indeed, in this chapter, Churchill recounts many conversations regarding the practices of surgery, occurring not only during dinner but also while sightseeing. His experiences correlate well with the modern-day surgical peer review, morbidity and mortality, and case conferences.

The first meetings Churchill recalls are those regarding the use of whole blood, initially misinterpreted by his superiors, as a treatment for septic patients. By this time, the US Army Medical Corps had become quite savvy in the collection and use of whole blood. The mortality of soldiers reaching the equivalent of Role 2 treatment facilities was effectively cut in half. This was largely due to the liberal use of whole blood and plasma transfusion. Contrary to the beliefs of his superiors, Dr Churchill (and presumably his colleagues) were using whole blood in a manner similar to how it is used today, as the fluid of choice for initial resuscitation as well as a means to prepare patients to withstand complex surgical interventions. Regrettably, following the Vietnam War, whole blood was almost universally replaced by component therapy based on the dual rationale that most patients do not need whole blood and that dividing donated units into components allows for the ability to treat more patients per unit of blood collected. However, as with many phenomena in medicine, whole blood has been "rediscovered" for the management of acutely bleeding patients, accelerated by the recent wartime experiences with warm fresh whole blood and low-titer type O whole blood (LTOWB) in Afghanistan and Iraq.

During Churchill's time in Rome, the topic of using specialized centers for the care of system-based problems resurfaced, particularly for specialties such as ophthalmology, otolaryngology, maxillofacial surgery, neurosurgery, and plastics. This model had proven successful in civilian practice in the continental United States during Churchill's era, especially in the care of nontraumatic pathologies such as various cancers, cardiac conditions, and pediatric illnesses. At the time of his writing, trauma surgery did not exist as a discrete, recognized field, and he alludes to the fact that surgeons of various niche specialties were displeased to perform the "jack-of-all-trades" work required for trauma care. On the other hand, Churchill hints that sub-specialization significantly degrades the broad surgical skills needed in combat.

Ultimately, the distributed model proposed by Churchill would require untenable and unsustainable resources, personnel, and logistical support, as noted in prior chapters and commentaries. Today, trauma centers where all specialists are gathered in a single facility, have repeatedly shown to provide the best outcomes for the full gamut of traumatic injuries. In a deployed setting, this correlates well to Role 3 facilities which afford complex patients the care they need in a timely manner.

SUGGESTED READINGS

DuBose JJ, Browder T, Inaba K, Teixeira PG, Chan LS, Demetriades D. Effect of trauma center designation on outcome in patients with severe traumatic brain injury. *Arch Surg.* 2008;143:1213-1217; discussion 7.

Gurney JM, Jensen SD, Gavitt BJ, et al. Committee on Surgical Combat Casualty Care position statement on the use of single surgeon teams and invited commentaries. *J Trauma Acute Care Surg.* 2022 Aug 1;93(2S Suppl 1):S6-S11.

Gurney JM, Tadlock MD, Dengler BA, et al. Committee on Surgical Combat Casualty Care position statement: neurosurgical capability for the optimal management of traumatic brain injury during deployed operations. *J Trauma Acute Care Surg.* 2023 Aug 1;95(2S Suppl 1):S7-S12.

King LS. Blood program in world war II. Medical Department, United States Army. *JAMA.* 1965;191:954.

Vanderspurt CK, Spinella PC, Cap AP, et al. The use of whole blood in US military operations in Iraq, Syria, and Afghanistan since the introduction of low-titer Type O whole blood: feasibility, acceptability, challenges. *Transfusion.* 2019;59:965-970.

29

V.I.P. Visit

On July 3, 1944, while I was in Algiers, I received a message requesting me to join a "Very Important Person" party in Rome at the earliest possible time. The Chief of Staff issued orders for my passage on a special plane that was leaving the next morning at 8:30. I packed up my records and files at the office and then returned to my billet where I stuffed my clothes into a valpak. After dinner at the Aletti I had a farewell drink *chez* Mairesse—the billet I had lived in since my arrival in Algiers on March 6, 1943. The next morning I left Maison Blanche and flew, first, to Caserta.

After the fall of Rome, A.F.H.Q. had moved from Algiers to Caserta. I hadn't as yet moved with it. Here, much of the royal palace—La Reggia di Caserta, located about twenty-two miles northeast of Naples—had been converted into offices. Portable living quarters for personnel had been set up in the gardens behind it.

As I have related in **Chapter 25** (From Capri to Typhus), I had been to the palace before, when it had been used as the headquarters of the Fifth Army Rear. Although I have given some description of it, it deserves at least a bit more. The palace, designed by the architect Luigi Vanvitelli in the neo-classic style, is one of the most magnificent palaces in the world, with four courtyards and a decor in marble that features the many varieties and colors of marble found in Italy. Adjoining the palace is a park with a magnificent fishpond, fountains, cascades and wooded hills, all of it breathtaking.

Although I walked through the interior of the royal apartments a few times, those parts of the palace not taken over for military offices were less familiar to me than the park. Cascades and fountains extended to the north to "Cascade Camp" where I had my billet. I drove back and forth along this stretch of road or walked along the fishpond every day. The fishpond was 475 meters in length and filled by water pouring from the throats of enormous dolphins. Cascades, waterfalls, rapids and fountains marked the descent of the water toward the palace.

Balustrades of pillars and statues of hunters and huntresses led finally— some 2,700 meters from the palace—to two large marble groups at the fifth cascade. One portrayed Diana and her nine nymphs, the other Acteon being attacked by the dogs. These groups arose from a large basin and stood in front of a veil of water fed by rapids that descended from above like a huge stairway.

From the basin where Diana was surrounded by her nymphs, one entered the English Garden—and one of the first portable houses behind large holly trees was my billet, which I shared with General Stayer. This garden was green with majestic plane trees and cedars of Lebanon.

In the English Garden there were large ravines, a small stream, a small lake with a chalet and a statue of Venus, ruins of a pagan temple in a subterranean passage, and artificial stones, statues from Pompeii, nymphs and fauns.

The medical offices were on the fifth floor of the palace, where 5,000 square feet of space had been reserved for both American and British medical sections. It so happened that *each* section had requisitioned this amount of space but the requests had been handled as *one*. A couple of our men were working on the problem of trying to obtain more space.

TRIP TO ROME AND NAPLES

On July 5, the Commanding General's plane took me to Rome. I sat in the cockpit with the pilot as we flew over the mountains close above Cassino and the monastery. In Rome I went to the Grand Hotel where, before I could even investigate getting a room, I was approached by General Stayer and Surgeon General Kirk, who had accompanied the V.I.P.—Henry Stimson, the Secretary of War. General Stayer's first reaction was: "Why did you come to Rome? I wanted you in Naples!"—but before the day was over he kept referring to why he had wanted me to come to Rome. I had already learned to hold my tongue when General Stayer was exploding. What really annoyed the General was that Secretary Stimson should be traveling with Norman Kirk as his personal physician. Kirk was a surgeon, and General Stayer knew he would not be dispensing pills to the Secretary and his traveling companions (**Figure 29.1**).

Kirk, Stayer and I paid a short visit to the 12th General Hospital where we had lunch and then made brief rounds with several of the staff—Mason, Allen and Langstrom. We then returned to the Grand Hotel where I was presented to Secretary Stimson. In his party was Harvey H. Bundy of Boston, Special Assistant to the Secretary of War (1941-45). The 33rd General Hospital was chosen for the Secretary to visit. He conducted his own rounds, refusing to be guided by anyone. Finally he went out to the tent wards in the July heat and dust, greeting each patient briefly, sometimes pausing to ask, "How were you wounded, soldier?" And this is when the incident I mentioned earlier took place.

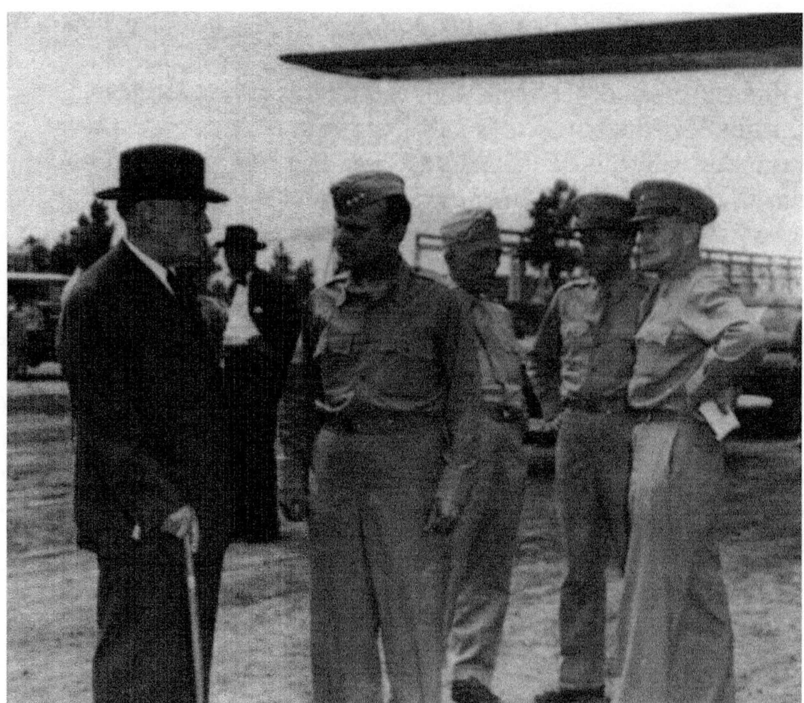

Figure 29.1 Secretary of War Henry Stimson during visit to Italy.

The tent ward for patients with venereal disease lay ahead, and despite Eldridge Campbell's trying to run interference the Secretary walked into the first tent. After I managed to tell him that these soldiers were not wounded but had "infectious diseases," he grasped the point and hurried along.

Kirk, General Stayer and I then went to the 6th General Hospital which had recently moved into the House of the Good Shepherd. Tom Goethals was waiting for us at the gate. We saw many of the surgical staff and as yet they had few patients. After brief stops at the 73rd Station Hospital and the 24th General Hospital we returned to the hotel where I obtained a room. I had a long talk with Norman Kirk and, when he had to leave to attend a formal state dinner, General Stayer and I dined in solitary grandeur.

An extract of a letter I wrote to my wife, relates the above events: "Accompanied the Surgeon General on his recent tour of inspection in this Theater, entering the orbit of *the elderly statesman* like a meteor scarcely visible to the naked eye. The SG was very appreciative of our work here and repeatedly introduced me as their best consultant in overseas theaters! Take *cum grano salis* as usual. At any rate, I thrive on appreciation so everything was rosy. Met your remote cousin (Bundy) who was with the party and remembered I had operated on his brother-in-law.

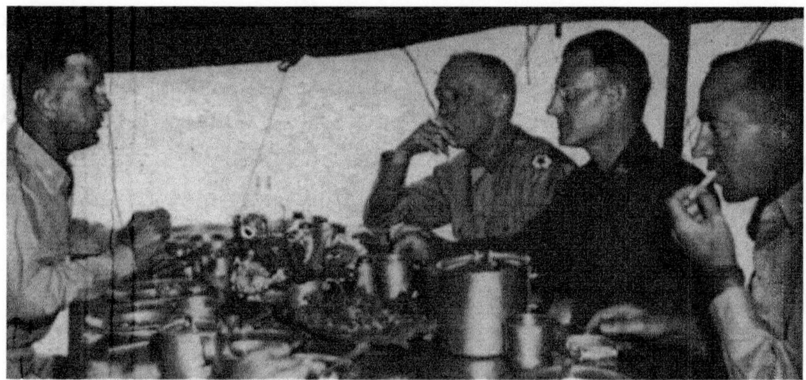

Figure 29.2 Left to right: Brigadier General Joseph Martin, Surgeon General Norman Kirk, Lieutenant Colonel Cato Drash, Major Howard Snyder.

The M.G.H. (6th General Hospital) is nicely settled but officers not too happy about living in tents. I don't know why, as I consider tents a great luxury."

The following day, Secretary Stimson and the Surgeon General went north to the Fifth Army (**Figure 29.2**) and I went south to Naples to arrange for a visit they were to make there. I went to the hospitals located on the fairgrounds to "demine" the route, which meant making sure that our visitors saw nothing out of order. My notes say: "Saw Cady at the 21st and Reyer at the 300th. In making rounds with Jim Kirtley, I was particularly impressed with the empyema patients Tom Burford had been curing with decortication and penicillin. Lined up several that will make a great picture to contrast with those photographed by Keller at the end of W.W. I." (See Chapter 30, Midsummer Madness, **Figure 30.1**.)

By the following morning, July 8, we were ready for Norman Kirk and General Stayer, who met us at the 21st General Hospital. Champ Lyons and Oscar Hampton were on hand and we all made rounds with Patton and Parker. Kirk was delighted to see so many battle fractures being treated by skeletal traction. Hurried visits were made to other fairgrounds' hospitals, and for lunch we were guests of Harry Jenkins at the 182nd Station Hospital overlooking the swimming pool.

At the 37th General Hospital we saw some amputation stumps closed by secondary suture that Kirk was not pleased with, being a staunch advocate of circular amputations closed by skin traction. Kirk, on his visit to the Fifth Army, had been very favorably impressed by our use of field hospital platoons for first-priority surgery. My diary says: "Thinks belly cases very remarkable—they are!"

After a very brief stay in Naples, Secretary Stimson suddenly decided to leave on the ninth. He had developed a diarrhea which the Surgeon General was treating with Epsom salts much to the annoyance of General Stayer. At any rate, the Secretary decided that Naples was no place to stay. With great scrambling, a fighter escort was obtained from Foggia because most of the squadron had gone off on missions. But, meanwhile, because he wasn't feeling well, Secretary Stimson decided to go back to Rome by train. On the way he suddenly asked where his luggage was. An aide explained that it had been sent by car and "will be in your room when you arrive."

"*You* hope," said the V.I.P.

RETURN TO CASERTA

After the departure of the Secretary's party I drove with General Stayer to Caserta. At the palace we found that the medical section had been allotted ample space on the ground floor. I then went to my house in the English Garden, a house that was divided into a living room in the center and a bedroom on each end. I was to live in that house for the duration of the war. The only defect was the lack of water seal traps on the drainpipes. A communal latrine was only a short distance away, and in the summer the fetid exhalations from drainage tile makeshift sewers backfired into the washstands.

Across from the house was a huge cedar of Lebanon—which, incidentally, was to be a landmark for me many years later. This was when, returning from a trip to the Middle East, I revisited the English Garden and was able to find the site of the portable house by locating that tree. Furthermore, an elderly Italian, working nearby, identified himself as the janitor who had taken care of the house when I had lived there—and he told me that it had been common gossip among his fellow workers that I was the son of Winston Churchill!

His ways of trying to please us, I recalled, were occasionally a bit foreign to our taste. One evening, while I had been reading, I noticed a large moth similar to the giant Cecropia on the wall. It was slowly opening and closing its wings as though recently emerged from the cocoon. It had been caught by the janitor, impaled on a pin and anchored to the wall for decoration. A DDT bomb soon brought its struggles to an end.

The senior officers' mess was in a huge glass-topped conservatory which housed tropical trees, vines and flowering oleanders. Long tables kept the military ranks separate and, after one or two meals with Stayer at the Commanding General's table, I found my appropriate level with the colonels and an occasional brigadier general. General Jacob Devers was the Theater Commander (U.S.A.) at that time.

A small prisoner of war orchestra—two fiddles, a zither and an accordion—gave the diners music for the evening meal. The repertory included the popular themes from Verdi's operas, and old favorites from World War I as well as new ones from World War II. World War I selections included: "It's a Long Way to Tipperary," "There Are Smiles that Make One Happy," "Katie, Beautiful Katie, I'll be Waiting at the K-K-K-Kitchen Door," "Pack up your Troubles in your Old Kit Bag," "The Caissons go Rolling Along," and, of course, the French "Alouette" and "Mademoiselle from Armentières." World War II favorites included, "Don't Sit under the Apple Tree with Anyone Else but Me," "As Time goes By," "Praise the Lord and Pass the Ammunition," "Wild Blue Yonder," "We'll Follow the Old Man, the Grandest Son of a Soldier of them All," "I'm Dreaming of a White Christmas," "Tropical Heat Wave" and "Nothing but Blue Skies."

Living in the same house with General Stayer, and enjoying the privilege of the senior officers' mess, had its drawbacks as well as advantages. I missed the close association with Perrin Long, Earle Standlee, Bill Stone and others at headquarters.

30

Midsummer Madness

Just as units are withdrawn from combat for a few weeks of recuperation, I now welcomed days free of looking at wounds, talking with the wounded and their surgeons, and looking over shoulders at operations. To live in more spacious quarters and in clean surroundings enabled me to think about what I had seen, to formulate future policies and to write.

As the midsummer heat hung over Italy the comfortable life at Caserta was interrupted only by an occasional trip to the Fifth Army and visits to the hospitals in Naples and Rome. It was easy to travel on the Blood Bank plane that made almost daily trips to the Fifth Army. On July 13, 1944, I left Capodocino on this plane with a cargo of blood at 1345 hours and put down at Cecina, just south of Livorno, at 1530 hours. Livorno, an important seaport, was still in German hands.

The following morning, after visiting the 8th Evacuation Hospital, I went with Joe Martin and Howard Snyder to the clearing station of the 34th Division, in the vicinity of Rosignano. The 2nd Platoon of the 33rd Field Hospital was attached. We then proceeded to the clearing station of the 91st Division in their first overseas setup. They were a fine-looking group, full of enthusiasm for their first experience in combat. Afterwards we went to the clearing station of the 88th Division with the 1st Platoon of the 33rd Field Hospital. This was in the vicinity of Montecatini.

At Headquarters of IV Corps (Advanced) we discussed the tactical situation with Major General Krittenburg and Major Henry Cabot Lodge. The plans were to outflank both Livorno and Pisa. At Fifth Army Rear we had a long discussion about surgical teams and I decided to return to Naples to make some changes. The 15th Evacuation Hospital was set up in a hospital on the outskirts of Grosseto. Ernst was just taking over from Frank Lever as Commanding Officer; Lever was to go to the 16th Evacuation Hospital. Before we turned in, Dan Mulvihill displayed his skill as a chef by frying fresh Italian eggs for sandwiches. Dan developed quite a reputation as a chef during the Italian campaign—he rarely ate a meal at the hospital mess.

On the fifteenth I made rounds with Manny Lichtenstein and made the following notation:

> *E.D.C. Comments:* "Badly mutilated young P.O.W. with larynx and esophagus shot away exposing the posterior pharyngeal wall. Doing well with tube gastrostomy and tracheotomy, but end tracheostomy must now be done to prevent mucous and wound secretions from running down trachea. Suggested also doing left cervical esophagostomy as dependent drainage of wound cavity and for possible antethoracic esophagus if he is ever able to swallow. Doubt this can be the case. *Jewish doctors and nurses working hard over this young Nazi.*

"At the Cecina airfield the Blood Plane was late but finally came in with penicillin, DDT and glucose aboard as well as a cargo of blood. Smooth flight back to Napoli in 1 hour 45 minutes, having wind off stern quarter. Rome looked small—as do all cities from the air. The Pontine marshes are still flooded and drainage is carrying silt into the sea. Perfect summer afternoon over the Mediterranean coast spread out below—Ischia, Cuma, Averno, Capri and old Vesuvius. To the Parco for a tub bath."

MIXTURE OF MEMORIES

The following afternoon I had lunch and a long talk with members of the staff of the 37th General Hospital. They were feeling low because of Surgeon General Kirk's discovery of a secondarily sutured amputation stump. Over at the 15th Medical Laboratory, according to my notes, I found Tracy Mallory excited by the appearance of the spleen in certain cases dying with anuria—it becomes stuffed with blood cells resembling the spleen in congenital hemolytic jaundice. At the 21st General Hospital I persuaded Drake to let Henry Schwartz exchange with Donald Wrock in the forward area for two or three weeks. Oscar Hampton was very enthusiastic about a recent visit he made to Barbara Stimson's fracture wards. He reported that she had done a remarkable job on some twenty-eight compound fractures of the femur with locally applied penicillin, oral sulfadiazine and minimal revision of the fracture site.

At the 300th General Hospital I had Sergeant Paul Showstack take photographs of the patients with infected hemothorax treated by Tom Burford with decortication and primary closure (**Figure 30.1**). As I had planned, we arranged them like Colonel Keller's in the Surgeon General's *History of World War I.*

There were about twenty-five generals and admirals at the high table in the mess—more stars, I noted, than MGM. After a walk through the grotto

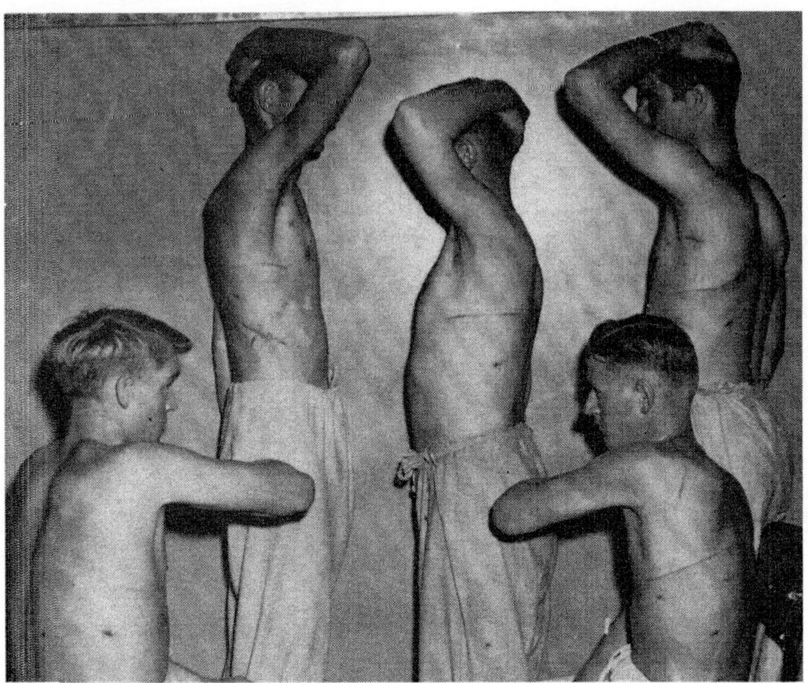

Figure 30.1. Patients with infected hemothorax treated by decortication of lung and pleura. (Posed to resemble Colonel Keller's photographs from World War I.)

I worked on my diary notes which I recorded were "up to date, hour and minute for the first time since July 3rd."

A division of Brazilians had come in the previous Sunday. General Devers suggested to me at breakfast that he wished me to check on the health and the sanitary discipline of the division. Bill Stone and I did so in the absence of General Stayer. Two hundred and ninety-five officers and 4,776 enlisted men arrived in Naples on July 16 after a seventeen day voyage from Rio de Janeiro. They were placed in staging area 3 in Bagnoli. Their immunization records were in order and they had been started on atabrine, six tablets a week, on debarkation.

Colonel Porto was the Surgeon of the Brazilian Expeditionary Force and he was busying himself translating our circular letters into Portuguese. Like U.S. troops this division arrived with the usual incidence of venereal disease—from the period spent in Rio de Janeiro prior to debarkation. These men were treated in our hospitals in Naples.

Strained relations between allies were inevitable when crowded together in the narrow peninsula of Italy. The compromising hand of General Eisenhower was no longer available and General Devers was by instinct a combat commander rather than a statesman. My diary records that: "There is increasing disaffection with the British at all levels. I heard it expressed in Corps, Army and here at A.F.H.Q." Basically it seemed aggravated by what many felt was their slowness and reluctance to pursue offensive action at the front. As for the French, DeGaulle was disturbed because the French Expeditionary Corps was still in line although it was not to have been used north of Rome.

REFLECTIONS ON THE WAR

The following is from my diary:

The concern in Fifth Army a few days ago, as an offensive for the Arno River Valley was being launched, was that a counter offensive might have to be faced if the right wing of our forces got too far ahead. The French E.C. must come out by the 20th for "Chorus" (my personal code name for "Anvil," the top secret designation of the invasion of southern France).

Field Marshal Alexander is desirous of operations that must lead inevitably to the Balkans—avowedly not an American field of interest. We are shipping supplies which the British have offered to distribute for us, but we have informed them that we will transport and distribute ourselves. The British have a small force in Chorus and repeatedly have tried to commit us to supply it for an indefinite period. They even insisted that transportation for their force be American.

The desire of the British to push to the east and their opposition to the landing in southern France displays their concern about Russia in the Middle East. Alexander's desire to reach the Po Valley, which would plug the entrance of Communism into Italy at Trieste, reveals the British intent to reduce Italy to a mandate and thereby secure the Mediterranean from future threats.

Optimism is growing about the end of the European war and "getting the boys home by Christmas." General Marshall in Rome promised "an early cessation of hostilities." Stalin is quoted by the BBC to have said that the Russians will reach Berlin in one thousand hours. Reports from the United States reflect the belief that the war is over. A P.O.W. lieutenant says that Germany has lost the war and is holding the western front only to negotiate favorable terms. Possibly these terms include protection from the Russians. Stalin's intent is said to be distribution of relief only to women and children and conscription of males into labor battalions to rebuild Russia.

(continued)

It is hard to know what to believe or what the next few weeks will bring. The invasion of southern France is rapidly being organized on a first priority rating. Certainly IV Corps has no immediate intention of storming the Apennines. The British will not move to the east without us along, and we have accomplished our objectives in Italy.

DIARY NOTE ON CLOSTRIDIAL INFECTION

Many surgeons (I wrote) were giving close attention to the clinical aspects of an aerobic clostridial infection (gas gangrene). Cases were observed with the proliferation of clostridia in blood clot without discernible invasive infection of living cellular tissues. This situation was attended by rapid pulse, high fever and delirium, although the patients were on penicillin. In four hours after giving antitoxin the pulse and temperature came to normal and the delirium cleared. Little is known about the action of the exotoxins that may be produced by clostridia.

Jergeson believes that the incidence of clostridial infection (myositis) in Fifth Army is now very low. In the two week period of the beachhead breakthrough, four hospitals on the beachhead and evacuees to P.B.S. after arrival, ran an incidence of about 3 per 1,000. In the 56th Evac. on the same terrain at an earlier date the incidence was about 10 per 1,000 if certain questionable cases are removed. In the 38th Evac. in P.O.W.'s with delayed evacuation and delayed surgery there was almost 100 per cent incidence of anaerobic cellulitis.

Careful watch should be kept in patients on penicillin therapy for those who may show symptoms from absorption of clostridial exotoxins and the clinical picture it may produce—destruction of red blood cells, fever, rapid pulse and toxic delirium. The symptoms of local invasive infection—pain, reduced blood volume and local wound pathology— may be lacking.

DIARY ENTRY ON SELF-INFLICTED WOUNDS—AND HEROES

Self-inflicted wounds are by no means always caused by firearms. A report from the 7th Station Hospital itemizes the foreign bodies intentionally swallowed by inmates in the disciplinary training center. Open safety pins, staples and needles comprised the list. And a station hospital in Corsica reports that a large GI had a rubber condom filled with beer obstructing the ileocecal valve!

On July 23 I returned to Cascade Camp in the cool of the evening through peaceful fields of hemp. The crop of grain and hay had been harvested and the fields were rolling yellow carpets. Peasants were hard at work—oblivious to world events. Their position seemed certain and accepted by them. My thoughts then turned to the many doctors. "More and more, I am impressed by the devotion of our doctors to work. Disciplinary problems practically do not exist. All are doing their utmost within the limits of their training and experience." In this kindly mood the number of misguided soldiers who swallowed safety pins seemed infinitesimal when measured beside the thousands of wounded in our hospitals and the dead in military cemeteries. *In Flanders fields the poppies grow between the crosses row on row. Ours not to reason why. Ours but to do and die. The world will little note or long remember what we say here. It can never forget what they did here. And gentlemen in England now a-bed shall think themselves accursed they were not here, and hold their manhoods cheap whiles any speaks that fought with us upon Saint Crispin's day.*

TWO MEMOS ON ONE SUBJECT

"Recently the rations as issued have contained local, said to be Lend Lease, supplies of salted fish. While these fish are probably safe as far as disease is concerned, the odor is extremely objectionable, no one will eat them, and they are absolutely unfit for issue to American soldiers."

—REGT. SURGEON

Indorsement:

"I concur . . . except for paragraph 6 regarding fish. A few men did eat the fish and I would not go so far as to state that 'they are absolutely unfit for issue to American soldiers.' In my opinion, the fish were suitable for human consumption but most of the troops of this command are not accustomed to a fish diet and their hunger was not great enough to overcome their objections to the odor. As a result, most of the fish issued to this command was wasted."

—LT. COLONEL, COMMANDING

PHILOSOPHY OF SURGERY IN WAR

A birthday party gave me the opportunity to explore Army philosophy with some of the young aides in the command group. They found working within the rigid framework of the Army to be quite trying, and also felt that they were losing valuable years from their chosen life's work in civilian society. They were *designers* by aptitude and training, feeling frustrated at becoming *operators*. I drew the analogy between the Army and a two-and-a-half ton truck started on a fixed-objective mission, for example the delivery of a load of ammunition.

The driver is to keep the machine going, repair simple defects but not redesign the truck. Were he to redesign the truck, all other drivers would require a new basic training and a shipload of new spare parts would be required.

Surgery, I pointed out, has developed and changed within the theater during the course of the war. But surgery had moved from civilian life to develop *within* the framework of the Army and in accord with the assigned mission of preserving manpower.

AN HONOR

During July, Champ Lyons worked hard in the Naples hospitals. On the twenty-fourth of that month he came to see me about the 37th General Hospital and I noted that he looked poorly and had been having some fever. On the following day I called Oscar Hampton and asked him to send Champ to a hospital for a checkup. It turned out that he had a severe attack of hepatitis. I saw Champ several times at the 300th General Hospital. On October 8 I made the following note: "Stopped at 300th to see Champ and Dick Chute—both with hepatitis. Chute leaves tomorrow for the Zone of the Interior. Champ has received the Legion of Merit and should go soon as promotion is impossible."

And on the twelfth: "He is now to be 'boarded' home."

On July 26, I received a note from Benoit in Algiers enclosing a clipping from the July 18, 1944, issue of *Echo d'Alger*.

> *"Le Commissaire à l'éducation nationale par arrêté en date du 20 Juin 1944, a approuvé une délibération du conseil de l'Université d'Alger, conférant le titre de Docteur 'honoris causa' aux savants; hommes de lettres, hommes d'action des nations alliées et amies, dont les noms suivent:"*

There followed a list of twenty-two names including: Brigadier General E. R. Boland, Dean of Guys Hospital Medical School, Perrin Long, James Bryant Conant and my own. In the press of my work I was unable to present myself in Alger on the appointed day—in fact I did not receive the sheepskin diploma until January, 1956. Recalling Orozco's mural in the library at Dartmouth College depicting dead knowledge, I planned to appear in an academic procession with a French gown and hood—but have never done so. The University of Alger was at the time the only free university in France, so I value this association highly.

CARE OF VETERANS

At a dinner in Cascade Camp on July 27, I had the opportunity to discuss the postwar care of the crippled and disabled with the new commander of the Veterans of Foreign Wars. I told him frankly what I thought of the surgical care of veterans, as I had seen it, and warned him that the doctors serving in this war who were devoting so much time to the soldiers over here, would raise hell if these soldiers were mishandled by the Veterans Administration. As it turned out, the Veterans Administration, as recast by General Omar Bradley and Paul Hawley after World War II, performed an enlightened service.

Bill Stone brought up an interesting aspect of the Medical Corps—postgraduate training in medicine or surgery before entering upon service with the regular Army can block a man from top assignments later in his career. This can happen because the man with postgraduate training may come into the service after other men of his own age; and date of rank in the group of officers of his age determines choice of assignment by seniority.

A "MAESTRO"

On July 29, taking Simeone along as an interpreter, I visited the Tuberculosis Institute in Naples. I inquired about Eugenio Morelli who, prior to the war, was at the Forlanini Institute in Rome. I had made inquiries about him in Rome but was told that he was not "at home" because of his Fascist activities.

Morelli had written a treatise on the treatment of wounds of lung and pleura based on experience in World War I. It so impressed Lincoln Davis of the M.G.H. and Frederick C. Irving of the Boston Lying-In Hospital that, after the Armistice, they translated the book into English.

No attempt will be made to transmit the flavor of this book, carrying, as it does, the reverence of the author for his "Maestro" Carlo Forlanini, and an exchange of compliments between translators and author.

In exploring the Treadwell Library of the M.G.H. during my days on the house staff, I ran across this book and was fascinated by Morelli's exposition of "pulmonary physiopathology." It awakened a lasting interest in thoracic surgery, at that time a terrifying undertaking by my "Maestros." It is true that the concept of the lung as portrayed by Morelli was oversimplified. In my Presidential Address to the American Association for Thoracic Surgery in 1949 I said: "The apparent homogeneity of the structure and function of the lungs is highly deceptive. They are not two gas bags suspended in a container." Morelli's model, as shown in his diagrams, was a gas bag suspended in a bottle.

James E. Wiseman, Thomas M. Scalea, and Elliot M. Jessie

Churchill's greatest contributions as consultant centered on three domains: whole blood transfusion for the treatment of hemorrhagic shock, surgical management of wounds, and casualty evacuation strategies. A thorough review of his writings shows he considered the precise and timely application of all three of these elements essential to preventing wound infections. We see evidence of this transformative philosophy taking shape in the present chapter.

As discussed in **Chapter 23: Gas Gangrene**, had emerged as a serious threat during World War I, with a mortality in the range of 50%. Sulfonamides and penicillin were discovered in the years following World War I, and under Colonel Churchill's leadership, the policy of the Mediterranean theater during World War II mandated that every soft tissue injury be treated empirically with one or the other. However, Churchill understood that antibiotics alone were not sufficient—the incidence of gas gangrene in his area of responsibility ranged from 0.3% to 1%, with delays in surgery increasing the rate of anaerobic "cellulitis" to 100%. This then sets the stage for his later work to improve medical evacuation strategies to minimize these delays. He similarly recognized that penicillin did not protect against the residual exotoxin even after eradication of the causative organism, an insight decades ahead of the prevailing medical knowledge of the era.

Later in the chapter, Colonel Churchill references a conversation he had with the commander of the Veterans of Foreign Wars regarding the surgical care of veterans. Churchill's interest in medical care for veterans was more than fleeting. In early 1946 he would serve as the chair of an ad hoc meeting on postwar research at the National Academy of Sciences. The meeting gave rise to what became the Committee on Veterans Medical Problems, of which Dr. Churchill was an inaugural member. This committee formalized a standing research collaboration between the National Academy of Sciences and the Veterans Administration that continues today.

In closing, two striking moments in this chapter deserve special treatment. The first comes in Colonel Churchill's discussion of a young German soldier with a devastating neck wound. Clearly his interest in the case is primarily technical, to document his recommendation for diverting cervical esophagostomy. We take note, however, of the last sentence of the paragraph, *"Jewish doctors and nurses working hard over this young Nazi."* With this observation, Churchill seems moved by the symbolism of persecuted people going to such great lengths to save the life of one of their tormentors.

A second, equally understated moment comes just two paragraphs later, in a reference to Dr. Barbara Stimson, a truly remarkable American orthopedic surgeon. The cousin of the Secretary of War Henry Stimson (**Chapter 29: V.I.P. Visit**), Dr. Stimson served under the British flag in the Royal Army Medical Corps since the US Army prohibited women from officially serving in the war. Again, Churchill's main interest is technical, as he purposefully points to the vital role of antibiotics in the treatment of compound femur fractures. But his comfort in praising a female combat surgeon is clearly progressive for this era. This theme of progress-leaning pragmatism proves remarkably consistent throughout his career. Indeed, the sophistication of his insights clinically, militarily, and personally remains stellar even by modern standards.

SUGGESTED READINGS

Buyske J. The Tale of Barbara Stimson: #ilooklikeasurgeon. *Ann Surg.* 2018 Jun;267(6): 1007-1008.

Churchill ED. The surgical management of the wounded in the Mediterranean theater at the time of the fall of Rome. *Ann Surg.* 1944;120(3):268-283.

Crews EM. *Colonel Edward Churchill's Transformation of Wound Care in the Mediterranean Theater of the Second World War. Valdosta State University MA thesis*; May 2012. https://vtext. valdosta.edu/xmlui/handle/10428/1135.

Haisley KR, Drexel SE, Watters JM, Hunter JG, Mullins RJ. Major Barbara Stimson: a historical perspective on the American Board of Surgery through the accomplishments of the first woman to achieve board certification. *Ann Surg.* 2018 Jun;267(6):1000-1006.

Moore FD. Edward Delos Churchill: 1895-1972. *Ann Surg.* 1973;177(4):507-508.

PART FIVE

The Last Phase

31

The Board for the Study of the Severely Wounded[1]

E.D.C. Comments: BY THE SUMMER of 1944 it was evident that although nearly two years of experience had enabled the theater to develop the procedures of resuscitation to a high peak of effectiveness, this was largely an accomplishment of the practical art and remained to a considerable extent undocumented by scientific evidence. If left in this status at the end of World War II, it would tend to be forgotten, as are many other practical lessons that emerge from the experience of war. Even the validity of the experience would be open to question. Bayliss, toward the end of World War I, had written: "On the whole it is remarkable that so little positive evidence is forthcoming as to the superiority of blood transfusions. Statements are made on the basis of general impressions, rather than on convincing proof. In the nature of the case, such proof would be difficult to provide." The question was often asked whether the experience in Italy was really accepted at face value and whether the precepts that had been formulated would be transferred to the conflict in the Pacific and to civilian needs.

EARLY STUDIES

"Some data of a precise nature had been obtained, but they were of a fragmentary nature. Lt. Colonel John D. Stewart, a member of the Consulting Surgical Staff of the Surgeon, NATOUSA, while on temporary duty with the Fifth Army in December, 1943, made arrangements with the Commanding Officer of the 2d Medical Laboratory, with the concurrence and support of the Surgeon, Fifth Army, to conduct a clinical study of the freshly wounded. A small mobile laboratory was set up at the 3rd Platoon of the 11th Field Hospital on 20 January, 1944. This platoon was situated near the 36th Divisional Clearing Station,

(continued)

---

[1]From: Churchill ED. Introduction. In: *The Physiologic Effects of Wounds.* Medical Department, United States Army. Surgery in World War II. Washington, D.C.; 1952.

northeast of Mignano, about seven miles behind the front. The objective was to study by formal biochemic methods certain aspects of shock, hemorrhage, and dehydration.

"A preliminary report was submitted under date of 17 March, 1944. Observations had been made on some 35 badly wounded patients immediately after admission, usually within 12 hours after wounding. A final report of this study, extended to include 100 desperately wounded observed during the first 6 months of 1944, was submitted on 2 January, 1945. The data indicated (1) absence of hemoconcentration in shock, (2) reduction of blood volume in shock, (3) greater reduction of red-cell concentration than of plasma protein concentration early after wounding, (4) lowering of both red-cell and plasma protein concentration later, and (5) frequency of later dehydration.

"During approximately the same period (11 February through 4 June, 1944) the Consultant in Anesthesia and Resuscitation, NATOUSA, and Captain Charles H. Burnett carried out an extensive study on the wounded at the 94th Evacuation Hospital, observing 557 cases on the Cassino Front (Mignano) and 2,296 cases on the Anzio Beachhead. In the latter site the position of the evacuation hospital bore the same relation to the front as a field hospital. While the greatest significance of this contribution lay in formulating procedure for the clinical management of resuscitation in the seriously wounded, in 37 of the most severely wounded fairly extensive laboratory observations were made. These confirmed the absence of hemoconcentration.

"Starting in March, 1944, in a field hospital platoon, Captain Joseph J. Lalich, 2nd Auxiliary Surgical Group, carried out a series of hematocrit and plasma protein determinations by the copper sulfate method. His findings, like those of the other workers, were quickly made available to forward surgeons and were submitted as a formal report on 12 November, 1944. Attention was called to the low hematocrit readings obtained from 3 to 5 days after initial surgery despite the very liberal use of blood transfusions in resuscitation. This was a phenomenon that was exciting interest in the general hospitals in Peninsular Base Section. For the success of the vigorous program of reparative wound surgery that was being formulated, it was found necessary to provide for the liberal use of whole blood transfusion at the base.

"There was need, however, for a far more comprehensive study. In the opinion of the Medical Research Committee of the Theater there was little doubt that the impetus of the tremendous program undertaken to provide so-called 'substitutes' for blood in World War II would be projected into the postwar period. It might be revived with any threat of a future war. It was essential, therefore, that the so-called impressions derived from experience be documented by hard, cold facts about the condition of a freshly wounded man. To this end, everything about a seriously wounded soldier that could be observed and recorded by precise measurement should be ascertained and recorded. The collection of data needed to be extended to a sufficient number of casualties to make the findings conclusive.

ESTABLISHMENT OF BOARD FOR THE STUDY OF THE SEVERELY WOUNDED

"The summer of 1944 in Italy was a period of readjustment to meet the over-all strategy of the war in Europe. Between mid-June and the end of July more than a division a week was withdrawn from the forces to train and stage for Operation Anvil, the attack in southern France executed on 15 August. Pursuit of the enemy to the north had brought the Allied armies up against the 'Gothic Line,' an elaborate defense system in the northern Apennines. Then on 10 September a general offensive was launched to break through into the Po Valley. As it became apparent that the Medical Service was to face a renewed heavy flow of casualties, the Medical Research Committee sponsored certain fact-finding tasks that required concentrated and carefully organized effort for accomplishment. One of these was further analysis of the state of the seriously wounded.

"More information was urgently needed regarding the problem of anuria. Kidney damage associated with crushing injuries sustained in air raids had been described as a component of the 'crush syndrome' by Bywaters *et al.* early in the war. Identification of damaged kidney function as a component of injury in the soldier seriously wounded by flying missiles on the battlefield came slowly, but experience had already suggested that it either was being overlooked or was subject to misinterpretation. Identification was slow because first of all it requires the coordinated effort of a wide variety of expert skills in the forward area to rescue desperately wounded soldiers and keep them alive until such time as suppression of kidney function manifests itself. This involves the activity of the entire medical department from the company aid-man in the field to the surgical team and nursing staff in a mobile hospital. When a gravely wounded man dies within 48 hours of being hit, the chances are that any suppression of kidney function will pass unrecognized.

"In the N.R.C. Conference on Shock held on 1 December, 1943, Dr. Donald D. Van Slyke had presented a communication on the 'Effect

(continued)

of Shock on the Kidney.' The concept was developed that the peripheral vascular constriction that compensated for a deficit in the volume of circulating blood in shock may practically stop the blood flow through the kidneys. Urinary excretion stops, and prolonged ischemia may be followed by permanent suppression of renal function. Although presented as a hypothesis, this concept brought a fresh point of view to a clinical problem that was beginning to be identified in the field. Under date of 16 February, 1944, a letter, from which the following extract is quoted, was addressed to Dr. Van Slyke by the Surgical Consultant.

> "By excellent forward surgery and the liberal use of whole blood transfusion as well as plasma, we are saving lives but also keeping certain men alive temporarily only to display the type of kidney damage you describe. This has been either complete anuria with death, or in one case a fall of urinary output to 200 cc. with ultimate recovery of kidney function. As you suggest, this phenomenon is not unique to the 'crush' syndrome but may occur in any wounded man who experiences a long period of greatly reduced volume flow.

"Delay in the identification of the problem of anuria in battle casualties was not solely a matter of organization or preoccupation with more pressing problems. Recognition of anuria depended on a close check of fluid intake and output, items that are difficult to secure even in well-run civilian hospitals. Chemical tests for azotemia were not available in the mobile hospitals. The terminal event of pulmonary edema from forcing fluids in order to correct supposed dehydration was subject to misinterpretation as a manifestation of blast injury or other result of direct trauma to the lungs.

"Even when suppression of urinary excretion was recognized, other causes than the specific effects of the injury required exclusion. In the earlier phases of the war medical officers were alerted to the effects of sulfonamide administration on the kidney. Early in 1944 the widespread usage of sulfonamides was still making it difficult to clarify the problem of posttraumatic anuria. This was referred to in the Annual Report of the Surgical Consultant (1943) as follows: 'Kidney damage is probably the most frequent and easily overlooked sequel of shock and is manifested by anuria or reduced urinary output. Information relative to renal damage produced by decreased volume flow of blood is particularly desired because of a close linkage with policies on sulfonamide therapy.'

"Even more important, however, was the use of blood transfusion in resuscitation. The question arose again and again how often blood transfusion itself might be responsible for kidney damage. To interpret posttraumatic anuria, blood given in transfusion must meet rigid specifications. It must be compatible both in type and iso-agglutinin titer. It must be collected and stored in a closed system to avoid contamination. When supplied in bulk in military operation, frequent checks must be made for free hemoglobin content both at the bank, in the forward hospital, and by examination of the recipients' plasma after transfusion.

"With the increased use of transfusion in the forward area and the distribution of preserved whole blood from the central laboratory in Naples, the identification of posttraumatic anuria became tangled with that of 'transfusion kidney.' Informal requests came from Anzio Beachhead for distribution of Type A blood for massive transfusions in this type of recipient. The policy of issuing only Type O blood in which the iso-agglutinins had been titered was adhered to. Blood with titer 1:64 or above was labeled 'for O-Type recipients only'; that with weaker iso-agglutinin titer was considered suitable for universal use. The problems of poorly preserved or contaminated blood encountered elsewhere in the field during World War II were not encountered in the U.S. Army, Mediterranean Theater.

"The basic conditions outlined above had been established in Italy by late summer in 1944. The medical department personnel were expert from long experience; penicillin had replaced sulfonamides in the treatment of the seriously wounded; the Theater blood bank was issuing a liberal supply of whole blood that met the required specifications. The total situation, both military and medical, was thus favorable for an intensive study of the seriously wounded soldier. Colonel William S. Stone and I conceived the idea of a mobile research laboratory and the Theater Surgeon recommended on 1 September, 1944, that a Board to Study the Treatment of the Severely Wounded be appointed by Lt. General Jacob B. Devers, Commanding General, NATOUSA. Such a board was established on 3 September, 1944. In retrospect, it is doubtful that this particular effort would have been feasible at an earlier date; even if undertaken it probably would not have been as productive, for reasons that have been presented.

"Selection of the personnel of this Board was a matter of vital importance. It was essential that medical officers be selected who were skilled in the techniques of clinical investigation that can be utilized without harm or discomfort to seriously injured patients. Different phases of the study required precise and critical observations in the laboratory, in the ward tents, and in the operating tent. It was essential that the members of the Board be familiar with the subjects

(continued)

to be studied—seriously wounded soldiers. Those finally selected had long experience in identification of the complex sequelae of wounds, and those in charge of the clinical aspects were experts in the practical art of resuscitation. Further, and most important, all had become expert in the art of overcoming, rather than being frustrated by, the retarding element of 'friction' ever present in a huge military undertaking.

"It is of more than passing interest to note that the minutes of the first meeting of the Committee on Transfusions of the National Research Council, already referred to, contain the suggestion 'that a group of men be allowed to work in the Army, freed from any of the obligations of Army officers, who would study cases of shock as investigators. This would give opportunity to observe shock on a big scale, an opportunity to get an insight into the nature of shock.' This was on 31 May, 1940. In May, 1945, as the Germans in northern Italy capitulated and brought the task of the Board to a conclusion, this objective had been accomplished—not precisely as visualized, but effectively. The members of the Board were in no way 'freed from any of the obligations of Army officers,' but were, on the contrary, selected because they were competent to assume the highest privilege accorded officers—the freedom of individual judgment and action. They were not a group that merely worked 'in the Army'; they were of the Army."

NEWS STORY

The following appeared in the *Stars and Stripes* on December 12, 1944. It was written by Sergeant George Bakim, staff correspondent on the Fifth Army front.

GI MEDICAL RESEARCH WORKS DEEP IN ITALIAN ZONE

Dec. 11 — High among the snow-capped Italian mountains, medical science has established its newest research outpost.

Deep in the combat zone, where blackout vigilance is nullified by the reflection on searchlights, shell bursts and flares, a group of Army officers have come in search of a clue and a cure.

Each of them an internationally known member of the medical profession, these front-line men in white are on the trail of an elusive kidney ailment, which has brought death to American soldiers who otherwise might have recovered from major combat wounds.

On a shell-shattered site, once occupied by an evac hospital, this unique research party has set up shop in a truck — a small but complete medical laboratory containing microscopes, spectroscopes and the dozens of other delicate instruments needed in their work.

The men who compose this strange wartime scientific expedition were handpicked for their two years of experience in the theatre and for their civilian backgrounds of distinguished medical service. To them has fallen the task of finding the "bug" in the otherwise smoothly running Army machinery for management of the wounded.

COMPATIBILITY

This distinguished group of Army medicos have two things in common. They're all "high" on research and they all come from Boston, Mass. What's more they all worked together in the hospitals of that city before the war. It's an ideal medical team, with the backfield composed of Lieutenant Colonels Henry K. Beecher, Eugene R. Sullivan, and Tracy B. Mallory and Capt. Charles H. Burnett.

Two enlisted men, in addition to a number of trained laboratory assistants, are also on this highly unique first team and hold down unique Army assignments.

S-Sgt. Paul Showstack of New York City, photographs the various phases of surgical operations, while T-Sgt. Louis Breslow, also of New York City, sketches in black and white or color the many details which escape the camera's eye.

This massing of medical talent up where only dough-foots dare to tread was precipitated by the discovery that the kidneys of certain severely wounded soldiers were clogged fatally by an unidentified pigment. It's a condition which is strangely confined to only those cases in which the odds of recovering are stacked heavily against the patient.

The job of these medically-wise pioneers and their mobile laboratory is twofold. First, they must discover the origin of the pigment. If and when they do, they must determine how to prevent its formation or how to keep it from being fatal.

LONG, HARD PULL

Working long hours under harrowing conditions, the researchers report some progress in the long and tedious processes of cause and effect and elimination. But, already, the search is narrowing.

(continued)

The first question they asked and answered was whether the medicants which were used to save these lives in the first place — plasma, whole blood, penicillin, sulfa drugs — were reacting against the kidneys. The answer was an emphatic no, as these medical bloodhounds swung over to another scent and scores of other questions. For example:

Why does the pigment appear only in the case of the most severely wounded? Does it result from a crushing of the muscles? . . . and so on.

This handful of researchers high in the Apennines, however, are not alone in their quest of the illusive "bug." They are constantly corresponding with leading civilian authorities in the U.S. who have gone right to work on their own carefully coordinated experiments.

One day the right question will be asked and the right answer found. Until then this handful of scientists will continue in their quest of a clue and a cure.

The Board for the Study of the Severely Wounded
COMMENTARY

Joel B. Elterman, Jeffrey A. Bailey, and Warren C. Dorlac

The first chapter of "Part Five" of *Surgeon to Soldiers* communicates a novel effort in 1944, establishment of a board of experts to study a particular observation among combat casualties that contributed to a significant number of deaths during the European campaign of World War II. The observation was that of renal failure among combat casualties. The exact etiology of renal failure was largely unknown at the time but hypothesized to be related to crush injury, widespread use of sulfonamides, sequela of shock, or the direct result of blood transfusion itself. Each theory included strong correlates but could not be explained in isolation. The board was established in September of 1944 and included three Army officers and two enlisted members who traveled to the Apennine Mountains of Italy in their "quest of a clue and a cure."

The downstream consequences of this effort cannot be overstated. At the time, the convened research team focused on a single relevant phenomenon. They selected qualified scientists regardless of military affiliation and placed them deep in the combat zone. They prioritized real-time data collection in combination with the application of scientific rigor. Similar efforts were later made during both the Korean and Vietnam conflicts, most notably the development of the Vietnam Vascular Registry. These conflicts identified the need for a trauma "system" to improve patient outcomes. The concepts quickly spread to the civilian medical community and led to the development of modern-day trauma systems in the United States and elsewhere. In the beginning of the 21st century, the United States found itself in what would become a 20-year period of sustained conflict in the wars in Iraq and Afghanistan. The further maturation of this effort came to fruition in the development of the Joint Trauma Theater System (JTTS) and the Joint Trauma Theater Registry (JTTR).

Implementation of the JTTS occurred in November of 2004 in collaboration with the surgeon generals of the US Military, the US Army Institute of Surgical Research, and the American College of Surgeons. One trauma surgeon (Trauma System director) and a team of six trauma nurse coordinators were deployed to theater to evaluate trauma system component issues.

The goal of the JTTS was to ensure rapid and comprehensive medical care for trauma patients from the point of injury on the battlefield to definitive care at higher-level medical facilities. A key component of the JTTS was the establishment of the JTTR. Scientific investigation conducted utilizing the JTTR resulted in 27 clinical practice guidelines and use of these clinical practice guidelines resulted in a significant improvement in mortality, producing the lowest combat mortality rates in recorded human history.

The subtle and perhaps extrapolated message that should endure from this chapter is this: Continuous collection, analysis, interpretation, and documentation of the injuries sustained by combat casualties as well as the therapies applied represent a crucial role for the surgeon in times of conflict. Moreover, failure to do so will result in a loss of knowledge and future generations will pay the same price with their lives.

SUGGESTED READINGS

Eastridge BJ, Costanzo G, Jenkins D, et al. Impact of joint theater trauma system initiatives on battlefield injury outcomes. *Am J Surg.* 2009 Dec;198(6):852-857.

Eastridge BJ, Jenkins D, Flaherty S, Schiller H, Holcomb JB. Trauma system development in a theater of war: experiences from Operation Iraqi Freedom and Operation Enduring Freedom. *J Trauma.* 2006 Dec;61(6):1366-1372.

National Academies of Sciences, Engineering, and Medicine. *A National Trauma Care System: Integrating Military and Civilian Trauma Systems to Achieve Zero Preventable Deaths After Injury.* The National Academies Press; 2016.

Concept of Operations for the Combatant Command Trauma System, October 2020. Accessed May 24, 2024. https://jts.health.mil/assets/docs/CTS_CONOP_21_OCT_2020.pdf

32

Invasion of Southern France

THE MIDDLE of August was hot in southern Italy. On August 13, 1944, I followed the Italian custom of a siesta after lunch and spent the blazing afternoon reading and writing. The zero-hour for Operation Anvil—the invasion of southern France—was close at hand. This had been planned at the Quebec Conference and D-Day was August 15. The invasion force was to move up the Rhone valley and join the cross channel forces near Dijon. The islands of Sardinia and Corsica, separated by the Strait of Bonifacio, had already fallen into our hands. Sardinia was seized on September 19, 1943, and Corsica had been taken by French troops a fortnight later. I had never been on Corsica, so when a message came on August 14 for me to meet General Stayer in Calvi, I took off immediately to join him on the "near shore" of another over-water assault.

CORSICAN PRELUDE

On board the private plane of the Chief of Staff, I took off from Marchinese at 11:00 A.M. flying up the coast and across to Ajaccio in an hour and three-quarters.

E.D.C. Comments: "After a snack lunch," my diary reads, "on to Calvi main—an R.A.F. field. Calvi claims to be the birthplace of Christopher Columbus and is the Corsican port nearest to France. The old town stands on a high rock, the modern town at its foot—a little over 100 miles across the sea from the southern coast of France." In a jeep borrowed from the 180th Station Hospital, three miles south of Calvi, I drove to Ile Russe where returning LST's were to dock with wounded from the assault. "Tony Vedala and Roulette," my diary continues, "were setting up a provisional receiving unit. I obtained a room at the Hotel Napoleon Bonaparte."

On August 15—the long-awaited day—I was awakened before dawn by the massive flight of the Airborne Division passing overhead. This was followed by wave after wave of heavy and medium bombers. Before it was light, the planes were breaking out recognition flares as they were over the island. Then all was quiet as the sun came up with its own colorful splendor.

At the 180th Station Hospital I made rounds with Rusbridge and Silver and saw a good case of fixation of a fractured metacarpal by wire pinning to the adjacent ones. Many Yugoslavs taken from Italians in Sardinia were now being used by us in labor battalions. One of them was in the hospital with a cast applied for a metacarpal fracture without displacement. What a world that lavishes such care on a minor injury, I thought, while only a few hundred miles distant, the Yugoslavs are being shot if wounded!

When I came back to Calvi, no LST's had returned. I described my feelings as like Tristan in Act III waiting for *ein Schiff!* Above our provisional hospital stood a rocky headland with an old signal tower. During lunch at the 180th Station Hospital the announcement of the landing came over the radio.

On the morning of D + 1 there was no news of arriving LST's "except for two British ones that may be in today." I went off to Bastia with General Stayer and Tony Vedala. The winding mountain road leveled off to cross the desert at the northern end of the island. After a stop at the advanced echelon of A.F.H.Q. we went by plane down the eastern coast and around to Ajaccio, arriving at lunchtime. Here we were taken by Brigadier General Rathay, Commanding General of the Northern Base Section (NORBS), to his requisitioned villa. The villa was at one time a residence of Napoleon III. Also at lunch were Lieutenant General Somerville and Undersecretary of War Robert F. Patterson—"V.I.P.'s viewing the landing," I noted.

I visited the 40th Station Hospital, which had received some casualties by LST. There were a number of prisoners of war whose boat had been hit. Their flash burns were not a serious problem. After a shower and dinner at NORBS, I heard that more LST's were docking on the other side of the bay. About 250 casualties from the first assault wave arrived. There was the usual dilution with extremely minor injuries and only fifteen seriously wounded or injured.

I made a long note in my diary about what I called the *dilution factor.*

E.D.C. Comments: "Among the special troops returned by LST from southern France arriving at Ajaccio on August 16, the low mortality rate was striking. There were many soldiers with minor injuries and scratches who in ordinary combat would never have left the divisional area. This is also observed with rapidly moving divisions." To illustrate this, the battle casualties admitted to hospitals in the Fifth Army were listed from the months of January to June, 1944. The deaths expressed in per cent varied from 3.0 to 4.8 until May, when the total number rose sharply and the mortality rate fell to 1.7 per cent. "With rapidly moving divisions," I noted, "many soldiers with minor injuries are left behind whereas normally 25 to 30 per cent return to duty from the Bn. Aid and Clearing Stations. When this mechanism is out of gear, dilution of hospital admissions is the inevitable result."

Considerable confusion reigned in the 40th Station Hospital, and I helped all I could to straighten things out. I made a list of the patients who could be evacuated to Italy in the morning by plane and, by so doing, reduced the surgical backlog. One patient was very ill with a compound fracture of the left tibia and "anaerobic cellulitis." He was badly in need of blood but transfusion facilities were not well prepared despite the lesson learned at the 35th Station Hospital on the island that summer.

There were about five patients with fractures of the os calcis and probable compression fractures of the vertebrae as the result of their boat hitting a mine. I watched the operation on a patient with a belly wound. The cecum was found to have a perforation of its anterior wall. The surgeon planned to do a cecostomy. I suggested that he should find the second hole but this he could not do. I then taught him how to mobilize the cecum by dividing the peritoneal reflection, rotating it to see the posterior side, and there was the other hole!

I was up early the next morning and out to the 40th Station Hospital. A visit was made on the P.O.W. wards and new cases examined. The ambulances were loaded with considerable confusion and a convoy traveled to the airfield. I rode the evacuation C-47 back to Naples—a two and a half hour flight. This plane was just back from the invasion—one of the doors was missing. A hospital ship below us, heading back from the invasion coast, was just clearing the Strait of Bonifacio headed for Naples. Our plane passed down the corridor along the east coast of Sardinia, then turned 90 degrees to Naples. Eighteen wounded on litters were aboard the plane.

This short stay on Corsica once again demonstrated the shortage of well-trained and experienced surgeons in the theater and the initial error in bringing a large number of station hospitals overseas and using them to receive battle casualties.

Great progress had been made, however, in the standards set for the care of battle casualties. As soon as medical units could be established on the beachhead, emergency surgical care was provided there. Parts of an official report dealing with the care of battle casualties transported on a hospital ship will follow. These wounded were evacuated from battle on the far shore. The greatly reduced incidence of minor injuries in the evacuation stream through hospital ships was striking.

STORY OF A HOSPITAL SHIP

A hospital ship was comparable to a station hospital as far as the surgical management of fresh battle casualties was concerned. In the Annals of Internal Medicine *21*:1, July, 1944, Ross T. McIntire, Vice Admiral, F.A.C.P., the Surgeon General of the Navy, wrote on the need for internists in the Navy. "On a hospital ship," he said, "we practice medicine in a different fashion. . . . . The internist becomes a fair surgeon; the surgeon learns again something about internal medicine." In the same article he recounts his experience on "one of our very large ships"—"one of the most modern we have." Here he "saw a highly trained cardiologist do a very difficult gangrenous appendix."

In the following account of the hospital ship *Chateau-Thierry*, it is to be noted that its intrinsic medical personnel was reinforced by an orthopedic surgical team on a short run to Naples. The account is an extract from a "Report to the Surgeon, NATOUSA, on an Informal Investigation Relative to the Handling of Casualties Aboard the U.S.A. Hospital Ship 'Chateau-Thierry' on its Voyage from Cape Draumont, France, to Port of Naples (August 16-18, 1944)." It was written by Richard Arnest and others.

The *Chateau-Thierry* sailed into the target area off Cape Draumont on the south shore of France on D+1 (August 16). The hospital ship commander had only a vague conception of what he might expect as to number or type of cases, his exact port of call, or the exact time that he would receive patients. From 0100 hours to 1900 hours on D+1, this ship received 421 battle casualties, not one of which had received definitive treatment. The first case to arrive aboard required enucleation of the eyeball which was done immediately as an emergency measure. Shortly thereafter, patients began to arrive from all types of small craft, and the ship and operating rooms were virtually deluged with casualties.

"Patients received were as follows: 278 litter; 142 ambulatory; 1 dead. 7 patients died aboard ship after admission to ship's hospital. One other died shortly after arrival in Port of Naples.

"The orthopedic team 59-4 performed 21 orthopedic operations. Team 59-3 and the surgical team from the hospital ship performed 27 other major operative procedures. In addition there were numerous débridements, applications of casts and other procedures, detailed data of which are not available.

"A triage team was set up which attempted to separate cases upon arrival into two large classes: the more serious, requiring immediate attention, and the less serious who, temporarily, could wait for operative treatment. 90% of all cases received were serious in nature, and in various degrees of shock. Three cases of penetrating abdominal, or combined thoraco-abdominal wounds were not operated upon.

"Operative procedures were stopped at 0200 hours on the morning of August 18 because it was felt that surgery would militate against possible chance of recovery, since movement from the ship to a fixed hospital was a matter of a few hours. The ship arrived in the port of Naples at 0618 on August 18.

"The U.S.A.H.S. 'Chateau-Thierry,' quite by chance, received patients from the fiercest pocket of resistance encountered in the entire beachhead. Attached surgical teams proved invaluable and the mass of casualties could not have been handled without them.

"Hospital ships going in with, or shortly after an invasion force, should have attached to them for duty, sufficient surgical teams to provide one working team for each available operating room, together with one or more relief teams. Additional clerical personnel is needed on such missions to permit more rapid cataloging and recording of patients. Officers experienced in triage work and shock therapy are most essential during such operations. The commander of troops should be briefed as to what type of casualties he might expect and given some specific information as to his mission."

INTERVAL BETWEEN CORSICA AND SOUTHERN FRANCE

On August 21, 1944, I went to Rome on the courier plane and checked in at the Ambassador Hotel. A stop at the 6th General Hospital the next day gave me an opportunity to talk with Horatio Rogers about surgical staffing problems. "The 6th G. H. has been pared thin compared with the original roster," my notes read. "Now Heine Faxon is ill. I went over his x-ray films with Don King and paid him a short visit. After lunch I looked over some chest surgical problems with Claude McGahey, who was doing a decortication in the morning, and then I went to learn something about eyes from Trygve Gundersen."

At the 33rd General Hospital I stopped to see an injured officer who had been impaled in a parachute drop. His urethra was ruptured and rectum torn. This is a nasty injury—deliberately produced in medieval torture and especially popular in Hungary. A sharpened pole was started into the rectum and the shaft was then planted upright in the ground.

While at the 33rd General Hospital I talked to Eldridge Campbell about a report received from Jason Mixter concerning neurosurgical injuries. My reply to Mixter about neurosurgery in our theater follows:

Dear Jason:

It was good to get your letter and the enclosed copy of your report. The latter represents the *first* information that has come to this theater relative to some of the problems encountered in our patients after transfer to the Z. I. This is not said in criticism—I have ceased being critical—but we would be only too glad to change procedures here in any way to meet the problems of reconstruction in the States.

Our cranio-cerebral wounds receive initial wound surgery in the evacuation hospitals—usually 5-20 miles behind the rear boundary of the division. So far we have been able to supply each evac. with a good neurosurgeon, and at times with two. Deep infection occurs in about 20% of cases débrided at the evac. and is almost always associated with retained bone fragments demonstrable by x-ray examination when the patients arrive at the base. The flat films of the evacs. during a busy period are not always of the best, and it has been suggested that improvisation of stereo films on a Bucky diaphragm may improve results.

The repair of dural defects is an accepted principle—usually with the use of living autogenous fascia or pericranium. Some neurosurgeons (not too experienced) have introduced preserved cadaver dura—but I am opposed to this on general principles as I fear that the scar reaction will be increased. We would appreciate any information you can send us on the fate of dural grafts or patches. I have given some fibrin film to selected surgeons for trial. If this is good for this purpose it should be made a regular issue item.

Peripheral nerves are, as you say, the prime problem and we have given a great deal of thought to the matter. I have discouraged the primary suture of nerves in the forward area. It is impossible to place them in the hands of experts—the neurosurgeon of an evac. cannot possibly leave his head cases to enter the surgery of the extremities. Also, focus of attention on the time consuming repair of nerves detracts attention from the primary function of forward surgery which is the saving of life and prevention of infection.

(continued)

It is an eloquent tribute to surgical standards that have been attained that secondary closure of wounds on or after the fourth day has become an accepted and routine procedure with success in at least 95% of cases. The possibility of repair of the nerve at this time has been studied. In most instances, however, swelling and contusion contraindicate interference at this period. We have also explored the possibility of nerve repair 2-3 weeks after secondary suture when healing by first intention has been attained. Some careful observers like Mike Mason and Henry Schwartz are working with this now. A second incision can be done if desired and the case covered by a course of penicillin.

As to the marking of the ends of the severed nerve with wire. We have given this matter considerable thought and at present are hesitant to advise it as a routine procedure. Having seen one patient come down with a black silk thread hanging out of the wound bearing a paper label "Median Nerve"—you cannot wonder at my conservatism. It seems to me that rough placement of the suture—piercing the end of the nerve and possibly approximation under tension or bridging a defect with a wire bowstring are all problems that would have to be faced as these and even unconsidered aberrations would almost certainly occur. Most of the men here are opposed to marking the nerve.

As to time of evacuation to the Z. I.—this is not by any means within control of the Medical Department. Recently there has been some limited plane evacuation set up and nerves, amputations, malignant disease and the blind been given priority.

I agree with your observation on plaster splints, and we have been trying to build light metal splints for this purpose.

There has been only one enthusiast for nerve grafting in the theater—a pupil of Klemme. I found him with a jam closet full of pickled nerves and quickly pinned his ears back.

You will find our Essential Technical Medical Data Report to the Surgeon General dated July 1, 1944, a discussion of cranio-cerebral injuries—from the evacuation hospital and the general hospital points of view—so I will not go into this question.

I feel sure that the hospitals of the Z. I. will gain a distorted opinion of the quality of surgery done in this theater as they only receive our worst cases. Personally I have quite the opposite point of view. The ability and capacity for work of the surgeons here have far exceeded my greatest hopes. They are doing a superb job with utmost devotion to high professional standards. New principles have been developed to replace clumsy and unsound procedures in vogue scarcely a year ago. I will admit the learning curve perhaps has been slow—but far more rapid than is usual in civilian practice. There is no quitting at 4:30 o'clock in the afternoon and Sunday is just another day.

. . . The M.G.H. group seem happy and have been busier—the two things are synonymous with Medical Officers.

Give my best to anyone at the M.G.H. who still remembers me.

Yours —
PETE

During this stay in Rome I called on the Professor of Surgery, R. Bastianelli. He was carrying on his surgical practice in a small private hospital known as his "Cancer Clinic." He was well known in the United States. He spoke vividly of the difficulties of living under a fascist regime; also of the decline of the university despite the ambitious program of new building construction. On August 24 I took Professor Bastianelli to the 33rd General Hospital for ward rounds and lunch. Horatio Rogers was invited to join us. It seemed important to me to promote such contacts between our surgeons and those of the nations in which we were but temporary residents.

SOUTHERN FRANCE

At a conference between Stalin, Roosevelt and Churchill held at Teheran in November 1943, Stalin agreed with the Americans that divisions from the Italian front should be used to land in southern France and develop an offensive up the Rhone Valley and thence towards the Vosges and the upper reaches of the Rhine. Churchill disagreed with this strategy, and I consider rightly; it removed ten divisions from Italy and thus made it impossible for an offensive from that country to be developed northwards. The war in Italy then became senseless; as Fuller wrote, it became 'A campaign with inadequate means, with no strategic goal and with no political bottom.' The invasion of southern France was, of course, exactly right for Stalin: it would keep the British and Americans well away from the Balkans and eastern Europe. I argued fiercely against it with Eisenhower when we were preparing the invasion of Normandy, but to no avail—the Americans were set on it. In my view it was one of the great strategic mistakes of the war, and I said so to the Americans in no uncertain voice.
—FIELD-MARSHAL VISCOUNT, MONTGOMERY OF ALAMEIN, *A History of Warfare*, p. 518.

If instead of the unnecessary landings in the south of France, which gravely weakened Alexander's armies without any corresponding effect upon the fortunes of the battle in this theater, the Americans had accepted the plan to move rapidly through the Ljubljana Gap, to occupy Vienna, and to secure a great part of what is now Communist Europe, the history of the world would indeed have been changed.
—HAROLD MACMILLAN, *Tides of Fortune*, 1945–1955, pp. xviii–xix.

With an early start to catch the Blood Bank plane from Naples, General Stayer and I left on September 16, 1944, for a tour of the Seventh Army in southern France. Flying high, we traveled up the coast, over Elba and crossed Corsica at Bastia, then over the Ligurian Sea to cross the French coast at Cannes. The Rhone valley was reached just east of Lyons after crossing the Dauphine Alps. Flying low below a ceiling of heavy clouds, the pilot followed a railroad to Besancon and put down on a grass field at 1300 hours. The clouds over Corsica and the mountains of France were unusually beautiful. A chill of autumn was in the air.

The plane carried 500 units of blood and also a French shipment of blood from Algiers. "R.A.F. fighters used Besancon field the day before," my notes say, "so it was closed to planes for evacuation. Our divisions are moving north toward Strasbourg. The French front is approaching Belfort—a strategically important pass or 'gap' in continental warfare." The next two weeks, it was thought, would clarify the situation on the Siegfried Line.

While waiting for transportation I looked at the patients being held in the Provisional Hospital for evacuation by air. About half of them were wounded Germans. Initial surgery had been carried out on all and they were being moved to the Marseilles area. From the airfield we went to the 11th Evacuation Hospital, where I made rounds with Wilson. The hospital was filled and closed to all but casual admissions. After supper J. D. Martin came over from the 43rd General Hospital and we had a long talk. Both Wilson and Martin said that whole blood transfusion had proved to be the greatest advance in forward surgery. In their eyes, plasma infusion was a temporary measure—a substitute for saline solution and other temporary measures of shock therapy used in the past.

The following day was a busy one because General Stayer decided to see all the front line hospitals. "After a breakfast of pancakes, coffee and meat-and-vegetable hash at the 11th Evac.," my notes say, "we found the 93rd in the vicinity of Rioz. Patients were seen with Currier and Howard Patterson." A patient with a lacerated popliteal artery had been repaired by suture and was doing well. He was a captain in the 179th Infantry Division who had been wounded by a shell fragment and operated upon seven and a half hours later. Both the artery and vein had been lacerated by the missile; the vein was ligated and the artery sutured with fine silk. A sympathetic block (L_1 to L_4) was performed and 1,500 cc. of blood given. Both the posterior tibial and dorsalis pedis arteries showed a palpable pulse and the foot was warm with good circulation.

Later, we saw Roy Cohn out in the driveway of the 59th Evacuation Hospital shoveling gravel. It was raining constantly and the mud problem increasing. The 59th Evacuation Hospital had no patients because it was just setting up.

Taking Roy along, we drove on to 6th Corps Rear. After lunch we went to Saulx to see the 1st Platoon of the 11th Field Hospital, which supposedly was backing up the 36th Division. This platoon was in a low-lying field full of water. After evacuating four patients they were preparing to move. We then drove Roy back to the 59th Evacuation Hospital and we moved along to the 9th Evacuation Hospital in the vicinity of Poligny. "It was good," I wrote in my diary, "to see the 9th Evac. in the field again instead of in the Naples fairgrounds." They had over 900 patients after a big push. This was a Sunday afternoon and a throng of French was visiting the hospital, bringing presents to the wounded. After a warming drink of rye we drove to Lons to the Seventh Army Command Post. General White, Chief of Staff, told us that General Bradley was holding General Patton in control. "If I were allowed to pick the hole," Patton had said, "I would be in Berlin in two days."

The B.B.C. broadcast gave the following appraisal of the war situation on September 17: The Fifth Army was headed for Bologna across the Gothic Line, and Kesselring was offering strong resistance to the Eighth Army at the Rimini end of the line. A breakthrough of the Siegfried Line was taking place near Aachen. The Russians were at Warsaw, but the fall of the city was not yet announced.

"Here in southern France," my notes read, "the Seventh Army has now arrived at a point of resistance facing Belfort gap. The 3rd, 36th and 45th Divisions are on the north next to Third Army. The French are moving across to the right flank. Paratroop teams are protecting the right flank of the Continental Base Section against three Italian and two German divisions in north Italy."

SCENE OF LIBERATION

Certainly I had never seen as happy a people or an army. I sat in my jeep during a traffic jam on the way down to Lons. Everyone was with a smile and a wave. The enthusiasm of the French populace was contagious.

The countryside was practically untouched by war from Saulx to Lons, though burned-out German vehicles dotted the road—one with brake linings still smoldering. The streets and houses were bedecked with French and American flags. Healthy-looking children were riding bicycles. It was quite a new phase of the war compared with the grim days in North Africa, Sicily and Italy.

On September 17, I wrote the following letter to my wife:

From Southern Italy to the cold autumn of France is a long jump. Aside from the cloudy skies and drizzling rain, however, it is very pleasant to be in a part of France that closely resembles Vermont. Even the green pastures with plenty of white and brown Swiss cows and an occasional flock of sheep—the pine woods and the clean little farms are reminiscent of home. On first stepping out of the plane the *smell* of wet grass was something I had not experienced since I have been overseas.

If you have followed the newspaper accounts of the progress of the 7th Army you will know the territory under my supervision. Having Frank Berry as Consulting Surgeon of the Army relieves me of any details, so I can just amble around and see what I wish.

The French have decorated their houses (and trees) with flags—American and French—and are all friendly and happy I suppose already beginning to split up into multitudinous political parties as usual.

As I landed up near the front, I shall in a few days go down the valley to the Riviera. Then perhaps back to Hqts as before long I should go up to Florence. This splitting of the theater activities poses problems in transportation, at least so long as the enemy sits in northern Italy.

Strange that I have little personal desire ever to go into Germany. The General says he will send me home very soon after the end, and let's hope that is not far away.

On September 18, I had breakfast at Seventh Army headquarters with Colonel Rudolph and then drove to the Seventh Army Rear. I found Frank Berry preparing a circular letter on tetanus because cases had developed in Germans and in French civilians. "Frank believes," I noted, "that gas gangrene is on the increase. If this is proven correct, it is probably a reflection of the wet, muddy weather. Frank and I agree that we would be willing to cut out the postoperative local application of sulfonamide, but just when an increase in wound infection is likely to occur is the wrong time."

I had lunch with Forsee and Sullivan at the 2nd Auxiliary Group detachment. Forsee was worried as to where his headquarters was officially located—in Fifth or Seventh Army territory. I suggested that he leave this matter in a confused state so each Army would think it had the headquarters. Forsee could then operate in both.

In the evening a noteworthy dinner was held at a small French restaurant, Chez Yvonne. It was deep in the foothills of the Jura, remote from tourist traffic even in peacetime and maintained the traditions of the French rural restaurant despite the period of German retreat and American occupation. It lay on the bank of the Ain—a simple dining room and a small kitchen presided over by large-busted Yvonne. In the kitchen was a small range with strings of mushrooms drying over it. All food served was from the immediate vicinity except the salt.

Taking seats around the table were General Stayer, Colonel Rudolph, Frank Berry, Lieutenant Colonel Oscar Reeder (in charge of hospitalization and evacuation), Lieutenant Colonel Ryle A. Radke (in charge of medical supplies) and myself.

The superb demonstration of *cuisine de pays* began with thick and slightly brown potato soup. This was followed by: potato salad ringed with tomatoes and covered with thick mayonnaise; a very rich pig liver and lard paté; large escargot served with apologies that no *truit* had been caught today; mushrooms with thick white sauce with a taste of sour cream; escalloped potatoes with cheese—rather thick and not too mealy; *poulet*—steamed and served with thin sauce; green salad—no olive oil, of course, and a dressing was made by adding chicken liver to bacon fat containing small bits of crackling. The wine vinegar was hardly detectable; cake and apples; *café nationale* with beet sugar. Wines were Chateau Neuf du Pape, 1939, and as a dessert wine the sweet and heavy Chateau Chalon vin de paille. The dinner was topped off by cognac.

My first note on the cold, gray morning of September 19 was that "the General didn't want any breakfast, but finally decided to eat an egg and pancake after drinking much water!"

We left Lons to go to Lyons but after pursuing the wrong road for thirty kilometers or so, we turned back. Oscar Reeder had loaded all baggage in the jeep which was to follow us. We lost the jeep and couldn't find it on the turn around near Louhans. Then the General found out that his baggage was in it! That was an unhappy hour or so for Oscar. To stall for time so that the jeep could get to Lyons before we did, he persuaded the General to go from Bourg via Ambérieu to see the air evacuation unit and a provisional convalescent hospital. The General turned his wrath onto the air evacuation and onto the mud surrounding the hospital, so the air cleared somewhat as we approached Lyons.

The city of Lyons was just pulling itself together after the jag of liberation. The French Forces of Interior (F. F. I.) were very busy there. General Tupper told me tales of having seen the collaborationists tortured—not a new event in the long and bloody history of this ancient city. Piles of broken glass windows littered the streets and barbed wire barricades were all about. DeGaulle was there three days ago and started the people to work picking up. Only two bridges remained and these were partly demolished. We drove into the railway train shed and crossed the Rhone on the railway bridge. The rails had been removed to make a truck route. The other remaining bridge had one span made of a Bailey. The sides of this bridge were jammed with pedestrians.

A platoon of the 15th Field Hospital was setting up in Lyons. German prisoners of war, looking young and scared, were cleaning out the building. A guard, leaning back in his chair with a rifle across his knees, looked like a squirrel hunter. There was no need to shoot to keep these prisoners from running out on the streets of Lyons. They would be torn into bits immediately.

Then we took the General window shopping, looking for perfume. Finally I found a bottle of Indiscrète and a box of Caron face powder and later a couple of bottles of Nuit de Noel. The prices were standard, but the saleswoman decided she was going to charge for the *flagon*! I gave her a pack of cigarettes (worth $80 a carton, by the way) so I more than squared accounts.

"In the evening," according to my notes, "I went to dinner with Oscar Reeder and Batch—our representatives in the Sixth Army Group. . . . After dinner I suggested to Oscar that he should inspect the mess and the chlorination of the table water, because the General in the morning would sniff for chlorine at breakfast. We went down into the kitchen to see the mess sergeant who insisted he put chlorine into the Lister bag, but he took a long time to produce any."

RHONE VALLEY

On September 20, General Stayer, Oscar Reeder and I made an early start south into the Rhone Valley. The valley had been swept clean by the retreating Nineteenth German Army and the pursuing U. S. Seventh Army. The villages showed little evidence of damage except where delaying actions took place. Near Montélimar the Air Force caught a transport column and the road was lined with burned-out vehicles, guns and a railway with two large railway guns.

From Avignon we turned left but soon found the bridges across the Durance impassable as the flood waters were sweeping over the pontoons. Back at Avignon, I saw what I suppose was the residence of the Popes. Then we crossed another railway bridge and went through fields and tiny Provence villages to regain the Aix road south of the Durance. An easy run through the Rhone delta brought us into the rocky pine woods of Aix. We reached the 27th Evacuation Hospital in time for supper. They had just evacuated all patients and were ready to move north. We visited the 36th General Hospital in a large sanatorium west of Aix where Jim Winfield was in charge of a large number of prisoners of war as well as American battle casualties.

We had a conference with the Continental Base Surgeon.

E.D.C. Comments: "He is hastily placing his hospitals where he can find buildings," I noted, "and has no clear-cut idea of the axis of supply. He wants a general hospital in Lyons, one in Dijon, etc., etc., as well as numerous station hospitals far up behind Seventh Army. I tried to explain the principles of evacuation from evacuation to general hospitals and keeping patients in general hospitals until they were ready for disposition. It was the same old evacuation panic. The deployment of general hospitals as if they were evacuation hospitals is basically wrong. Evacuation by air will be shut down increasingly by winter weather and provision must be made for rail and ambulance movement of patients from Army. This should be on the Epinal-Dijon-Marseilles axis—not on the Besancon-Grenoble-Beach axis. The latter will soon fade out of the picture as the French move into Belfort."

The next morning, September 21, saw a heavy cover of ground fog in the low areas, not unlike Cape Cod on an autumn day. We made an early start along the main highway to le Muy and then south to Ste. Maxime where a clearing platoon was still acting as a holding hospital. Before turning south at le Muy, we went north a short distance to Draguignan to visit the 51st Evacuation Hospital which was also getting ready to move north.

At St. Raphael the 78th Station Hospital was temporarily set up in the Golfe Hotel—formerly Seventh Army Headquarters. I made rounds there. At Cannes I stopped and bought some children's books and a pin for my wife. Between Cannes and Nice we had a long delay until a French tank convoy passed, but we arrived at Nice by midafternoon. The city was quite deserted. This flank of the Seventh Army had been turned over to forces under General Fredericks, supposedly to hold a line back at le Muy. They had pushed ahead, however, to the Italian border just beyond Menton.

At the Alhambra Hotel I met someone I knew from Airborne Force Headquarters and spent a good deal of time getting the facts on the problems the force was having in the Maritime Alps. The plan was to pull back these troops about D+5 but they had been in active ground combat since D-Day. It was too bad to use specialized troops in this manner.

I spent the night at General Fredericks' villa in Nice. There, I jotted down some of the facts I had heard about the Airborne attack. They are as follows:

The Germans had set up glider defenses in all open flat fields. These were heavy posts about twelve to fifteen feet high, connected by wires to booby trap grenades or artillery shells. These defenses were not picked up by aerial photographs, and were not recognizable even now, when it was known what to look for. The staff of the Airborne Division had come over from the States five weeks before D-Day. Despite planning to pack a surgical hospital in gliders and take it in, no opportunity was found to carry the plans through.

The Airborne force in the southern France landing included 5,000 parachutists and about 1,500 glider personnel in 376 gliders. The first echelon medical service went in with the jumpers at 0430 to 0500 hours. The clearing component went with the gliders. The gliders started at 1500 hours and the medical company came in about 1800 hours. They had picked out their station from aerial maps but it was too close to the command post and caused traffic confusion. Contact with ground forces was made at 1500 hours on D+2. Two hundred and thirty-seven casualties, including prisoners of war, were evacuated from the clearing company. There were 57 deaths in two days, 15 to 20 in the aid station. Glider landing injuries were numerous, typically of head and face, upper extremity and chest. In a total of some 300 casualties there were between 87 to 90 gunshot wounds.

The booby trapping of the defenses had not been completed and many of the poles put in by the French were loosely set. Captured vehicles were used in collecting the injured. Many parachutists caught in trees had been shot or bayoneted.

E.D.C. Comments: "The experience suggests," I noted in my diary, "that a portable surgical hospital be designed. When stripped down, this hospital should be of a size to be mounted in not more than six gliders. A full airborne medical company should drop with parachutes—except the vehicle drivers—they should follow early. All vehicles—artillery movers and others—should be fixed up to be converted into litter carriers, as many have little to do after their primary job is completed and can be released for collection of the wounded and injured."

After an early breakfast at General Fredericks' villa, we started on the long drive to Lyons. The perfume center—Grasse—was approached by a narrow detour around a demolished bridge. From there the Napoleon Bonaparte Highway took us to Grenoble through the Dauphine Alps. As we neared Grenoble the rugged Pelvoux Massif came into view. We had planned to spend the night in Grenoble but, after looking about, decided to push along to Lyons which we reached about 6:00 P.M.

The following morning, September 23, General Stayer was nursing a cold, so Oscar Reeder and I went to Sixth Army Group Headquarters. We found little to do there, so we walked around the city, looking at the shops and otherwise killing time until the General recovered from his cold. "E.T.O. plans to take over the Seventh Army and Sixth Army Group in another month," I wrote in my diary. "At that time I can go home."

CONTINUING THE TOUR

General Stayer went back by way of Marseilles that afternoon and I borrowed a jeep and driver and headed back toward the front. The only jeep I could get had no top and the weather was cold with a constant drizzle. I reached Besancon about 6:00 P.M. and looked up the 46th General Hospital, which was just setting up. Hot coffee, bread and jam restored my spirits effectively and I spent the night in a hotel where the officers of the hospital were living temporarily.

The weather was still cold and rainy on the following morning. The 46th General Hospital had about 150 patients and the rest of their equipment was being trucked up from the beaches. The headquarters of the Seventh Army was at Vesoul, so I pushed along through the rain and fog to reach that city. Frank Berry was at headquarters and had just received a promotion to full colonel. This called for a celebration, so we set off for the 9th Evacuation Hospital, which was about two miles south of Plombiers in a sea of mud and fog.

Jack McKittrick was doing a débridement and another surgeon a midthigh amputation for "gas gangrene" on a prisoner of war. My note on the latter case was: "Really believe this was 'anaerobic cellulitis' in the dead leg with dissection of a little gas upward along normal tissue planes. This misinterpretation may account for the fact that so-called gas cases following arterial obstruction do so well following amputation. The surgeon is dealing with the putrefactive changes in the dead tissues rather than the invasive infection of 'gas gangrene.'"

A cold night in Jim Thompson's tent was punctuated by artillery fire in the north. The cold and constant rain continued as I headed north through Remiremont with a stop at a platoon of the 11th Field Hospital just south of Plombiers. Gordon Madding had been left in charge of some thirty nontransportable wounded. One patient with ligation of the common femoral artery needed amputation, and a man with a spinal cord lesion as well as one kidney out and the other damaged, needed suprapubic drainage. The cord injury may have been only a contusion although the patient showed hyperesthesia and complete loss of motor power.

North of Remiremont I found another platoon of the 11th Field Hospital that had been set up during the night. Two artillery shells had dropped in the hospital area that morning. The site was near the bank of the Moselle and our artillery was still on this side of the river shooting across into the Vosges mountains. The forward troops were about six miles across the river. The surgical teams of this platoon had found a warm and dry room in a nearby house. It was warmed with a battery of some fifteen electric heaters.

The return to Vesoul in the rain was made more tolerable because my driver acquired a bit of tarpaulin in Bescancon with which the jeep had been converted into a "closed" car. In this contrivance I put in at 2nd Auxiliary Group Headquarters. By the following morning I had a full-blown edition of the General's cold with pouring sinuses.

Headquarters of the 2nd Auxiliary Group in Vesoul provided a large schoolroom with a small stove, so I holed up there for a couple of days. Henry Beecher showed up for a few minutes. Later in the afternoon, Tech. 4th Gr. Melvin Shaffer, from the Museum and Medical Arts Service, arrived—an excellent photographer.

One of the surgeons showed me an article he had just completed on war injuries of the chest. It was full of new entities such as "the wet lung of trauma," "hemithoracic empyema," and "traumatic thoracotomy." My reaction was worded:

E.D.C. Comments: "The thoracic surgeons obviously think I am too critical of their writings but I know of no area where the effects of narrow specialism are as glaring as in chest surgery at the present moment—particularly in trauma. Chest surgeons have spent so much time in sanitariums and on elective thoracic surgical operations that their lack of background in trauma is pathetic. They are busy 'discovering' things that they did not know existed. Being 'chest surgeons' they think no one else knew about the reaction of the lung to traumatic injury!"

By September 28, both my cold and the weather were much better. My predictions about the end of the war were becoming more realistic.

E.D.C. Comments: "It looks like the weather is closing down too early to bring the war to an end this fall," I noted. "Certainly opinion over here and as reflected from SHAEF is not too optimistic. The airborne landing in Holland has failed or is but a limited success. There are no rumors of Germany cracking and it is thought that we will have to fight our way in for military occupation. The Russians are said to be holding off in order to preserve the industrial facilities of Germany which they expect to use."

The following day I was on the road again. At the 59th Evacuation Hospital I made rounds with Matheson and Cohn while Shaffer took photographs. A young German soldier had a bullet through his spine; another with "toxemia" from residual blood clot showed mental apathy, fever and rapid pulse but no sign of reduced blood volume. This patient complained bitterly of pain, completely relieved by the evacuation of clot. "What is the significance of pain as a symptom of infection?" I asked myself. "In the last case at the 9th Evac. I thought it might be attributed to the associated femoral thrombophlebitis. Is it possibly a muscle cramp or spasm?"

At Vesoul, I saw Barker of the 12th General Hospital, who came in on the Blood Bank plane. "He reported," I noted, "that Naples is becoming a ghost city and the fairgrounds seem deserted with the 9th Evac., the 33rd G.H. and the 21st G.H. moved out. The 37th has been flooded out and is moving into the buildings of the 33rd. Barker hates to see things breaking up, as we all do. We had three bottles of champagne in lieu of cocktails before dinner at Seventh Army just to cheer us up."

French headquarters was in Besancon, and on the last day of September, Courtillet came up to see me to clear again certain policies of wound management. The 95th Evacuation Hospital was in the vicinity of Saulx, so in the afternoon I dropped over to make rounds with Grantley Taylor and to take some photographs. "Dutch" Ludwig—Seventh Army psychiatrist—and Frank Berry joined me for dinner and we had a long discussion about the Italian campaign. Ludwig came back to the 2nd Auxiliary headquarters for the night. We were beginning to have more neuropsychiatric cases (N.P.'s) as a result of men being a long time in the line and the coming of cold weather.

On October 1, Frank Berry and I visited the 46th General Hospital and obtained photographs of two patients with abdominal wounds, both being examples of errors in judgment. At the 2nd Convalescent Hospital I picked up a couple of German helmets for my sons—there was a great clamor among the young at home for these helmets. At Evacuation Hospital No. 415 (French) I saw Pierre Stricker. Pierre's home was formerly in Mulhouse so he was getting near home although he seemed doubtful about ever getting there. Like other Frenchmen he was like a little boy who has hauled off and hit a bully in the eye and is waiting—a little scared—to see what happens next. Everything had happened so suddenly that they couldn't believe it was real; many believed that the Germans would be back.

"Dinner with Joe Still, Berry and Robinson—Still just returned from Paris," I recorded in my diary. "Rumor has it that the war must be prolonged so that E.T.O. may enjoy a winter in Paris! The Medical Section has built up a tremendous headquarters with all officers in blouses instead of field uniforms and 'spit and polish' formalities. All are completely vague about Seventh Army—where it is and where it came from. The show in the big tent will start in another month and our little curtain raiser in North Africa—Sicily—Italy and southern France will be forgotten."

ACCUMULATING MORE DATA

I have referred to the sensitivity to criticism of the forward surgeons. It amused me in making rounds at the 11th Field Hospital on October 2 to find them upset by an account published in the August issue of the *Army Medical Bulletin*. An observer, referring to field hospitals, had written that "some are really good." I spent the entire day at the 11th Field Hospital platoon and the clearing platoon of the 36th Division accumulating case records on all but about six of their patients. In the late afternoon I went to Epinal to find the new headquarters of the 2nd Auxiliary Group. It was set up with a machine records unit in a schoolroom. The room made a cold bedroom for Joe Still and me. The following morning I visited another platoon of the 11th Field Hospital, which was joined with the clearing station of the 45th Division. I made rounds with Fred Jarvis, Carlton, Swingle, McMillan and others. We had a discussion about the value of a brief delay period in resuscitation.

My notes read in part: "Beecher, who was present, believed that in the age group we are dealing with, surgery should merge with resuscitation and be undertaken as soon as the patient is warm, shows good peripheral circulation and the blood pressure has improved and is showing improvement. Further delay can be obtained only at the expense of further 'external support,' that is—more blood or plasma. Massive amounts of blood are hazardous in themselves, so delay for any reason should not be countenanced.

"Many of the 2nd Auxiliary Group surgeons—Jarvis, Sullivan, and others — believe that an added two to three hours, even if obtained at the expense of the very slow infusion of plasma or blood, is important in 'establishing' the patient so he is better able to withstand anesthesia, surgery, moving and putting to bed.

"This is an important controversy, but perhaps more theoretical than practical when blood is being used and is available in liberal amounts during and after surgery. It is possible that Jarvis and others still are thinking in terms of resuscitation with plasma only. However, they insist that blood pressures will drop if patients are hurried to surgery."

Many interesting cases were passing through. A patient who died with anuria was autopsied by Ed Cantlon, and I obtained photographs of the kidney and a complete record. I took moving pictures of Swingle performing an amputation on an elderly French civilian; also of a thoracoabdominal penetrating wound operated on by Jarvis. A tent fire caused some excitement but was promptly extinguished by Cantlon. Much to their surprise I led a chorus of French children in a rendition of "Avec mes sabots." After dark, back at Epinal, Sullivan dug up some stoves from bombed-out houses and made a warm room.

The next day I learned that a radio message had come through from Caserta, requesting my return. I went to Luxueil, again in the rain, and found an air evacuation plane just about to take off. We left about noon. After landing in Dijon the plane went down the Rhone valley to a huge field at Istris. With the commanding officer of the 162nd Medical Battalion, I drove to Aix for a 12th Air Force courier plane out of les Milles.

I had dinner with Ira Ferguson and other friends at the 43rd General Hospital, and afterwards we made rounds with Ira and J. P. Martin. Two prisoners of war had tetanus—there had been nine cases in the hospital in this location and seven had died.

E.D.C. Comments: "We talked about German surgery as Ira Ferguson saw it when he took over this place from the Germans," I noted. "It is very bad. The men are poorly trained. The practice in blood transfusion is to select a type specific donor from dog tags and use a direct syringe (Unger) method. A pause is made after the first 10 cc. to watch for a reaction. It is rare for the Germans to give more than 250 to 300 cc. and they were amazed to see a 1,000 cc. transfusion in addition to 2,500 to 3,000 cc. infusion. They are quick to advise amputation and unsound in indications. As Ira remarked: 'War surgery can be very grim in the hands of untrained surgeons.'"

On October 5, I left les Milles at 0900 hours. It was foggy and cloudy out at sea. The plane rounded the tip of Corsica and put down at a field south of Bastia, then to Grosseta with time out for chow. I left Grosseta at 1300 hours in a storm with strong wind from offshore. We put down at Tarquinia just north of Civitavechia for five minutes. After a stop at Lido Roma and Napoli, I arrived at Capodochino in the rain.

EPILOGUE

In an address on the surgical management of the severely wounded given at a meeting of the Yale Medical Society on March 13, 1946, I described two cases that illustrate the high level attained by the surgeons of the Mediterranean Theater in the autumn of 1944.

E.D.C. Comments: "On the last day of September, 1944, a mortally wounded American soldier was brought to a small forward hospital in southern France. He was in severe shock, but following three units of plasma and a transfusion of whole blood, his condition slowly improved. An x-ray examination was made and he was taken to the operating tent. Ether-oxygen anesthesia was induced and an intratracheal tube inserted, as it was planned to open the chest cavity. Operation was started just seven hours after the shell-burst that produced the wounds.

"The tenth rib on the left side was resected, and the chest cavity opened widely. A fragment of shell coming from below had perforated the diaphragm, pierced the pericardium and lodged in the wall of the heart. A sharp projection of the fragment extended through the wall of the ventricle into the chamber of the heart. The missile measured 2 × 2 × 0.5 centimeters. It was removed and the torrential hemorrhage controlled by the index finger of the surgeon which readily entered the left ventricular cavity. The wound of the heart was repaired with silk sutures. The pericardium, that had been opened to give access to the heart, was closed, leaving a 2.5 cm. opening for drainage.

"The diaphragm was then incised and a ragged tear of the spleen and its pedicle disclosed. Splenectomy was performed. Perforations on both anterior and posterior walls of the stomach were sutured. Two large perforations of the colon required mobilization of the bowel and exteriorization through a separate incision in the abdominal wall. The lower pole of the kidney had been lacerated by the missile, and after careful inspection was managed by an exteriorizing drain placed through an incision in the flank. After the diaphragm and major incision were sutured, wounds of the back, thighs, and legs were treated by excisional surgery.

"During the operation, eight pints of whole blood were given by transfusion. The condition of the patient at the end of the operation was better than when it started. The pulse rate was 100 and the blood pressure 120/70. Penicillin therapy was instituted. On the fourteenth of October the patient was transferred to a general hospital in excellent condition. On the first of November the exteriorized segment of colon was repaired and replaced in the abdomen. On the eighteenth of November the patient was walking and his wounds were healed. Six weeks after wounding he was sent back to the United States.

"The case of this particular soldier is admittedly dramatic, partly because the missile reached the heart. Aside from that it may be taken as representative of emergency forward surgery in World War II. In no way can it be passed by as a single lucky episode or stunt.

Here is an extract from a letter received by a forward hospital in Italy from a medical officer still farther forward in an artillery battalion.

"I want to commend the work of the surgeons and nurses who treated Corporal A. who was admitted to your hospital on 1 January, 1945. When this soldier was brought into the battalion aid station, he had a hole in his belly big enough for a canteen to go through. There was a perforation through the diaphragm, through which a blowing sound was heard with each breath, indicating a punctured lung. His right forearm showed several deep lacerations and a compound fracture or two. His left arm presented a compound fracture—dislocation at the elbow.

"After he was evacuated, his commanding officer called me about the severity of the case. I told him nothing short of a miracle could save that man's life. I am happy to hear that the miracle was performed and that Corporal A. is now coming along fine in the . . . General Hospital, all limbs having been saved."

Matthew D. Nealeigh, Gordon G. Wisbach, and Matthew D. Tadlock

In this chapter, Churchill is perpetually in motion—visiting, discussing, learning, listening, teaching. He travels by courier plane, evacuation C-47, blood bank plane, and Jeep to monitor the advancing front in Southern France. He describes various casualty evacuation modalities: by ground via ambulance and train, by fixed wing airplane, and by sea in both US Navy Tank Landing Ships (LST) and hospital ships (**Figure 32.1A-C**). Therefore, this chapter is quintessentially about *logistics*. At this point in the war, the Allies had well-established logistical chains providing far forward whole blood, appropriately sized surgical capability and capacity, and patient evacuation.

At the beginning of World War II, the US military had only two Navy hospital ships; by war's end, it operated 39 (15 Navy, 24 Army), including one that transported Churchill home at the war's end. In the European and Mediterranean theatres, US and British Armies preferred casualty evacuation by hospital ship because of Geneva and Hague convention protections. Despite these protections and clear markings, the British lost six hospital ships to Axis aerial attacks in the Mediterranean. Conversely, the US Navy preferred medically augmented LSTs for their practicality of casualty receiving during amphibious assaults and the short distances traveled in the Mediterranean (**Figure 32.1C**).

During the invasion of Southern France, the US Army utilized 12 evacuation hospital ships such as the *Chateau Thierry* (**Figure 32.1A**), Casualties were first treated by a landing barge shock team before a boom lift with a double-decker cradle hoisted them onto the ship for further treatment and evacuation. Throughout most of World War II, particularly in the Navy, hospital ships were generally utilized as "scoop and sail" ambulances. It wasn't until the 1945 invasion of Iwo Jima that they were utilized to their full capability as combat surgical hospitals.

Chapter 32 is now two years past the New York Times article prompted by Churchill, supporting whole blood services. While whole blood is nearly ubiquitous in theatre on both land and sea, he continues to proselytize, but—importantly—he does this from the front. He records one conversation with surgeons who tell him, "whole blood transfusion had proved to be the greatest advance in forward surgery." Despite relearning whole blood's value in recent wars, current availability is limited and the US military is largely dependent upon component therapy and the "walking blood bank" model,

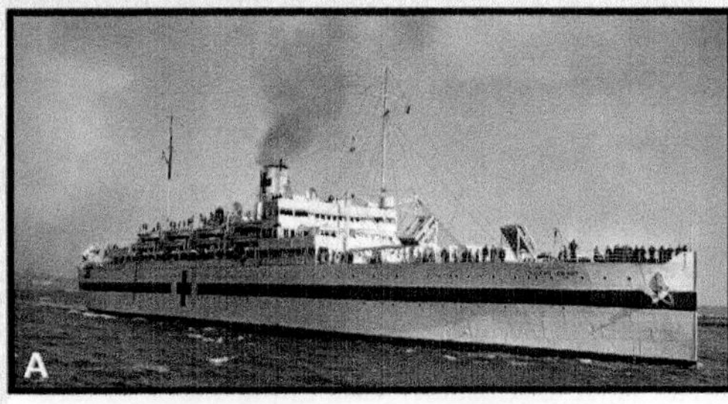
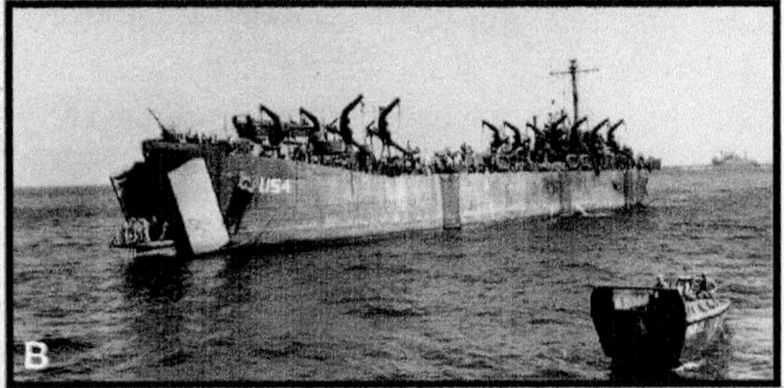
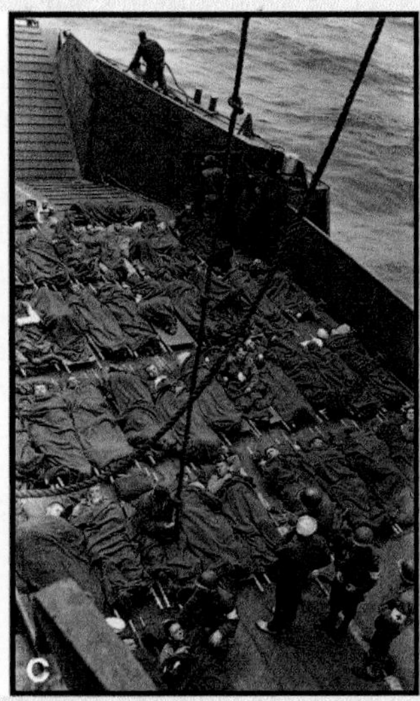

Figure 32.1 (A) US Army Hospital Ship *Chateau Thierry*, named after the location on the Marne River where American forces won their first definitive victory in World War I. Here it is pictured near South Boston, Massachusetts, March 1944. (Provided by OHA 343 U.S. Army Signal Corps Photography Collection. Otis Historical Archives, National Museum of Health and Medicine. Used with permission) (B)* USS LST-4 approaches the shore at Yellow Beach, Pampelonne, Var, on August 16, 1944, during the Southern France Invasion (Courtesy of Naval History and Heritage Command, obtained from the National Archives.) I. (C)* Example of casualties on an LCT (Landing Craft, Tank) being brought to an LST (Landing Ship, Tank) for evacuation during the 1944 Normandy Invasion (Courtesy of the Bureau of Medicine and Surgery Archives.) *B, C: Government photos, not in copyright.

particularly on aircraft carriers, casualty-receiving amphibious warships, and its two Navy hospital ships.

At the time of this commentary, the specter of future Large-Scale Combat Operations (LSCO) is ever-present. The Russia-Ukraine war is ongoing and the People's Republic of China is a significant pacing threat. Despite this, Military Medicine continues to focus on deploying small single surgeon teams, commonly used during the last 20 years of war. Viewing this strategy through a World War II lens, General Omar Bradley's quote, "Amateurs talk strategy, professionals talk logistics," comes to mind. In future LSCOs across Europe or the Indo-Pacific region, contested airspace will force us to reestablish the sophisticated logistical chain used in World War II to support long-range whole blood delivery, surgical capability and capacity for forward and large-scale casualty evacuation by land and sea.

SUGGESTED READINGS

Gurney JM, Jensen SD, Gavitt BJ, et al. Committee on Surgical Combat Casualty Care position statement on the use of single surgeon teams and invited commentaries. *J Trauma Acute Care Surg.* 2022 Aug;93(2S):S6-S11.

Lane DA. Hospital ship doctrine in the United States Navy: the Halsey effect on scoop-and-sail tactics. *Mil Med.* 1997 Jun;162(6):388-395.

Massman EA. *Hospital Ships of World War II: An Illustrated Reference to 39 United States Military Vessels.* McFarland; 2015.

Remondelli MH, Remick KN, Shackelford SA, et al. Casualty care implications of large-scale combat operations. *J Trauma Acute Care Surg.* 2023 Aug;95(2S):S180-S184.

Tadlock MD, Gurney JM, Tripp MS, et al. Between the devil and the deep blue sea: a review of 25 modern naval mass casualty incidents with implications for future Distributed Maritime Operations. *J Trauma Acute Care Surg.* 2021 Aug;91(2S):S46-S55.

33

Escort to a Congresswoman

For Many Years Edith Nourse Rogers, of Lowell, had represented the Massachusetts Congressional district that includes Belmont, where I live. A message had been received at Caserta that she was to visit the Mediterranean Theater. This was the reason for the request that I return to headquarters from southern France. I was to act as escort in her visits to our hospitals. Mrs. Rogers was in the E.T.O. and would be coming to Caserta. I had a few days to catch up with affairs at headquarters and in Naples.

Dick Shackelford, of Baltimore, for instance, had recently arrived in the theater as a "casual replacement" and I immediately began to look for a spot for a surgeon of his experience and ability. Doug Kendricks had come to Italy from the Surgeon General's office to study the blood transfusion problems. Champ Lyons and Dick Chute were still patients in the 300th General Hospital with hepatitis. Both were to leave for the Zone of the Interior.

On October 8, 1944, Perrin Long and I were on our way back from Naples when we stopped at the French Croix Rouge. The Fascist regime had brought a large number of boys from Tunisia to Italy. They were mostly of Italian parentage but of French citizenship. The Croix Rouge was rounding them up and taking them back to Tunisia. "How highly the young male animal is valued in Europe!" I jotted in my diary.

Meanwhile, the Veterans Administration and the greatly expanded role it would play after World War II had become a subject of growing interest to many of us. One day, a general told me that all doctors employed by the Veterans Administration had been commissioned in the Army by presidential order. This had been done despite many protests. It was done, "in order to make them veterans and thus enable them to hold their jobs against returning men now in the service."

A WHIRL AROUND ITALY

Mrs. Rogers was at dinner in the palace mess, accompanied by Lieutenant Colonel Storer Humphreys and Lieutenant Commander Harold K. Latta as escorts. I was to accompany the party to Rome. The following morning we left Capodoccini in a B-25 for a forty minute flight. We were met by the Commanding General of the Rome Area Command, and by Ambassador Alexander Kirk. After a brief visit to the 73rd Station Hospital, we went to a cocktail party in the Barbareni Palace, now the U. S. Embassy, where Mrs. Rogers was to spend the night. At the party were Mr. Myron Taylor, the personal representative of President Roosevelt to the Vatican, Charles Poleti and many others. I was invited to remain for a quiet dinner with the Ambassador and his secretary, Mr. Horn, who had been with Kirk in Arabia. Horn had paid a visit to Ibn Saud in the desert. Telephones were installed in Saudi Arabia only after the Koran had been read over once to demonstrate that it was not the work of the devil.

An appointment for Mrs. Rogers to be received by Pope Pius XII was at 10:00 A.M. on October 17. We met Mr. Taylor punctually and followed his car into a rear gate. An elevator took us to the papal offices. Our party then passed through about fourteen rooms in which stood guards and then dignitaries in an increasing order of importance until finally there were those with whom we were expected to shake hands. Ultimately we were seated in a throne room in which hung a portrait of Il Papa. A clock was mounted on an enormous amethyst crystal and on the floor was a silken rug with the papal crown pointing toward the golden throne. This recalled the orientation of prayer rug patterns in Islamic countries which point toward Mecca. We sat uneasily on red gilt chairs waiting to see what was to happen next.

Finally Mr. Taylor went in—then Mrs. Rogers. Then Mrs. Rogers came out and we three escorts went into the adjoining room. The Pope shook hands with each of us in turn, asking where we were from and whether we had families and he blessed them all. He asked me whether I would like to have a souvenir and took a small medal from his desk for me. His Holiness appeared tired and older than he seemed at public audience.

We then went out, past the dignitaries, the flunkies and the Swiss guards, leaving the Vatican at 11:30 on the dot.

From the Vatican we escorted Mrs. Rogers to the M.G.H. unit. There, at the 6th General Hospital, she visited the wards and was simple and direct in her approach to the sick and wounded.

Excusing myself from a dinner at Ambassador Kirk's villa, I hopped on a plane back to Naples and had a dinner meeting with General Stayer at Caserta. Returning to Rome in the morning, I joined the Rogers party at the airport and took off in a Hudson 109 with a British crew, expecting to put down in Florence at 10:00 A.M. sharp. There was no hole in the heavy fog that filled the valley of the Arno, so after circling several times we went to a landing field near Cecina that was used by a bomber group. I made some telephone calls and arranged an alternate schedule, which meant going to Leghorn and driving over the road to Florence. When we were ready to push off to Leghorn in a command car, we learned that the field at Florence was open. After more telephoning we flew to Florence, arriving at 1500 hours. The plane was met by a lineup of nurses and Wac's, with Joe Martin, the Fifth Army Surgeon, and Joseph P. Sullivan, the Quartermaster, officially welcoming her.

In a convoy of sedans, and accompanied by a battery of photographers, we were shown the activities of the quartermaster department—salvage—dumps—diets and bakery. Then at Lightening Rear, Mrs. Rogers had tea with nurses and Wac's—and her escorts had rum with Sullivan. Someone in our group told a story of a soldier being court-martialed for calling his officer an S.O.B. The witness to the incident was certain the soldier had referred to that officer because he was the "only s.o.b. around here."

On the following morning the convoy reassembled to leave at 0800 hours. Highway 5 took us to the defenses of the Gothic Line in the Appennines—barbed wire, mine fields, tank ditches and gun emplacements. Finally we arrived at the Command Post at 1000 hours and were met by General Mark Clark. After a review of the guard we went into a hut where the tactical situation was explained with the aid of maps. That day an attack was being concentrated on Mt. Grande, which General Clark believed was the key to the present situation. Mrs. Rogers was invited to present a Legion of Merit medal to a public relations officer of the Fifth Army.

We then visited the 8th Evacuation Hospital and the 94th Evacuation Hospital at Monghidoro. The 94th Evacuation Hospital had just moved to this site and shells had fallen in the motor pool that morning. Here we called on our research group—Harry Beecher and Tracy Mallory. Showstack and Breslau, of the Museum and Medical Arts service, were with the research group. Breslau had done some excellent watercolors of hospital scenes.

After lunch at the 94th Evacuation Hospital, we drove forward into the divisional area. The "bomb line" for guidance of our bombers was marked with white to keep our bombers from dropping their eggs on our forward units. Well beyond a little village of Loiana we reached an observation point that provided a wide view of the front. Shells whistled overhead—outward bound; a few shells well over on the right were incoming. A smoke screen protected a bridge and antiaircraft bursts marked the course of a plane.

Returning to press headquarters, Mrs. Rogers held a conference. She was urged by public relations officers to tell the people back home that the war was not won by any means. The attitude of the public relations officers reflected the feeling of the Fifth Army that theirs was now "the forgotten front."

We went back to Florence and had dinner with Edgar Erskine Hume at "Villa Vittoria." The dinner, arranged by the Allied Military Government Occupied Territory (AMGOT), City of Florence, was in the usual style of

Hume, the AMGOT governor of the city. It was replete with printed menus and place cards bearing the seal of the city. Consommé was followed by paté of salmon, roast beef, peas, potatoes, tart Florentine, cheese and coffee, apéritifs, red and white Chianti and cordials.

On October 20 we drove to Firenzwola on the road to Imola. This had been the main axis of attack against a steep pass. Trees had been blown off the top of the pass by our artillery creating a tangle "like that in the Connecticut valley after the 1938 hurricane." The 16th Evacuation Hospital was at Firenzwola and had kept out of the mud by using ammunition boxes as sidewalks. Harry Blesse provided lunch at the 56th Evacuation Hospital near Scarpena and we reached Florence at 1230.

There, we were taken to the old palace where "with trumpets, banners and a mace under the arm of Edgar Erskine Hume," Mrs. Rogers signed The Golden Book of Florence. We reassembled at the Hotel Excelsior and reformed the convoy to the airfield. General Clark dashed up in a Cub plane; General Eaker made an appearance; a bouquet of flowers was presented by Wac's and nurses; then we took off. I slept most of the flight to Naples, where we arrived at 4:45 P.M. It was a clear day, with Naples harbor looking as it should. Then we went to Caserta with Mrs. Rogers, who went off to a tea. That night we had cocktails at the Grotto Club and dinner as guests of General Crane and General Pence, following which Mrs. Rogers went to Ambassador Kirk's villa on Posillipo for the night.

The morning was gorgeous, with full sun on the balcony overlooking the bay of Naples from Posillipo. I met Mrs. Rogers there at 0900 hours and took her to the 15th Medical Laboratory in the fairgrounds. Humphrey and Latta took off for Pompeii. We then saw other medical units still in Naples, hiding a nurse with her newborn baby at the 300th General Hospital—an example of "demining" the tour of a V.I.P. After lunch in the mess at Caserta we visited General Noce in the War Room for another briefing. Major Colman of the Wac's then took charge of Mrs. Rogers until it was time for the party to reassemble for mess. Mrs. Rogers took off for the United States early the next morning.

"I am utterly exhausted," I wrote to my wife, "after a whirl around Italy with our congresswoman from Lowell. I was her escort—she brought two others down from Normandy but they did not know the ropes here. She was particularly interested in hospitals, having been overseas with the Red Cross in the last war. I was glad to get acquainted with her as probably she will be chairman of the veterans' legislative committee in the next congress and it is important to try to keep veterans' benefits straight so far as hospitalization and surgical care are concerned.

"She is really quite a person—not too savvy but willing to listen and learn. For years she has been criticized every time she has voted for a new cruiser, particularly, she says, by a strong pacifist group in Belmont. Her mail is already beginning to shift in that direction again.

"I am glad I voted for the lady as for many years she has not had an opponent of real stature according to her escort from Concord. She puts a great deal into the post from her private resources."

I saw Edith Nourse Rogers several times in Washington, D.C. after the war when I was working with the Army and also the Veterans' Administration. On one occasion when I took my sons to visit the Capitol, Mrs. Rogers took them to her desk on the floor of the House while it was in session.

Edith Nourse Rogers died on September 10, 1960.

34

Christmas at Home

I Received the following orders toward the end of November:

Restricted
Headquarters
Mediterranean Theater of Operations
United States Army

APO 512

AG 201-P-Churchill, Edward D. (O)

27 November 1944

Subject: Orders.

To: COLONEL EDWARD D. CHURCHILL, 0-199980, MC, Medical Section, AFHQ.

1. The above named officer will proceed on or about 28 November 1944 from present station to a United States airport, thence, by indorsement on these orders to Washington, D.C. for temporary duty at the *War Department* with the *Office of the Surgeon General.* Travel to be performed is in connection with temporary duty.

2. Colonel Churchill is cautioned against the compromise of classified military information and is advised of his responsibility in preventing unauthorized publication of personal information of value to the enemy. He will cooperate with authorized and properly identified intelligence officers representing the United States, both overseas and after arrival in the United States.

3. Mode of transportation and baggage allowance authorized:

    a. Within Theater and to United States: Aircraft. APR II NAP (C/S, AFHQ)

    b. Within United States: As prescribed by CO, U.S. Port of Arrival

c. Return to Theater: Aircraft. (APR USNA-2-2813-MEDJAN)

d. A baggage allowance of sixty-five (65) pounds and an excess baggage allowance of twenty (20) pounds for official documents is authorized while traveling by aircraft. Colonel Churchill is on a special mission which makes it necessary for him to carry classified material.

*   *   *

4. Upon completion of temporary duty at Washington, D.C., a leave of absence for twenty-one (21) days, exclusive of authorized travel time, is authorized Colonel Churchill at Boston, Mass. At expiration of leave, he will report to the proper U.S. airport for return to his organization.

BUSMAN'S HOLIDAY

My commission in the Army of the United States dated from January 9, 1943, and I had been in the overseas theater since early February of the same year. The above leave of absence enabled me to attend the meeting of the Southern Surgical Association at White Sulphur Springs, West Virginia. I would also be able to spend the Christmas holidays at home. In many respects, however, the trip was a busman's holiday, for I not only visited the wounded in Army hospitals but gave many talks about their surgical care in the North African-Mediterranean Theater.

A plan to further the work of the Board for the Study of the Severely Wounded (see Chapter 31) was also on my agenda. This was described in the following letter which I drafted for General Stayer to send to the Surgeon General:

DRAFT

Dear General Kirk:

Colonel Churchill has undoubtedly told you about the investigative work being carried out in this theater on the treatment of shock in the severely wounded. The study of the anuria cases occurring in this group has been particularly interesting. It is believed that a conference between shock investigators of this theater and those in the U.S. would greatly aid further progress in developing methods of treatment for these cases. We believe that a pooling of ideas with the establishing of understanding and direct communication between the investigators involved would do much to coordinate the work here with the work at home. We have

(continued)

the advantage of observing and working on actual shock cases but are handicapped by laboratory and other investigative facilities. While investigators at home must work as a rule with laboratory animals instead of human cases.

It is also believed desirable to arrange for some of the investigators at home to visit this theater and work with the Theater Board. The individuals concerned and the time could be worked out by those participating in the conference.

I am planning to send Lt. Colonels Tracy, Mallory, Beecher, Simeone, and Sullivan to the U.S. on TD to represent the theater. Col. Mallory will be at the Museum consulting with Col. Ash in the hepatitis problem and he will be able also to participate in the shock discussion.

If there is a N.R.C. meeting on shock during March it would be an opportune time for general discussion of the problems. However we feel that much could be accomplished if individual discussion could be held between the MTOUSA Board and the workers in New York, Philadelphia, Baltimore and Boston. It is particularly desired to confer with and get the advice and help of the individuals named on the attached list.

Such contacts as may be advisable with other similarly trained and experienced individuals are also desired. The list submitted is not meant to be selective for it contains only the names of investigators known to the Board as possibly being available for a conference on shock and anuria.

We feel that there is a chance to make real progress in the treatment of the serious conditions encountered as a result of prolonged shock and we would appreciate any help you can give to aid us with the problems.

Sincerely,
M. C. S.

The names on the "attached list" were: Donald VanSlyke, Lieutenant Commander Robert A. Phillips and Lieutenant Commander Vincent Dole, of the Rockefeller Institute; Walter B. Cannon, Chairman of the Shock Committee, N.R.C.; Dr. Oliver, New York Hospital; Homer Smith, New York University; A. N. Richards and C. F. Schmidt, University of Pennsylvania; C. H. N. Long, Yale University; Magnus A. Gregersen, Columbia; John P. Peters, Yale Medical School; George Thorne, Charles Janeway, Edwin Cohn, Howard Armstrong, Oliver Cope, Joseph C. Aub, of Harvard Medical School; Alfred Blalock, of the Hopkins, and Eugene Stead, of Atlanta.

Far from seeking guidance in the technical aspects of wound surgery, the theater was desirous of information from chemists and physiologists on the physiologic effects of wounds.

An outline schedule of this trip will precede a more detailed account of certain episodes.

ITINERARY

Date	Hour	
28 Nov. 1944	1135	Depart A.T.C. Terminal, Naples
29 Nov. 1944	0840	Depart A.T.C. Term., Casablanca
1 Dec. 1944	0235	Arrived A.T.C. Term., New York
2 Dec. 1944	1700	Signed In, Surgeon General's Office, Washington
8 Dec. 1944	2300	Signed Out, Surgeon General's Office, Washington
9-11 Dec. 1944		3 days leave, Special Order #294
12 Dec. 1944	0830	Signed In, Surgeon General's Office, Washington
21 Dec. 1944	2300	Signed Out, Surgeon General's Office, Washington
22 Dec. 1944		21 days leave, par. #5, MTOUSA
11 Jan. 1945		orders.
12 Jan. 1945	0830	Signed In, Surgeon General's Office, Washington
28 Jan. 1945	1030	Signed Out, Surgeon General's Office, Washington
	1230	Depart A.T.C. Term., Washington
29 Jan. 1945	1950	Arrived A.T.C. Term., Casablanca
30 Jan. 1945	2330	Left A.T.C. Term., Casablanca
1 Feb. 1945	1000	Arrived A.T.C. Term., Naples

The transatlantic flights were via the Azores, Stevensville and Monkton.

SURGICAL CONFERENCE

The meeting of the Southern Surgical Association, scheduled for the fifth and sixth of December, 1944, was preceded by a program at the Ashford General Hospital, White Sulphur Springs. Colonel Daniel C. Elkin was Chief of Surgery and Colonel Clyde M. Beck the Commanding Officer. Elkin had converted the Ashford General Hospital into a center for vascular injuries, and a wealth of aneurysms, arteriovenous fistulas and other bizarre effects of wounding were assembled here. Important contributions had been made to the placement of incisions for exposure of the damaged vessels. Elkin's interest in vascular injuries had stemmed from his years in Atlanta, where he had treated many patients who had been injured by knives and ice picks. At that time Elkin cited 150 cases treated surgically with no loss of limb or evidence of circulatory inadequacy. Block of the sympathetic ganglia had been abandoned and dependence placed on time alone for reestablishment of collateral circulation.

In my talk to the Southern Surgical Association on December 6, I told the story of the private in the 92nd Infantry Division whom I had seen on ward rounds at the 38th Evacuation Hospital.

"'I certainly am glad,' he had said to me, 'to get back with my *folks*'—meaning the medical officers and nurses of this hospital from Charlotte, North Carolina. We are usually acutely aware of where our *families* are located but in the present turmoil it is hard to know on which side of the world our *folks* are likely to be found. Most of you here this evening would feel at home in Italy because you have both family and 'folks' there."

"I only wish I could express how much it has meant to me to have the privilege of working for the doctors and hospitals that are overseas. If my faith in the surgical profession had ever been lacking, it would have been restored by my daily contacts with the surgeons of my theater. Many of them are well known to you."

"From the south we have had the 56th Evacuation Hospital from Baylor; the 38th Evac. from Charlotte; the 8th Evac. from the University of Virginia; the 300th General Hospital from Vanderbilt. I saw Colonel Reyer the day before I left Italy. He was preparing his annual report—numbers of patients admitted, operations performed and so on. The startling item was that 58 miles of two pound loaves of bread had been sliced by hand. That means over 6,000,000 slices. This may be taken as a plug for a mechanical bread slicer on the Table of Equipment!

"There's the 45th General Hospital from Richmond, with Guy Horsley now succeeding Steve Graham as Chief of Surgery; the 24th General Hospital from Tulane; the 64th General Hospital from L.S.U.; the 43rd General Hospital from Emory, with Ira Ferguson and the Boland boys; the 21st General Hospital from Barnes Hospital, St. Louis; the 70th General Hospital from St. Louis University. In the smaller semimobile evacs., Charlie Wasden and Dick Shackelford are Chiefs of Surgery. In station hospitals are the Hughes brothers of Memphis, and Harry Jenkins of Knoxville. Among the forward surgeons of the Auxiliary Group are Luther Wolff, Larry Hunt, Jim Mason, Gene Caldwell, Paul Dent, Dan Williams and many others."

"These men not only exhibit loyalty and devotion but treat GI Joe with the same sense of responsibility they might show to private patients at home."

"I also pay tribute to another group—the officers of the regular Army Medical Corps. Echoes of the conflicts of 1918 are no longer heard. These men deserve our highest praise and admiration. The distinctions between 'regulars' and reserve officers grow less apparent every day as mutual trust and help develop. The 'regulars' know how to run the machine—supplies, personnel and planning for future actions. We look forward to extension of this association under the leadership of General Kirk."

"I was told that I must tell you about the surgery of the North Africa-Mediterranean Theater. First, just what does the consultant to an overseas theater do? I would like to have you picture the consultant as a Koussevitzky or a Toscanini out in front of an orchestra. A large number of general surgeons form the section of strings. The specialists are the other groupings of instruments: the chest surgeons—woodwinds; the orthopedists—the brass and percussion; the neurosurgeons—the flutes and piccolos, and so on.

"A consultant really is a grumpy old music critic who sits comfortably in the front row of the balcony and gets up before the performance is over to go home and pound a typewriter."

"The basic task of military surgery lies in phasing the steps in the management of an individual wounded man passing through many hospitals and cared for by as many different surgeons. His progress extends halfway across the globe from the first aid dressing under enemy fire to final discharge as a patient from a hospital in the U.S.A. or return to duty from some point along the way."

"A high quality of forward surgery is the keystone to the successful management of the wounded. It not only saves lives but minimizes complications and resulting disability...."

"The 300th General Hospital that set the record in bread slicing has closed 13,552 wounds ranging from one to 52 per patient. The average number of wounds per patient was three...."

Loyal Davis read a communication on peripheral nerve injuries—one of the subjects that provoked active discussion throughout World War I and subsequently. To the layman, the problem would be like that of splicing two severed cables, each of which has hundreds of individual wires to be brought together as they were originally. My discussion of Davis's paper follows:

"Surgeons in an overseas theater are acutely aware of the difficult problems in peripheral nerve reconstruction that are being returned to the United States. I can only assure you that we have not been complacent about the matter, and many conferences have been held in an attempt to find a solution. At the present time the policy relating to the surgical management of anatomical severance of a nerve is as follows:"

"(1) The forward surgeon at the time of the initial débridement makes a careful record of the injury as he observes it. Preoperative appraisal of nerve injury notoriously is difficult and inexact in patients with multiple wounds, particularly if they are suffering from shock. The most precise information comes from anatomic observations at operation. Here

(continued)

again, it may not be desirable to embark upon a painstaking dissection with extension of the field of operation beyond the zone of devitalized tissues. (2) Dusting of the wound with sulfonamide may be omitted—certainly in the area of the nerve trunk. (3) Exposed nerves are covered with muscle so that the dry fine mesh gauze used as a filler is not in contact with the nerve. Petrolatum gauze is not recommended. (4) The joints above and below the point of injury are immobilized to minimize retraction of the nerve. (5) A firm pressure dressing supported by a plaster of Paris shell is designed to reduce wound exudation. (6) Penicillin therapy is maintained by the systemic route. (7) On reaching a general hospital the original dressing is removed under aseptic precautions in the operating room. This usually is possible on or shortly after the fourth day after injury. The depths of the wound are revisioned and the nerve injury reassessed. Electrical tests may be made if desired.

"Oftentimes a more deliberate examination will correct or supplement the initial notes made in the forward area. Appraisal at this time is based on the ultimate functional restoration of the extremity, taking into consideration muscle damage and bone or joint lesions in relation to the nerve injury. Procedures such as muscle suture or even shortening of the limb by removal of devitalized comminuted bone fragments may be carried out at this time. The divided ends of the nerve may be approximated by a single fixation suture. The wound is closed if sepsis is not present, or if further excision of sequestrating tissue adequately prepares the wound for closure. Closure of the skin may be staged, or if a large skin defect exists a skin graft is applied at once or as a staged procedure. (8) When first intention healing has been secured—and this results in 80 to 95 per cent of cases—formal suture of the nerve is undertaken. This should be feasible in many cases during the third or fourth week after injury.

"Throughout the course of reparative surgery, the patient is protected from the hazards of invasive infection by systemic penicillin therapy. We do not consider that the local usage of sulfonamides contributes to the success of the program—and, until further evidence of its efficacy is presented, choose to use penicillin by the intramuscular route rather than as a topical application."

"During the staged operations of a program of reparative surgery, the red cell volume of the patient must be kept at normal levels by repeated whole blood transfusions."

EXCHANGE OF LETTERS

The days in Washington flew by, filled with conferences, visits to nearby Army hospitals (Walter Reed, Newton D. Baker at Martinsburg, West Virginia), Edgewood Arsenal and other places where research on military problems were being pursued at a feverish pace. I had conferences, for instance, with Fred Rankin, Nick Carter, Mike Debakey and Al Shands. On the twentieth of December I attended a meeting of the N.R.C. Committee on Shock and Burns; the following day I heard a report of the Division of Surgery by John S. Lockwood, the chief of this division. Unable to enter active service because of physical disability, John Lockwood, one of the ablest surgeons of his generation, did a magnificent job in this position.

At the time I was in this country, Lockwood and John Fulton, also of Yale, were having a difficult time with each other. As I recall, the sum requested by Fulton was astronomical. Selections from an exchange of letters follow. They are inserted to preserve a record of these two vivid personalities.

January 2, 1945

Dear Colonel Churchill:
I am taking the liberty of forwarding to you herewith a copy of my letter to Dr. John F. Fulton, Secretary of the Conference on Wound Ballistics. Some thought is being given to the question of establishing a unit to investigate in animals some of the problems connected with the management of injuries of muscle, bone, nerves and brain produced by missiles of varying mass and velocity. As you see, I have made some "extrapolations" based on your recent discussion of wounds and I hope I have interpreted your views correctly. Any comments you would have to make on the subject would be very much appreciated.

Sincerely yours,
JOHN S. LOCKWOOD, M.D.
Chief, Division of Surgery

• • •

January 2, 1945

RE: PROJECT ON MISSILE CASUALTIES

Dear Doctor Fulton:
The desirability of obtaining additional knowledge of the nature of missile wounds is obvious. The project appears as an especially timely one in view of the new knowledge derived at Princeton concerning the predictability of the physical characteristics of tissue distortions produced at the moment of impact of the missile with the target. The objective of

(continued)

the proposed study would be, in general, to define in biological terms the immediate and late significance of the traumatizing effects produced in different tissues by missiles under conditions subjected to careful physical control. The ultimate objectives of the investigation would be: a. to assist the military surgeon in understanding the special characteristics of missile injuries, b. to provide a rational basis for present and future surgical treatment, c. to develop new apparatus which would aid the military surgeon in the care of fresh casualties, and d. to aid in designing protective devices against specific types of missile injuries.

However, it is not enough thus to state that the project is important and timely, and that the general objectives appear to be desirable ones. Before actually proceeding to establish such a project, some thought must be given to the questions of the attainability of these objectives through investigations in animals and of the specific plan of research. I would like, therefore, to open discussion on the following points:

1. In terms of practical treatment of casualties, of what value would be data based upon injuries produced in animals under carefully standardized conditions? As I conceive them, war wounds are largely random injuries produced under conditions which are completely variable in respect to mass, shape, and velocity of projectiles at the moment of impact, anatomical region or regions of injury, associated foreign bodies and bacterial contaminants. Would the data provided by such a carefully controlled study aid in teaching the military surgeon anything he can use in treatment which he does not already know?

2. Surgeons who are thoroughly conversant with basic principles of wound surgery, such as Col. E. D. Churchill, Chief Consultant for the Mediterranean Theater, seem inclined toward the belief that the present problem in respect to war wounds is not so much one of developing new methods, as of obtaining prompt and adequate general application of what is already known and practiced, whenever possible, by the best qualified forward surgeons. Present principles of wound management may be based to some extent on empirical grounds, or even on false hypotheses, but nevertheless, according to Col. Churchill, the incidence of serious wound complications is negligible when present rules of sound treatment are practiced.

3. The experimental production of localized tissue infections in animals which are at all comparable to wound infections seen in man is fraught with great difficulty. This fact would serve greatly to limit the validity of any findings derived from long-term management and study of missile wounds in animals.

4. The organization of the entire project can only be satisfactorily arranged if it is focused on certain *very specific* questions, the answers to which are urgently required by the armed services. Only such a project could attract and hold the interest of the superior types of investigators who would be required. No program should be approved unless these conditions can be satisfied.

Before proceeding further with specific plans for the project under consideration, I believe we should obtain from qualified military surgeons of practical experience their constructively critical comments on the points which I have raised in this letter. This letter is, in fact, a consequence of my lack of success in attempting to reduce a desirable general objective to terms sufficiently specific for preparation of a sound proposal for contract.

I will discuss this matter with Col. Callender at my earliest opportunity. Copies of this letter are being sent to Dr. Weed, Dr. E. N. Harvey and Col. Churchill for their comments."

Sincerely yours,
JOHN S. LOCKWOOD, M.D.
Chief, Division of Surgery

● ● ●

3 January 1945

RE: MISSILE CASUALTIES SURVIVAL PROJECT

My dear Dr. Lockwood:
This will acknowledge your letter of 2 January 1945 concerning the proposed long-term study of missile casualties. I thoroughly agree with the aims and objectives outlined in your first paragraph, and I am also very glad of the opportunity to discuss the four points raised in the body of your letter.

1. *Probable value in terms of practical treatment of casualties.* I believe that information of immediate practical value from the therapeutic standpoint could be obtained from a broadly conceived program of study in which the end results of specific missile wounds are studied. Information is needed on two points, namely, (a) the closure of infected wounds, and (b) the viability of tissue.

(continued)

a. *Closure of infected wounds.* I realize that a few theater surgeons are closing infected flesh wounds with the aid of penicillin and other chemotherapeutic agents. The results have been surprisingly good but I believe that it is still contrary to official instruction to close such a wound and there are many surgeons, both our own and among the British, who refuse to deviate from the old-time concept of leaving every potentially infected wound open to drain and heal by secondary union. During the first two weeks of December I had opportunity to discuss the subject at some length with Sir Howard Florey who has been in close touch with operations in North Africa and the Sicilian campaign, in Normandy and more recently in New Guinea. Those who have used penicillin to assist in closing locally infected wounds have had remarkably good results; but he is under the impression that few actually are taking full advantage of penicillin for local application. Wounds similar to battle wounds can be produced under carefully controlled conditions in animals, the interval between wounding and closure varied and clearcut evidence obtained as to feasibility of closing infected wounds with penicillin.

b. *Viability of tissue.* An experienced surgeon is said to know at a glance when tissue is viable and when not. My impression is that this is far from the truth in view of wide differences of opinion with regard to débridement. I believe that through survival studies in animals such as monkeys and chimpanzees direct evidence can be obtained concerning tissue viability and a valid rule of thumb developed to guide military surgeons in dealing with injured tissue. A special case in point is that relating to peripheral nerve which we have already discussed at some length. This morning I received a further letter from Commander William Livingston of the U.S. Naval Hospital, Oakland, California, under the date of 29 December. I believe that through experimental study of high velocity missile wounds in the extremities of animals, data would be obtained which would provide a direct answer to his questions and would guide neurological surgeons with regard to whether or not it is wise to resect the nerves which have apparently degenerated following wounding by high velocity missiles.

2. *Application of existing knowledge.* I have little comment on the point raised by Colonel Churchill beyond saying that he is one of the most skillful of all our surgeons and I would expect his results to be of the best but I am sure that Colonel Churchill would be the first to welcome information concerning the actual mechanism of wounding since this inevitably places therapeutic procedure on a more rational basis.

3. *Infections in animals.* It is true that dogs and cats behave very differently to infection than man but this has not been our experience with laboratory primates. I find that during the past fifteen years we have carried out more than 5,000 surgical procedures on monkeys and chimpanzees and while we have had very few postoperative infections attributable to operative contamination, we have had considerable experience dealing with infection following fights, accidents in catching a postoperative animal, etc. The behavior of both the monkey and the chimpanzee so far as infections are concerned is so closely similar to that of man, that I think that valid deductions could be drawn from their use in the ballistic study.

4. *Specific questions.* I heartily agree that the project should be developed on the basis of such specific questions as have been outlined in paragraph 1, above. I should be much interested in learning what you hear from Dr. Weed, Dr. Harvey, Colonel Churchill and of your interview with Colonel Callender.

Very sincerely yours,
J. F. FULTON, M.D.

• • •

(The following is from the letter, referred to by Dr. Fulton, which had been sent to him by Lieutenant Commander William Livingston):

RE: NERVE RESECTION FOLLOWING MISSILE WOUNDS

I value Van Wagenen's opinion and shall quote his observations recorded in his letter. He says that he is exploring all his cases that meet the following criteria:

> If the course of the missile could have injured the nerve.
> If an adjoining fracture could have injured it.
> If the area is badly scarred from infection or tissue loss.
> If there is no evidence of recovery in four months.

He says, "We have not analysed our figures on negative explorations and do not know percentages. My impression is that we have about 15 per cent negative explorations, that is, the nerve is intact after dissecting away scar. Resections are never done unless *gross* damage can be demonstrated. Each nerve is stimulated with a Hinsey-Geohegan stimulator at the time of exploration."

(continued)

A report of this kind from a man of Van Wagenen's experience must be given a great deal of weight, and there appears to be too great a discrepancy between his observations and ours. There is, but the discrepancy is not as great as these surface facts would indicate. In the first place, we may be over optimistic about spontaneous recovery and the subsequent history of our cases will undoubtedly reveal cases of complete nerve division that have been overlooked. When we explore we usually find more pathology than we had anticipated finding. But the essential factual observations remain true, and as such are worth recording. The principal motivating force behind the paper was the fact that I had had to reverse my own conviction that all these cases should be explored early. I was opposing the establishment of a "policy" that would make it incumbent upon all surgeons in front areas to explore *all* cases in which a nerve lesion *might* be present. The reason I had come to oppose such a policy was that most surgeons, including myself, wouldn't know what to do with "lesions in continuity" in which there was no response to electrical stimulation at the time of operation. I could see the possibility of a great number of resections in nerves that might better be left alone. I am certainly not enthusiastic about the end-results of resection of nerves in humans, and I am greatly impressed with what some of these badly damaged nerves may do if left alone. Denny-Brown's work also demonstrates clearly that in experimental animals a "pseudo neuroma" may persist for many weeks and that until the local damage has been repaired the nerve peripherally will not respond to maximum stimulation because the fibers have degenerated. I have only seen personally one instance in which a good surgeon had explored a nerve and left it alone though feeling doubtful as to its ability to overcome the damage, in which subsequent resection was necessary. There may be more of these cases later, but in contrast to this I have seen a large number of resections done on the basis of findings which are to me entirely unconvincing of the necessity of this procedure.

The essential facts in our paper I *know* to be true. I have no desire to criticise the policy of early exploration in the hands of experts, although even they may learn something that will modify their views from Denny-Brown. But I would oppose the policy as it imposes an obligation to explore early for less well qualified men who may light-heartedly undertake resections on inadequate grounds."

• • •

25 January 1945

Dear John Lockwood:

It is difficult for me to comment on the Project on Missile Casualties as you request in your letter of January 22nd. In general, the interpretation of my point of view in paragraph 2 of your letter addressed to John Fulton is correct in so far as the problem that confronts the Medical Corps. Here education in the application of existing knowledge is a major task. Quite obviously, however, emphasis on the needs for a constant educational program within the Medical Corps should in no way be interpreted as criticism of sincere efforts to extend our knowledge about the pathology of wounds.

The letter from John Fulton to you, relating to the Missile Casualty Survival Project, can be looked upon only as the response of a physiologist to being placed on the defensive regarding the probable value of a research program in terms of practical surgical treatment *before* even preliminary experiments have been undertaken. Far from being critical of Fulton's statements, I must express admiration that he accepted the challenge at all, mixed with regret that he walked into the trap. It is not surprising that his information on the applied surgical level is incomplete—as a matter of fact it is no more incomplete than that of many surgeons. I think it is for us as surgeons to seek the application of any basic concepts that such a study may unfold—not for Fulton to predict them even before his studies are initiated.

Sincerely,
EDWARD D. CHURCHILL
Colonel, Medical Corps

A TALK AT THE M.G.H.

On December 22 I reached Boston to spend Christmas with my family. After January 1, two weeks were consumed in social engagements and special appointments. I recall an evening at the Bronson Crothers' with Salvemini and George LaPiana; dinner at the Jason Mixter's; Grand Rounds and talks with the house staff at M.G.H.; luncheon at the Somerset Club arranged by Phillips Ketchum; a meeting with the wives of the staff of the 6th General Hospital; an appointment with President James B. Conant; and a visit to Cushing General Hospital.

On January 4, 1945, I gave a talk in the surgical amphitheater at the M.G.H. A few extracts follow: "We look on ourselves as a 'detachment' of the M.G.H., working at a distance. This is true whether we are grouped together as the 6th General Hospital, or whether we are scattered and work as individuals. Someone has described Algiers as resembling Harvard Square!"

"I am known at the M.G.H. as a 'reformer' as many of you know, but took a firm vow that I was not going to reform the Army. This was a good resolution because the Army has reformed me."

"When younger officers are impatient because they can't get this or that, or the Army is doing this or that, I ask them if they have ever traveled from Boston to New York on a boat of the old Fall River line. After supper, passengers could walk on a narrow metal runway and look down into the engine room. A tremendous flywheel revolved slowly. From time to time a mechanic walked by on a shiny steel catwalk and reached over to the eccentric and gave a grease cup a small turn. The Army in combat acquires a momentum like a flywheel. Nothing must be done that might jeopardize the turning of the wheel. If you can from time to time tighten a grease cup or put on a few drops of oil, it is all a single individual can accomplish.

"An army works toward a limited objective; the Trustees and Staff of the M.G.H. work toward an objective that is not limited either in goal or time. In civilian life one can be a designer; in the Army one is an operative."

"An army does not speak of education; it refers to training. A man is trained to reach a specific objective, not educated to attain a broad and perhaps ill-defined goal."

"An army in a long campaign has to deal with a series of specialized situations and unforeseen occurrences. On the basis of the experience of a specialized situation there is likely to be a great hue and cry to redesign the Army. This is resisted and then critics speak of the conservative attitude of the slow and ponderous machine. After the battle of Tunisia, everyone knew we needed this and that; after Sicily and its new situations, the same critics were heard; now in Italy what pertains in summer is not satisfactory in winter...."

"The Army is like a mule. After it has learned a formula, the only way to get it to unlearn that formula is to knock it in the head."

I also made an appearance on January 9 at the Harvard Medical Society in the amphitheater of the Peter Bent Brigham Hospital. My subject was, of course, "The Care of the Wounded in the Mediterranean Theater." I was introduced by Oliver Cope with the words: "We have two legends; in one of the legends there is substance—Dr. Churchill." To this I responded: "The other legend is not here unfortunately. I saw him a little over a year ago in Italy (Dr. Elliott Cutler)."

In this talk I explained that "military surgery" was an adaptation of the science and art of surgery to the movements of an army in combat and the care of wounded men. I then discussed the problems that faced us in North Africa, Sicily and Italy and described how they were met.

A few more days in Washington and then departure from the A.T.C. terminal at 12:30 P.M. on January 28, 1945. The return route was via Stevensville, the Azores, Casablanca, Algiers and arrival in Naples on February 1 at 1000 hours.

Accompanying me on the flight back to Italy was Mike DeBakey, who with Nick Carter had been the mainstay of the Surgeon General's Office. For the first time he was to be introduced to an overseas theater. I carried with me a sheaf of notes: information about patients from the theater seen in stateside hospitals, as well as technical information that might be useful to our laboratory and research workers.

On my first night back I had a highball with Fred Hanson, Gene Sullivan, Oscar Hampton and Mike DeBakey, followed by dinner at the palace mess. Obviously my mind had been refreshed by the trip for I jotted down the following "thoughts for development" in my diary:

"(1) One is aware of the strength and personality of certain men on entering their domain even before meeting with them. Just as a traveler senses the nearby mountain range as he traverses the foothills although the high peaks are as yet unrevealed."

"(2) The focus of diagnosis as taught has been on the categories of disease, rarely emphasizing the necessity to diagnose the *normal*. Increased emphasis on therapeutics also obscures the normal. Hanson now believes that the leakage from combat of nonbattle casualties is four times greater in the psychosomatic group than in simple N.P.'s. Doctors are not willing to assume the responsibility for making the diagnosis: normal. The problem is simpler in the Army than in civilian life where the patient will seek other doctors until he finds one who 'understands' his case and 'does something for him.' This is made clear in military medicine by the uniform age, sex group and the simple and obvious nature of the situation from which the man is trying to escape. The surgeon is the last to join the procession because of (a) the emergency nature of his problems, and (b) his reliance on objective findings which may be present but inconsequent."

I also jotted down some of the things Hanson, Sullivan, Hampton and I had talked about at dinner.

". . . Finally, for the edification of the new arrival—DeBakey—the discussion turned to the walled city of Casablanca and the practical view of the French toward prostitution by wholesale. Sullivan who had been with the 6th G.H. in Casablanca described the nude, insane inmate who customarily smeared herself with feces. Some patrons enjoy an insane prostitute, so they are kept in residence. Babies that are born in the city are cared for and adopted by Arab families who are anxious to obtain them."

Kirby R. Gross, Luke J. Hofmann, and Stacy A. Shackelford

This chapter chronicles Colonel Churchill's return to the United States after having been deployed for nineteen consecutive months (February 1943 through November 1944). His schedule included 24 days of leave and an additional 38 days devoted to communicating the situation in the theater with colleagues. Two major themes dominate the communication between Colonel Churchill and his stateside colleagues: (1) gaining new knowledge (research) and (2) ensuring the application of current knowledge. These two points are as relevant at the time of this reprint as they were in Churchill's day.

As an academic surgeon, Colonel Churchill thrived in the realm of clinical investigation and also had many colleagues with productive basic laboratories. He recognized that limited research funding demanded active engagement between investigators and deployed military surgeons to prioritize research questions relevant to forward surgery. In his correspondence reflecting on the conflict between clinical surgeons and basic scientists, Churchill concluded that the guiding direction for research investments should come from clinical leaders. Ultimately, the research community strongly supported efforts to improve battlefield care, a fact that remains true today.

Trauma systems, trauma centers, and the specialty of trauma/surgical critical care were all undefined entities in the World War II (WWII) era. Practice patterns for trauma in civilian practice were likely of great variability, and war wounds proved dramatically different from injuries the deployed surgeon encountered stateside. Guidance for managing war wounds was generated in theater, and the surgery consultant was responsible for distributing knowledge and assessing compliance—not easy tasks in the austere environment of WWII. In many ways, Colonel Churchill was the forefather of the Joint Trauma System (JTS), which fulfills these functions today. Yet, even with the infrastructure of the JTS and processes to generate clinical guidance based on data gathered in the deployed trauma registry, the implementation and dissemination of that knowledge still proves very difficult. Today's military surgeons also face a deployed practice that differs greatly from civilian or in-garrison practices, while the continued trend of sub-specialization in surgery noted by Churchill further conspires to make *military surgery* a discontinuous specialty. These challenges should motivate future military surgical leaders to identify durable solutions.

Colonel Churchill's time away from theater was hardly a vacation. He tirelessly engaged with stateside colleagues and clinical leaders to educate all on the state of the art in combat casualty care and to identify the issues for which new knowledge was required. These efforts ensured that projects undertaken were directly relevant to the most important and pressing challenges and questions in the combat theater. As Colonel Churchill stated, "A high quality of forward surgery is the keystone to successful management of the wounded. It not only saves lives but minimizes complications and resulting disability."

SUGGESTED READINGS

Blackbourne LH, Baer DG, Eastridge BJ, et al. Military medical revolution: military trauma system. *J Trauma Acute Care Surg.* 2012;73(6, supp 5):S388-S394.

National Academies of Sciences, Engineering, and Medicine. *A National Trauma Care System: Integrating Military and Civilian Trauma Systems to Achieve Zero Preventable Deaths After Injury.* The National Academies Press; 2016.

Joint Trauma System. Clinical practice guidelines. Accessed October 7, 2023. https://jts.health .mil/index.cfm/PI_CPGs/cpgs

35

Rome Congress of Army Surgeons

PROFESSIONAL MEETINGS for the open discussion of experience continued to be held in overseas theaters during the war. From February 12 to 16, 1945, a Surgical Congress of the Royal Army Medical Corps (Central Mediterranean Force Army Surgeons) convened in Rome.

The Congress was organized by Brigadier Harold C. Edwards, Consulting Surgeon A.F.H.Q., who had long before succeeded Weddell with whom I had made my first trips around Algiers and southern Tunisia. Major General W. C. Hartgill, Director of Medical Services, A.F.H.Q., had followed Major General Sir Ernest Cowell, the D.M.S., who had greeted my arrival in Algiers two years before by saying he was glad that I had arrived before the war was over. General Hartgill had gained and warranted the respect of both medical sections in A.F.H.Q.

The Congress was held in the Eastman Dental Clinic in Rome and some forty to fifty medical officers of the U. S. Forces attended as guests. I subsequently sent a full report of this Congress to the Surgeon General in Washington as "par. (C) Surgery in Essential Technical Medical Data." In this report I added my personal comments to indicate any differences in the procedures of the British and Americans. Complete freedom of speech was the rule of the Congress and the opinions of individuals found free expression.

The following is extracted from my report.

PAPERS AND COMMENTS

MAJOR H. W. BURGE, R.A.M.C.—"The Primary Operation in Battle Wounds of the Limbs." Progress in the management of the wounded was described from the days in North Africa when casualties were brought to the operating table with anesthesia already induced but before the patient had been undressed or washed. He believes that the R.A.M.C. has not stressed sufficiently the removal of foreign bodies, and hopes that in the future radiography can be made available for the preoperative examination of extremity wounds. He suggests that a "Fourth New Principle" of the initial operation be *preparation of the wound for delayed primary suture* by mobilization of the skin, and states that all fragments of bone in a compound fracture of a long bone should be left in place. Devitalized and detached fragments act as grafts.

E.D.C. Comment: U.S. surgeons have been asked to *record* the amount of actual skin loss as a guide to the surgeon who will perform delayed suture. It does not appear wise to transfer mobilization of skin, to the forward surgeon. This should be a carefully studied procedure with the application of the principles of plastic surgery. U.S. surgeons prefer a more radical policy in eliminating contaminated, devitalized fragments of bone.

Major G. H. Wooler, R.A.M.C.—"The Primary Treatment of Wounds." In a paper on the same subject of forward surgery the need was stressed to limit the *duration* of the initial operation because of deterioration in the condition of the patient. If the condition deteriorates, he advises transfusion, oxygen and delay in further procedures until the patient can withstand completion of the operation.

E.D.C. Comment: U.S. surgeons, in contrast, stress the necessity of *maintaining* compensation by continued transfusion, and merge surgery and resuscitation as one indivisible procedure. A possible explanation of this difference is found in the "Interim Report on the Work of the British Traumatic Shock Research Team, British War Office, Miscellaneous Report #215 (#8708)," where the following statement appears: "Inferior quality of blood reduces the proportion of blood used because medical officers choose rather to run the risk of a low hemoglobin than the very real risk of a bad blood transfusion. This has been our own experience. For, with injuries and transfusions comparable with those of our civil experience, we have in the field met with a much greater incidence of reactions during blood transfusion, of subsequent jaundice and of later gross renal disturbance. *We hesitate now to give massive stored blood transfusions for resuscitation or even small transfusions for the later correction of anemia.*" It is obvious that an abundant and safe supply of whole blood is one of the cornerstones of forward surgery. This has been attained in MTOUSA. Major Wooler stressed the need to follow the missile tract by *vision* rather than palpation.

(continued)

> *E.D.C. Comment:* This is very difficult to impress on the forward surgeon. (See Circular Letter No. 26, 19 April, 1944—"The operation on a wound is an anatomical dissection and should never be made to resemble a digital pelvic examination.") It is Wooler's custom to apply penicillin powder to the surfaces of the wound following débridement, beginning with the deepest recesses. Aqueous acriflavine is employed as an irrigant.

LIEUTENANT COLONEL C. J. B. MURRAY, R.A.M.C.—"Delayed Primary Suture of Flesh Wounds." There are two essentials: first, getting the wounds sutured and, second, protecting against infection until this can be done. The period of hospitalization has been reduced 50 to 60 per cent. In suture of soft tissue wounds with penicillin therapy, 458 of 500 were successful; with acriflavine powder, 174 of 229. Suture is performed on the fourth to sixth day, preferably on the fourth.

MAJOR SCOTT THOMSON, R.A.M.C.—"The Role of Penicillin in War Wounds," a paper referred to by the Chairman, Brigadier Harold Edwards, as "the best contribution so far made in the assessment of penicillin." This paper was an abstract of a long report by the essayist and Lieutenant Colonel F. H. Bentley entitled "A Survey of 1000 Wounds in Respect of Chemotherapy, Bacteriological Flora and Healing" made to Director of Pathology by the Penicillin Control Team, C.M.F., 30 November, 1944.

> *E.D.C. Comment:* It is important to have a clear understanding of the definition of terms as given by Major Scott Thomson.
>
> "Clean"—No reactive changes of inflammation.
> "Dirty"—Surface of wound covered by tissue exudates.
> "Infection"—Not a state of disease but a bacteriologic demonstration of staphylococcus aureus or hemolytic streptococcus present in the wound.
> "Septic"—Looked dirty and proved infected.

The summary and conclusions of Scott Thomson's paper follow:

1. One thousand and four were examined on admission to hospital from casualty clearing stations. From 25 to 50 per cent were found infected by *Staph. pyogenes aureus. Strep. pyogenes* (hemolytic streptococcus) was found in 6 per cent.
2. The majority of wounds infected by pyogenic cocci were clinically clean. The rates of infection were higher in dirty than in clean wounds.

3. The proportion of wounds infected by pyogenic cocci was found to be dependent upon three factors:
    a. The interval that elapsed between time of wounding and operation at a C.C.S. Wounds operated upon under 12 hours had a lower incidence of infection than those operated on between 12 and 24 hours.
    b. The application of penicillin-sulfathiazole powder to the wound at a C.C.S. Compared with sulfanilamide, the reduction in incidence was from 43 to 25 per cent.
    c. Dressing of wounds between operation at C.C.S. and operation in hospital, increased the incidence of infection.
4. No evidence was obtained that delay between C.C.S. and general hospital influenced the rates of infection.
5. A number of wounds received no application of a bacteriostatic at C.C.S. The incidence of infection was not greater than that found in wounds treated by sulfanilamide but a much larger proportion of them was clinically dirty. It appeared that the virulence of an infective process is controlled by bacteriostatics before the bacteria are destroyed.
6. The success of wound suture depended less upon the appearance of the wound than on the presence of pyogenic cocci. Wounds infected with these organisms obtained "Grade 1" union in 80 to 85 per cent—whether they appeared clean or dirty. Wounds that were infected, even if appearing clean, had a much lower rate of success.
7. The presence of staphylococci with some measure of resistance to penicillin did not influence the results of suture when penicillin was employed locally in the wound.

OTHER PAPERS AND OTHER DAYS

The Proceedings of the Congress make a 150-page paperbound book, so it is impossible to continue to summarize the presentations of the many R.A.M.C. officers who appeared on the program. The entire first day was devoted to "The Treatment of War Wounds." In the evening there was a reception by the British Ambassador, Sir Noel Charles, K.C.M.G., M.C. On the morning of February 13, a special audience was granted by His Holiness the Pope.

In the afternoon session the subject "Wounds of the Chest" was covered by the presentations of Lieutenant Colonel A. L. d'Abreu, Major W. F. Nicholson, Captain F. Hodgkiss, N.Z.M.C., and Major Maxwell Telling.

On the morning of February 14, the subject was "Abdominal Trauma." A visit to the 10th British Convalescent Depot occupied the afternoon. Some old friends—Lieutenant Colonel D. S. Poole-Wilson and Major R. V. Battle—spoke in the morning. Then there were papers on protein metabolism by Somers H. Sturgis and Harwell Wilson, of the U.S.A.M.C., and Major Garden of the R.A.M.C. The afternoon was devoted to "Vascular Injuries." "Short Papers" filled the program of the final day. The papers may have been "short" but the experience was "long," as when Major Patrick Clarkson, R.A.M.C. spoke on "The Treatment of a Thousand Jaw Wounds."

The closing address was by the Surgeon, Mediterranean Theater of Operations, U.S.A.—General Stayer—who spoke movingly of his participation in wars since 1898, and the amazing advances made in the care of the wounded.

FREEDOM OF THE FLOOR

During the first session of the Congress, I was introduced by Harold Edwards and given the freedom of the floor. My remarks follow:

As spokesman for the surgeons of the United States Army Medical Corps, in this theater, I wish to express our deepest thanks for being included as guests in this meeting.

We have in the United States a publication known as the *Congressional Record.* In addition to the formal speeches of our congressmen and senators, privilege is granted for the incorporation in the *Congressional Record* of a large number of miscellaneous items, many of which are not suitable for debate on the floor of Congress. At least some of these have the purpose of framing the remarks of congressmen so that their place in history is preserved for students of the future. Possibly this is the origin of the expression "keeping the record straight." I offer two items, neither of which is debatable, for incorporation in the records of this congress so that the students of wound healing fifty years from now will know that we had some idea of our place in surgical history. The first of these appeared in 1918 in Paris in a publication of the Red Cross known as *War Medicine* and was written by Rene Block:

> The best moment for delayed primary suture is the fourth day after operation; this is the time at which, in the service of Dr. Lemaitre, we do the first dressing of wounds which have not been sutured, provided the patient is without pain or fever and the bandage has not become soiled at an earlier date. If the wound is not sufficiently clean, it is best to delay suture for several days more; it may be practiced as late as the twelfth day.
>
> The operative technique is identical to that for immediate primary suture; rather than suturing the whole *en masse* with silkworm gut, it is better to suture layer by layer with fine catgut in order to re-establish the anatomical layers, and especially to make possible the natural gliding of the tissues.
>
> For those who know how to effect a good ablation and who have the technique of delayed primary suture well in hand, the possibilities of this procedure are infinite. Thus between the fourth and the twelfth day we have been able to close wounds with extensive gas gangrene, even when accompanied by fractures, in which cases the best of results have been obtained.

The second item goes back a bit further—in fact, to Lord Lister. It is of interest that this particular quotation was carried forward into the *British Medical History of the War of 1914–1918* as if surgeons at that time were a bit confused by hypochlorinated solutions, Bipp paste and iodine, and were seeking to clarify their place in history.

> If, for example, a pair of forceps is handed to the operator with the intervals between the teeth occupied by dry septic pus and a portion of this dirt becomes detached and left in the wound, the evil cannot be corrected by any antiseptic wash that is now at our disposal or that the world is ever likely to see.

The first quotation was merely a mild deflation of both British and American officers for the great to-do about delayed primary or reparative suture. Actually, this was rarely carried out in World War I, but the concept was proposed by Rene Block. The quotation from Lord Lister was more barbed, for the British surgeons were fond of putting sulfonamides, acriflavine and penicillin into wounds. Local or topical application of medicaments largely had been given up by U.S. medical officers.

On again reading the Proceedings of the Congress in Rome after a lapse of over twenty years, I was impressed by how completely absorbed we were with wounds. Like Rudyard Kipling with Boots, boots, boots—with us it was Wounds, wounds, wounds. The tendency to regard the wound as an entity apart from the body is discernible. We were not far distant from the medieval wound surgeons. To us wounds had personalities. They "obtained" A-Grade healing for themselves and were described as "simple" or "complicated" and as "clean" or "dirty." It was high time the war was over.

AFTER THE CONGRESS

On February 17, following the adjournment of the R.A.M.C. Congress, the American officers met to discuss our policies as of that date. Since the record of this meeting points out views on several controversial subjects toward the end of World War II, it is included here. The minutes were taken by Lieutenant Colonel Rolland R. Best, M. C.

MINUTES OF SURGICAL CONFERENCE OF 17 FEBRUARY 1945

Colonel Edward D. Churchill, Presiding

Meeting called at 0900 hours, Saturday, 17 February 1945, Excelsior Hotel, Rome, Italy, following adjournment of the R.A.M.C. Surgical Congress the preceding day. Major General Stayer and 30 officers present.

(continued)

After short discussion on hospitalization and evacuation it was concluded the present program was quite satisfactory.

Vote taken as to a method for discussion of material presented at the Congress—by anatomical division or by papers presented. Discussion by papers carried. It was suggested by Colonel Churchill that meeting continue until 11:00 A.M. and then, if necessary, time would be extended.

The question of dry, fine mesh gauze or petrolatum gauze in wounds discussed. When put to vote the evacuation hospital group expressed the preference for dry, fine mesh gauze.

The question of sulfonamides locally in wounds was discussed and when put to a vote the army and base hospital groups expressed the opinion that with exceptions wounds should not be frosted with sulfonamides.

Inquiry as to the desirability of using penicillin locally in wounds revealed several were experimenting with it but nobody wished to propose its universal use as an experiment.

Discussion of compound fractures:

(a) Lt. Col. Cox proposed wider use of posterior counter drainage in extremities. Emphasized the necessity in cases where débridement had not been as meticulous as desirable because of treatment of concomitant wounds of the head, chest or abdomen which had been time consuming and shocking to the patient.

(b) Removal of bone fragments. Lt. Col. Duncan expressed the opinion that he was inclined to remove all loose bone fragments. Major Cahen believed all larger fragments should remain unless grossly soiled and when fragments are not removed posterior drainage should certainly be done. If posterior drainage was not accomplished at the primary débridement it should be done at the time of secondary closure. Lt. Col. Snyder conformed to leaving all clean looking bone with any periosteal attachment. Lt. Col. Lichtenstein favored radical removal of bone and only leaving larger fragments of clean attached bone. Colonel Churchill stated that from information and his observations in some of the hospitals in the Zone of Interior too radical removal of bone fragments had not been done in this theater. This was supported by the fact that sequestra were being removed. Also, he added that no criticism had been offered by surgeons in the United States.

The subject of amputation stumps was discussed and there was a general dissatisfaction with the present regime regarding secondary closure. Lt. Col. Rogers expressed the opinion that more stumps should be secondarily closed. After further discussion Colonel Churchill proposed a question for a vote. This stated that amputation with short flaps at the lowest level followed by secondary closure partial or complete would be a more satisfactory method for the management of amputations. There was a unanimous opinion expressed for this method of management.

In the discussion on secondary closure it was proposed that more advancement and undermining flaps would result in better closures.

On chest wounds no discussion took place and there was general concurrence with the methods expressed at the British Surgical Congress.

Liver wounds were discussed and there was a general feeling that liver wounds should be explored. If a wound of the diaphragm was present, it should be repaired and repeated emphasis made on subcostal drainage to prevent a pleural biliary fistula. Location of wound in liver should determine location of subcostal drain. Removal of 12th rib and drainage was favored. Colonel Churchill mentioned fibrin foam and stated that it was now available at medical supply depots. He suggested placing this substance in the liver wound and draining down to this area. In a discussion on the use of a pack in liver wounds the Penrose drain was considered better than the large pack by several of those discussing the subject.

The colostomy problem was reviewed and free mobilization of colostomized or exteriorized segments emphasized to prevent any tendency toward tension. Warning was expressed against the use of cecostomy or partial exteriorization to divert the fecal stream for rectal wounds. As to technique, keeping the mesentery toward the medial side and the use of catgut sutures was mentioned. Colonel Churchill reviewed the new directive on colostomies which is to appear at an early date. He remarked that the long spur would not be necessary in future colostomies. Lt. Col. DeBakey remarked that in the Zone of Interior it was believed that a colostomy for a wound of the rectum should have the stomas separated regardless of the difficulty later encountered in the restoration of the intestinal continuity. He mentioned impactions, fistulae and retraction of the colostomy. Further discussion revealed a tendency by this group not to separate the stomas.

There was some discussion on the ileocolic and right colon exteriorization for wounds of this region and although an opinion had been expressed that many of these cases had offered difficulties in closure and were not being closed as frequently in this theater, questioning revealed that this was probably incorrect. Formation of sufficient spur and early crushing was discussed. There were a few remarks on closing

(continued)

the smaller anterior wounds of the cecum. Lt. Col. DeBakey was asked to express an opinion of surgeons in the Zone of Interior regarding ileocolic exteriorization. He stated there was a preference for bringing the ends out of separate incisions. Lt. Col. Snyder and Lt. Col. Best favored present ileocolic exteriorization. After some interrogation by Colonel Churchill it was the opinion that in general the present plan of management was quite satisfactory.

At 11:00 A.M. Colonel Churchill asked for an expression on continuing this discussion and it was favored.

Introduction of the subject of wounds of the bladder and urethra brought no comments.

Vascular injuries were then discussed. It was felt that if there was a suspicion of arterial injury, the artery should be exposed. Lt. Col. Snyder proposed more attempts should be made to close wounds of the arteries. Lt. Col. Lichtenstein discussed blind end suture for the conservation of vessel wall tissue as in a case of his he was able to save a collateral vessel. The general discussion favored more attempts to suture wounds of arteries.

Colonel Churchill brought up the question of suturing nerves at time of primary débridement in selected cases because of the general dissatisfaction of delayed nerve suture in the States. This early suture was to be reserved for those cases where the surgeon was not working under pressure at the time, where the tissue damage was minimal, the time element was satisfactory and technical facilities were adequate. Lt. Col. Snyder expressed the feeling that he desired to have nerve suturing done only in base hospitals.

The use of concentrated plasma was considered not rational but several favored using it in view of some of the clinical results. Lt. Col. Payne registered some enthusiasm and favored its use as a result of his experience in treating several body and inhalation burns on air pilot patients. Tracheotomy had been necessary in a number of cases and offered him the opportunity to observe the improvement which he believed the result of concentrated plasma injection. Other discussers felt that the improvement in such cases was probably due to other factors in the treatment.

Colonel Campbell introduced the subject of repair of skull defects. He did not believe a foreign material should be placed in these wounds at the time of primary débridement. Waiting a few weeks to rule out infection was favored.

Meeting adjourned at 12:00 noon.

Danielle B. Holt, Juan A. Asensio, and Norman M. Rich

In this chapter of *Surgeon to Soldiers*, Colonel Churchill first highlights the multinational exchange to preserve the hard-earned surgical lessons learned from combat casualty care—a meeting of the Surgical Congress of the Royal Army Medical Corps (RAMC) and delegates from other allied services from February 12 to 16, 1945, three months prior to the end of conflict in the Mediterranean theater. This multiday conference in Rome summed up the Allied experiences with war wounds, availability of a safe supply of whole blood, chest wounds, abdominal trauma, and vascular injuries, reflecting many of the same challenges that persist with modern-day care of the combat injured. Indeed, the fledgling concepts of damage control surgery can be seen in his description of the initial lifesaving, reparative, and reconstructive phases of war surgery.

The following day, February 17, 1945, Colonel Churchill presided over a "hot wash" of the RAMC Surgical Congress with 30 US medical officers at the Excelsior hotel in Rome. Attendees of this meeting formed the nucleus of what would become the Excelsior Surgical Club over the subsequent year. In recognition of Churchill's singular contributions throughout the war, he was named the club's first and only "honor member." The keynote address at the inaugural US meeting in Boston in October 1946 was named in his honor, and now the American College of Surgeons (ACS) Edward D. Churchill lecture is delivered at the annual Clinical Congress. The Excelsior Surgical Club became the Excelsior Surgical Society in 1951, and annual meetings of this convivial group continued until 1986. In 2014, the creation of the Military Health System Strategic Partnership with the American College of Surgeons (MHSSPACS) revitalized the Excelsior Surgical Society in 2015 as an official society and the home for military surgeons within the ACS.

Formal military-civilian partnerships (MCPs) first arose in World War I with military medical units assembled by the Red Cross and War Department within academic medical centers. As the John Homans Professor of Surgery at Harvard Medical School, Churchill personified the bidirectional learning between academic medicine and military surgery and worked to reignite this ethos during World War II. A similar collaboration is now embodied in the collaboration between MHSSPACS and our nation's military medical school, Uniformed Services University (USU). The new ACS Military Clinical Readiness Curriculum (mCurriculum) provides just-in-time trauma readiness modules for deployed surgeons and represents one example of the tremendous benefit of this partnership. Clinical MCPs have also proliferated in recent years now involving approximately 20% of US trauma centers. These partnerships help maintain the surgical readiness of military surgeons and surgical teams. The Clinical Readiness Program developed at USU then monitors clinical readiness as measured by each surgeon's combat-relevant knowledge, skills, and abilities acquired and maintained through clinical practice in a military treatment facility and/or MCP site. The MHSSPACS has published *The Blue Book: Military-Civilian Partnerships for Trauma Training, Sustainment, and Readiness* that details best practices in MCP development, governance, and sustainability. MHSSPACS and the Excelsior Surgical Society reflect the enduring spirit of Colonel Edward D. Churchill's relentless pursuit of optimal care for the injured and preservation of military surgical lessons of war.

SUGGESTED READINGS

Asensio JA, Petrone P, Pérez-Alonso A, et al. Contemporary wars and their contributions to vascular injury management. *Eur J Trauma Emerg Surg*. 2015 Apr;41(2):129-142.

Elster EA, Bowyer MW, Knudson MM. Assessing clinical readiness: a paradigm shift in medical education. *JAMA Surg*. 2021 Nov 1;156(11):999-1000.

Gurney J, John S, Whitt E, et al. Data-driven readiness: a preliminary report on cataloging best practices in military civilian partnerships. *J Trauma Acute Care Surg*. 2022 Aug;93(2S):S155-S159.

Holt DB, Hueman MT, Jaffin J, et al. Clinical readiness program: refocusing the military health system. *Mil Med*. 2021 Jan 25;186(Suppl 1):32-39.

Knudson MM, Elster EA, Hoyt DB, et al. *The Blue Book: Military-Civilian Partnerships for Trauma Training, Sustainment, and Readiness*. American College of Surgeons; 2020.

Knudson MM, Elster EA, Woodson J, Kirk G, Turner P, Hoyt DB. A shared ethos: the military health system strategic partnership with the American College of Surgeons. *J Am Coll Surg*. 2016 Jun;222(6):1251-1255.

Rich NM. Military surgeons and surgeons in the military. *J Am Coll Surg*. 2015 Feb;220(2):127-135.

Royal Army Medical Corps Muniments Collection. Proceedings of the Congress of Central Mediterranean Force Army Surgeons, 12-16 February 1945. Accessed December 28, 2023. https://wellcomecollection.org/works/w3pmmssn

36

Grand Opera and Brain Surgery in Florence

OTTO AUFRANC, Gene Sullivan and I went to Rome on March 19, 1945 — the 6th General Hospital was celebrating the departure of Tom Goethals with a farewell party. The next day Sullivan and I continued north on Highway 2, making a detour to Orvieto to see the bas-relief on the cathedral that portrays the creation of Eve. This is one of the few portrayals of this event that pictures God acting as a technician. He is bending over Adam and grasping the rib. Orvieto, as seen across the valley, was one of the finest cities of Italy, untouched by the war and by the industrial age. There was not a factory chimney on the skyline and the valley contained the vineyards that produce the sweet, white Orvieto wine. We were disappointed in our call on Eve, for the bas-relief was packed away behind a bombproof ramp put up to protect the lower facade of the cathedral.

Highway 2 leads over Radicofani at the top of the pass — the impertinent stronghold of an ancient robber baron. My notes read: "In Florence to the Excelsior Hotel where we joined Hugh Cairns and Allen Stammers for dinner. After dinner, Shoreston invited a few of us to hear Tito Ruffo sing. In my college days I had heard Tito Ruffo in his prime as a member of the Chicago Opera Company. This concert was offered by the Maestro as a token to Shoreston for some professional courtesy."

Somewhere in Florence we entered a small apartment with a portable Victor phonograph on the center table. Ruffo, then a man past seventy with white hair, played Red Seal records made by his full, rich baritone voice 30 or more years before. He first sang Faust in Covent Garden in 1901!

Tito Ruffo leaned over the disc and listened intently to every phrase. At times his lips moved noiselessly. How fortunate, I thought, to be able to recapture at such an age one's own performance at the prime of life! Surgeons make their "recordings" on more perishable material than wax.

NEUROSURGICAL CONFERENCE

The stimulus to come to Florence at this time was a neurosurgical conference which opened on March 21 at the 24th General Hospital. Meetings of surgeons or physicians were always called "conferences" or disguised under some equally trite army term. The term "study group" would be scarcely fitting, I recall thinking, because it implies that there is still something to be learned — a poor public relations term for a surgeon! If anyone had been familiar with the real meaning of *symposium*, this would have been admirably descriptive of what really went on: "a convivial meeting for drinking, conversation and intellectual entertainment" (Oxford Dictionary). At the conference Wrork read a paper urging the more extended use of primary suture of peripheral nerves. Wallie Ritchie and Air Commodore Ironside, R.A.F., talked on the same subject.

In the discussion period I tried to present the problem of peripheral nerve injury from the standpoint of the function of the extremity as a whole — bones, muscles, joints and blood vessels. I used my favorite quotation from Oliver Cromwell: "My brethren, I beseech ye by the bowels of Christ, to consider that ye may be wrong!"

The gist of what I said was: Lesions of the peripheral nerves cannot be dissociated from the total problem of wounds of the extremities. Examine the problem before you as a pathologist examines a microscopic slide. First, under *low power,* one becomes aware of shock, of associated injuries, of the need for prevention of infection and of other effects of wounding that endanger life as well as limb. Then, under *high power,* the components of extremity surgery are examined. (These I covered one by one.) Only after these needs are met may the microscope be changed to the *oil immersion* objective and the peripheral nerve injury be examined.

Hugh Cairns spoke on wounds of the spine. These, he said, differ from ordinary accidents which result in displacement and deformity that require reduction and immobilization. He did not agree with Weary on the advisability of radical operation. The major goals are to prevent sepsis and a spinal fluid leak. Without a wide laminectomy it was difficult to do anything that might promote cord conduction.

Shoreston emphasized that the general aspects of spinal wounds were dealt with according to the principles of débridement. Torn dura must be repaired — anterior defects may be closed by grafting. The neurologic aspects of the wound should not influence the decision to operate. With complete transection (no sensory perception after thirty-six hours) no patient has recovered any useful function. Absence of motor power plays little part in prognosis.

The 24th General Hospital entertained at dinner in the evening. Joe Martin spoke about the Fifth Army, and Dick Shackleford told about his experiences in the Pacific.

The following day, March 22, Shoreston gave an excellent paper, illustrated by diagrams drawn by Breslow. Both Shoreston and Peter Ascroft gave mature and thoughtful papers dealing with mechanisms rather than a reporting of statistics. (Later I wrote in my diary: "I fear that most of the experience assembled from this war will be reportorial — what happened rather than a correlation of observational data to point out new relationships. With few exceptions our medical officers are in the statistical phase.") Ascroft's paper was on: "Causes of Death in War Wounds of the Head." He was an R.A.M.C. officer who had examined the dead on Italian battlefields as they were being assembled by the Graves Registration Service. The disfigurement caused by the explosive action of high-velocity missiles striking the skull was so horrible that he was forced to take a leave of absence after his harrowing experience.

Captain Tribee, of the 2nd Medical Laboratory, had examined about 1,000 bodies of soldiers killed in action. He had collected some interesting data, but little that would provide the N.R.C. Ballistics Study group with what they were clamoring for. There were many variables in studies on those killed in action — for example, mutilations inflicted by shell bursts after death.

FURTHER TOUR

After lunch I went with Simeone to his laboratory and then to San Miniato al Monte on the hill across the Arno. In the sacristy were soft-colored murals portraying scenes from the life of Saint Benedict by a fourteenth century artist, Aretino. One painting in particular had attracted Simeone's attention as an early portrayal of the crush syndrome. The devil pushed a wall onto an ancient frater who was then restored to health by the good saint. I obtained a set of postal cards, the product of Nazi propaganda. The cards portrayed the destruction of the Monte Cassino Abbey and one of the cards bore the statement, credited to the Vicar of the Abbey, that there were no German troops in the Abbey.

Returning to Florence, I went to the Palazzo Vecchio to see General Hume. Hume, an avid stamp collector, gave me some German postal stamps for my sons. He had obtained them in Aachen at the time of its capture by the Americans. These were supposed to be the first German stamps "liberated" in Germany.

On March 24, at Pistoia, I made rounds at the 70th General Hospital with Stewart, Woolsey, Burford, Shorbe and Jensen. I found Bob Boardman, the son of a family friend, looking well and convalescing from a chest wound and soft-part wounds of the legs.

That afternoon we drove through the beautiful spring Italian countryside to Lucca, deciding to spend the night in the country at the 170th Evacuation Hospital instead of pushing on to Livorno (Leghorn). Fireplaces in the pyramidal tents for the chill of spring evenings were the specialty feature of Pel Glasier and the 170th Evacuation Hospital. Pel's tent was known as the "Powder River Lodge."

Lucca is enclosed by bastioned walls and a moat, and its Piazza Puccini is a tribute to the composer born in this hill town. We drove down the valley toward Pisa. "The first view of the Leaning Tower should be from this approach," I noted in my diary, "for it stands in the foreground of the city and the cathedral and so is not dwarfed by them." (I have seen the Tower "loom" in a ground fog like a ship at sea.) We drove through the corner of the city to pass by the Leaning Tower, then on across the temporary bridge that spanned the Arno, and through the enormous Army supply dump and vehicle park that lined the highway for miles, to reach Livorno. "I have yet to see," I noted, "anything interesting or beautiful in this bedraggled seaport." A comfortable night was provided by Colonel Nylon in the 33rd General Hospital, where I occupied Eldridge Campbell's vacant bed.

The 12th General Hospital was close to the 33rd and just beyond it lay the 7th Station Hospital. At the 12th General Hospital I made rounds with Mike Mason and checked on the distribution of patients in specialty wards. Both here and at the 70th General Hospital I saw many excellent results of thoracoabdominal wounds and considered this problem well solved. The incidence of empyema was low; Tom Burford, when I talked with him at the 70th General Hospital, said he hoped to hold it to 6 per cent.

After lunch I drove back to Rome and spent the night — March 26 — at the 6th General Hospital, where Marshall Bartlett was Acting Commanding Officer. On the following day I reached Caserta.

The day after my return, my notes read, "I was asked by the C.G. to come to General Nelson's office for a demonstration of body armor. Major Bates, Doriot's representative in M.T.O., showed a field jacket with inserts of doron — a new material to stop low-velocity shell fragments. The Navy has a jacket in production." The idea seemed to be a promising one and it was suggested that this type of body armor had a place "in specialized situations." This was a favorite Army cliché meaning that one was unable to see application for a new gadget but it might come in handy sometime. General Nelson suggested a protective vest for special issue by a combat unit rather than by general issue. Moving on to another subject, Major Bates, according to my diary, "is convinced that protective measures (dry socks and shoepac) as well as foot discipline have kept the trench foot incident in Fifth Army during the past winter well below what might have been expected."

The organization of the Army Medical Corps was now a favorite conversation piece at headquarters. On the evening of March 28, I stopped in Bill Stone's hut for a long discussion on the subject. Otis Benson was also on a committee appointed by General Stayer to draft a report on the matter in view of the experience in war. We reconvened in Benson's hut in the Air Force camp at 6:00 P.M. and sampled a wide selection of liquors from Paris followed by dinner at the Air Force mess.

The following day we met again at Stone's hut seeking to formulate some method of setting up a permanent committee or advisory group to work for and with the Surgeon General on personnel and professional education in the peacetime Medical Corps. Actually this discussion found fruition after the war in a group assembled by Secretary of War Patterson. As we discussed the needs in Italy, it was difficult to find an administrative formula that might compensate for lack of intelligence and inadequate experience.

Esmond Long, the tuberculosis authority from Chicago, came in to see me on March 30. On Easter Sunday — April 1 — I took Long to Cassino and on the way we had a long discussion on pulmonary lobectomy for tuberculosis. This was a subject I had written about just before coming overseas, since I thought it might be important in the treatment of World War II veterans.

As we drove along the familiar Highway 6, the earth seemed to have swallowed all traces of the war, just as the sea. A slower process for the land but just as inevitable and complete.

Bradley A. Dengler, Rocco A. Armonda, and Alex B. Valadka

Churchill begins this chapter by describing his travels to Rome to attend the farewell party for Tom Goethals, who was the outgoing commander of the 6th General Hospital. Of interest, Tom Goethals was the son of the famous Army Engineer Major General George W. Goethals, who was responsible for building the Panama Canal. Churchill then visits a cathedral in Orvieto that features a bas-relief of the creation of Eve, and he points out the rarity of seeing a depiction of God "acting as a technician" as he removes a rib from Adam. In Florence, Churchill visits an acclaimed but elderly opera singer who played phonograph records of his powerful voice from the prime of his career. Churchill notes that surgeons "make their 'recordings' on more perishable material."

He next describes a neurosurgical conference. He draws on the delicate nature of opera as he summarizes his discussion of wartime peripheral nerve injuries. "Lesions of the peripheral nerve cannot be dissociated from the total problem of wounds of the extremities," and "the problem of peripheral nerve injury [must be evaluated] from the standpoint of the function of the extremity as a whole—bones, muscles, joints and blood vessels." These basic principles remain unchanged even though modern weaponry causes more severe extremity and peripheral nerve injury and complex tissue loss. Churchill's principles are currently described as "functional limb restoration," which aims to restore function and stability and minimize neuropathic pain. Sufficient time is required for devitalized tissue to be resected, infections treated, and vascular damage repaired. Multidisciplinary planning facilitates soft tissue coverage with tissue flaps and improved function with tendon transfers. Nerve repairs are still done by "primary suture" as described by Churchill, although with some caveats. Blast injury and higher-power weapons may cause larger peripheral nerve disruptions that require suturing of cabled nerve grafts from autologous sural nerve to bridge gaps and provide a tension-free repair.

The conference continues with a presentation by Hugh Cairns on spinal cord injuries. Churchill specifically references how these wounds "differ from ordinary accidents which result in displacement and deformity," which is clearly a reference to military penetrating injuries. Cairns advises against radical operations while prioritizing the goals of preventing sepsis and spinal fluid leaks. Wide laminectomy to "promote cord conduction" is also described. Little has changed in contemporary management of wartime spinal cord injuries. Clinical practice guidelines continue to advocate for repair of cerebrospinal fluid leaks and thorough decompression; instrumentation and complex operations are avoided if possible because of high rates of infection after intra-theater hardware implantation. Wide laminectomies for incomplete injuries are still widely recommended, potentially with rapid decompression, expansile duraplasty, and spinal cord perfusion pressure monitoring.

Despite the passage of nearly 80 years since the end of World War II, and the advent of modern weaponry with increased morbidity and mortality, the general principles described at the conference in Florence have not drastically changed. Although nerve injuries have become more complex, they continue to be managed with the primary focus on limb function. Surgical principles for the management of spine injuries, namely wide decompression, cerebrospinal fluid leak repair, and avoidance of overly complicated surgeries, continue to be the recommendations of experts.

SUGGESTED READINGS

Lambrechts MJ, Issa TZ, Hilibrand AS. Updates in the early management of acute spinal cord injury. *J Am Acad Orthop Surg*. 2023 Sep 1;31(17):e619-e632.

McCulloch I, Valerio I. Lower extremity reconstruction for limb salvage and functional restoration—The combat experience. *Clin Plast Surg*. 2021 Apr;48(2):349-361.

Neal CJ, McCafferty RR, Freedman B, et al. Cervical and thoracolumbar spine injury evaluation, transport, and surgery in the deployed setting. *Mil Med*. 2018 Sep 1;183(suppl_2):83-91.

37

Paris, London, Berlin—Home

THE FOLLOWING are extracts from three letters I wrote to my wife. The first was dated April 15, 1945.

"Back in my little hut after touring the world. After an overnight stay in Paris I went on to London for a quick tour of some of the hospitals that were situated in that general area. London is well picked up and not as badly hurt as I had expected. The English countryside is beautiful in spring—much greener than we have grown accustomed to in Italy.

"On my way back I went to Heidelberg and Frankfurt. With Gus Christler of Memphis I went through a large warehouse of reserve medical and surgical supplies, and close up behind one of the advancing armies visited forward hospitals.

"The devastation from air bombing is great in any sizable city and there is little apparent effort to clean up old wreckage. Tombstones have been erected in the rubble of brick and mortar. The roads are lined with 'liberated slave laborers.'

"Two impressions: (1) Germany is removed completely as a menace to the modern world; and (2) if the Nazis had been given two or three years to develop Europe and complete their armament of planes and bombs, England and America would have looked like this.

"To Paris for a day and a half where I crossed Mike DeBakey's trail. He had left the Mediterranean Theater shortly after we had watched the 10th Mountain Division take Mt. Belvedere. A New Orleans friend—Charlie Odum—was Surgical Consultant to George Patton's Third Army and Patton sent Mike to Paris in his own plane. Mike lived with General Patton for six days and found him a charming person. One evening the beef was not cooked correctly by a new chef. On this occasion he exploded with his famous bad language. His mess was a small group—Codman, Odum and one or two others. On this trip Mike was collecting data for Beebe on medical logistics and pursuing his own collection of data concerning vascular injuries. Fifth Army had a high rating in the Surgeon General's office because of its efficiency in the use of hospitals and medical personnel.

"In Paris, DeBakey told Elliott Cutler of the E.T.O. wastage in the usage of personnel. When questioned by Paul Hawley he cited data to prove the point. Hawley welcomed the opportunity to show his Army surgeons how they could economize. When Mike returned to Washington he gave the data he had collected to Beebe. It was published in 'Health' which was distributed to all commands.

"General Bradley read the article and raised hell with his surgeon who had his promotion withheld.

"Paris was untouched directly by war, but a bit distrait. Saw Elliott Cutler and many other friends. Visited some of our hospitals in the area. Stopped for a moment at Notre Dame in passing—as I did in Westminster in London. Then back to Italy where I am collecting my wits.

"Events are rolling by so rapidly in the closing phase of the War! It is difficult to keep up or comprehend the news. No idea yet about when I can get away. Perhaps two months or so after V-day in Europe is declared unless some new assignment is given me. I have no desire to go elsewhere and no reason to believe I will be requested to do so. Will try to wind up commitments here and retire to private life."

• • •

28 April

"Since returning from E.T.O. I have been working at my desk instead of participating further in the Götterdämmerung operation as it is fittingly termed. I do not recall history having recorded such an example of national insanity and suicide.

"I haven't much ambition to travel about these days. Suppose that I must visit the Po Valley before long—but will wait until the confusion quiets down a bit. As far as Germany is concerned—I should prefer not to see any more of it."

• • •

8 May

"There has been so much surrendering during the past week that everyone including myself is dizzy. And now it is all over. Strangely enough there is very little celebration and little emotion expressed over

(continued)

here. Work goes on as usual through it all. That is the only way we have of blowing off steam!

"The speeches I have been listening to today are a bit pompous and self conscious. All except the Prime Minister with his real expression of feeling in 'Advance Brittania!' Everyone else I have heard is trying to say something equal to the Gettysburg Address—and no one has been equal to the occasion. Truman's speech was almost entirely an admonition to keep at work until Japan is defeated. A little more joy and enthusiasm could well have been included. Perhaps joy is not the right word. Possibly everyone is just too exhausted. Their 'thanks to God' do not ring quite sincere, or perhaps they are a bit off key."

INVITATION TO BERLIN

On April 30, 1945, at 3:30 P.M. Adolph Hitler shot himself. On May 2, Prime Minister Winston Churchill announced in the House of Commons that over a million Germans in northern Italy had surrendered unconditionally. The war was over on the Italian front. On May 7, Germany surrendered to Eisenhower at 2:41 in the morning. The Third Reich of Adolph Hitler that was to last a thousand years was at an end.

General Stayer had gone to Berlin on General Lucius Clay's staff. By August many of the details of demobilization had been taken care of and I received a letter from General Stayer extending an invitation to join him there.

He wrote:

"I'm having amazing times looking over this area. It is beyond description. Heidelberg is untouched and the medical school is ready to start when permission is given. I have talked to various people and when you can get away I would like to have you come up and go over the medical schools in this area and give me your advice as to what should be done. The Germans are very willing to do anything we ask and I believe they can start at an early date. General Clay is very insistent that the medical schools be opened as soon as possible."

I had not been in Germany since 1926-27, when, on a Mosely Travelling Fellowship, I had spent a few months in several of the important surgical centers, particularly those in which thoracic surgery was being developed. Ferdinand Sauerbruch had been in München at that time; and now, at the end of the war, I recalled his interest in artificial limbs and thought it important to find out about developments in the rehabilitation of amputees by so-called cineplastic operations. It was fortunate that

Oscar Hampton decided to come with me on this junket because of his knowledge and experience with orthopedic surgical problems. We drove up the Brenner Pass to München where I tried to find the Pension Helios in which I had lived in 1926, now reduced to rubble. "Up there is where I once slept," I told Oscar Hampton, pointing toward the blue sky. I know München well—or thought I did. It was 75 per cent ruined by bombing and it was estimated at that time that it would take ten years to clear the rubble.

At Nüremberg we saw the amphitheater in which Hitler had harangued his followers. In Wiesbaden we called on Rudolph Brauer with whom I spent some time during my Mosely Travelling Fellowship. He was a physician who took up the surgery of pulmonary tuberculosis because he could not persuade a surgeon to do a thoracoplasty in the manner in which he knew it should be done. In 1945, Brauer was a senile old gentlemen dressed in a worn frock coat and wing collar. He was living with his books and hardly aware there had been a war and that the war was now over. His greeting was warm and kindly.

THE SAUERBRUCH HAND AND ARM

Frank Berry joined us in Frankfurt and we spent more than a week traveling by car through Stuttgart, Augsburg, Würzburg and other cities in Germany. Leaving Frankfurt by air we signed in at Berlin on August 31. We called on Sauerbruch the following morning and were assured that he would gather together some patients and demonstrate his operations for amputees on September 3. In the meantime we viewed the "sights" of the bombed city with bulldozers at work scooping up the rubble and trucks carrying it outside the city. Women were hard at work gathering firewood from the debris.

Sauerbruch had been able to assemble a few patients for us to examine, so we were able to see examples of the Sauerbruch hand and arm. One patient in particular was employed in the Charité hospital where he could be used as a demonstration case. Sauerbruch also performed one or two of the operations required to convert the forearm muscles into motor mechanisms to move the articulated elements of the prosthesis and provide the amputee with a grasping function. The patient he demonstrated could use a hammer, grasp a nail and use a screwdriver.

We discussed the "lobster claw" hand, examples of which we had seen elsewhere in Germany. It was not a hand but a conversion of the two bones of the forearm into a pincher-like appendage. It was used only for patients who had lost their eyesight as well as both hands, and enabled them to pull up the bedclothes or carry out other grasping motions.

Over a midmorning cup of ersatz coffee Sauerbruch disclaimed all knowledge of the atrocities of the Nazi concentration camps. This was a common introduction to a conversation with anyone in Germany at that time. It was accepted at face value; perhaps it was literally true, or possibly it meant no "official" knowledge or merely, "One sees what one wishes to see—no more and no less."

Sauerbruch, like other prominent Germans, was investigated by our forces. Frank Berry obtained a copy of the charges and as deputy in charge of Health, Education and Welfare on General Clay's staff, wrote a defense for him. Most of the charges were labeled as ridiculous. He received a high income as Professor at the Charité. He had cared for von Hindenburg and had been the senior surgical consultant to the military. He was cleared first by the British and thus automatically by the United States.

According to Berry, Sauerbruch missed Havana cigars as much as the equally unobtainable surgical periodicals. A present of cigars warmed his heart. He told Berry of his sixty-ninth birthday party the previous year. Many of the guests were high-ranking Army officers who despised Hitler— some thirteen were involved in the July 1944 plot against Hitler and were executed. Among these was General von Beck, formerly Chief of Staff of the Reichswehr. Sauerbruch had operated on him some years previously for carcinoma of the sigmoid.

During his birthday party Sauerbruch heard the group talking and asked what it was all about. One of them—von Beck—said: "Keep your nose out of this. You are a doctor and a surgeon, and don't belong in these matters. You are important where you are. Stick to your own work."

In August, 1938, von Beck had written: "To make our position clear in the eyes of future historians, and to preserve the name of the High Command of the Army untarnished, I, as Chief of the General Staff, wish it to be known that I refuse to countenance any National Socialist policy that might endanger peace."

These and other episodes made Sauerbruch's life miserable during the Hitler regime. His friends and patients were of an earlier generation and by temperament he was a Prussian of World War I and the Kaiser's time.

Sauerbruch died on July 2, 1964, one day before his seventy-sixth birthday.

On September 4, 1945, Oscar Hampton and I left Berlin at 11:15 A.M. by plane and reached Frankfurt at 1:15 P.M. The following day we drove back to the Brenner Pass and left Germany behind at 5:00 P.M.

HEADING HOME

During the two-and-a-half years of war we had grown accustomed to the wreckage of cities from bombs and shell fire. From our viewpoint as surgeons this had become the backdrop of the stage on which the tragedy of World War II was enacted. From Casablanca to Berlin it was the same. Displaced people, motherless children, prisoners of war, the mass graves of concentration camps were also familiar to us. Our parts as surgeons in World War II were with the wounded, with the crippled, the maimed, the suffering and the dying. This aftermath of the Nazi regime can never be measured or expressed in statistics. Johann Holst, Professor of Surgery in Oslo, said: "Es liege eine grosse Unsinn über Deutschland." ("Germany is possessed by the Devil.")

I returned to Caserta, gathered a few belongings into a duffle bag and, with diaries and records packed in two wooden boxes, left for home on the next hospital ship.

It is quite impossible to describe the emotions that welled up on leaving Italy. I shall let a letter from Eldridge Campbell, Professor of Surgery at Albany, speak for all of us.

> We are off at last and by sundown have cruised past many familiar spots on the shore line. Tomorrow at 4:00 we reach Leghorn—load patients—then turn westward. Thus will end but not close one of the most interesting and in many ways satisfactory chapters in the lives of many of us. What the future holds for us no one knows, but be it what it may, I am sure that most of the surgeons of this theater will meet it, better prepared.

Aboard the hospital ship as we neared Gibraltar I recalled the story of Hercules and the following passage:

> After traversing various countries Hercules reached the frontiers of Libya and Europe, where he erected two pillars: CALPE and ABYLA on the two sides of the Strait of Gibraltar, which were hence called the Pillars of Hercules. Throughout classical times the Pillars of Hercules represented the end of the known world and the limit of civilization.

The Statue of Liberty was a welcome sight in the morning sun as the ship entered New York harbor. We were met by the usual brass bands playing "Roll Out the Barrel," and the shrill screams of tugboat whistles as we slowly—oh so slowly—came to berth at the Hoboken pier. The war was over.

Rathnayaka M. K. D. Gunasingha, Mary J. Edwards, and
Matthew J. Bradley

"One sees what one wishes to see." Colonel Churchill uses this statement to describe Ernst Ferdinand Sauerbruch, a highly respected German surgeon, who reported personal ignorance of the atrocities in Nazi concentration camps. However, one could also use the statement to describe Churchill's own apparent acceptance of this "ignorance," and the general medical community's dismissal of Sauerbruch's involvement with the Third Reich.

Churchill and his contemporaries recognized Sauerbruch as a talented surgeon who contributed to numerous surgical advancements. He served in World War I as the consulting Staff-Surgeon-Major to the Prussian Army, and his experience with the wounded drove him to develop a functional limb prosthetic. In 1927, Sauerbruch became the Chair of Surgery of the Charité Hospital and professor at the University of Berlin, a major intellectual center in the world at the time. Prior to World War II, Sauerbruch gave an invited lecture at the American Medical Association and observed the daily operations of the Mayo brothers' clinic.

Churchill met Sauerbruch in Germany while on a traveling surgical fellowship many years before and now sought to follow up on Sauerbruch's advances with artificial limbs. Churchill described Sauerbruch as miserable under Hitler's regime—inasmuch as he "missed Cuban cigars and surgical journals." Sadly, Churchill was either woefully ignorant or intentionally dismissive of Sauerbruch's actions and associations during World War II. These include his public support of the National Socialists, as reflected in a scientific speech calling on the audience to support the will of Adolf Hitler. Sauerbruch also signed the *Vow of allegiance of the Professors of the German Universities and High-Schools to Adolf Hitler and the National Socialistic State*, which banished independent academic freedom from higher education in Nazi Germany. Finally, he served as state chancellor and surgeon general under the Nazi regime and headed the *Reichsforschungsrat* (Reich Research Council). In this capacity, he would have approved research projects on those in concentration camps. This information was notably not included in his investigation and subsequent exoneration by the Allies. Thus, history suggests Sauerbruch at best overlooked the Nazi agenda or at worst served as a willing instrument for the Nazi party's agenda.

Sadly, Sauerbruch was not alone in this ignominy. By 1942, 45% of German physicians had joined the Nazi party, the highest rate of any profession. Nazi physicians administered cruel research programs, led euthanasia programs (*Aktion T4*), and served as the selectors for the Final Solution (the killing of all individuals of non-Aryan blood). While *United States of America vs Karl Brandt, et al.* (the Nuremberg Doctors' Trial) prosecuted 23 Nazi physicians and found the majority guilty, hundreds or even thousands more enabled these heinous crimes yet went unpunished.

In a shocking epilogue, shortly after World War II, Sauerbruch killed multiple patients through a combination of his own mental and physical decline and a medical community unwilling to remove him from clinical practice. This appalling end to Sauerbruch's surgical career, otherwise marked by numerous innovations and well-deserved accolades, illustrates the grave but predictable outcome when a surgeon betrays the solemn responsibility we have both to our patients and to our profession. In the face of such betrayal, we must have the discipline to see what we do not wish to see and then the moral courage to act in response.

SUGGESTED READINGS

Cherian SM, Nicks R, Lord RSA. Ernst Ferdinand Sauerbruch: rise and fall of the pioneer of thoracic surgery. *World J Surg Springer*. 2001;25:1012-1020.

Dewey M, Schagen U, Eckart WU, Schönenberger E. Ernst Ferdinand Sauerbruch and his ambiguous role in the period of national socialism. *Ann Surg*. 2006;244:315-321.

Ernst E. Commentary: The Third Reich—German physicians between resistance and participation. *Int J Epidemiol*. 2001;30:37-42.

Sidel V. The social responsibilities of health professionals. *JAMA*. 1996;276:1679-1681.

Trunkey DD, Botney R. Assessing competency: a tale of two professions. *J Am Coll Surg*. 2001 Mar;192(3):385-395.

APPENDICES

Cranial and Peripheral Nerve Wounds

I HAD a long session with John Martin on October 29, 1944, at the 12th General Hospital in Rome. The discussion was about head wounds. From November 8, 1942, to November 7, 1944, John had cared for 232 penetrating wounds of the brain. Most of these were at the 12th General Hospital and some at the 70th General Hospital in Oran where he worked on temporary duty when the 12th General Hospital was closed. Forty-four of the cases were from North Africa, 14 from Sicily and 161 from Italy; 13 were nonbattle casualties.

Of the battle casualties, 2 were caused by land mines, 25 by bullets, 187 by shell fragments, and 5 by other missiles (grenades, secondary missiles). Seventy-two (32.9 per cent) did not heal primarily on the basis of liberal criteria; of these, 32 gave evidence of deep cerebritis. The series of dural patches is too limited to give convincing evidence on various methods: in 12 cases with pericranium patch there were 5 abscesses; 11 patched with fresh fascia developed 4 abscesses; 6 patched with preserved dura developed 4 abscesses; 1 closed with temporal muscle and fascia healed without abscess.

Not a single patient, so far as Martin knew, returned to A Grade duty status. A few were boarded as such but "bounced." Ten went to B Grade duty. There were 3 deaths in the battle casualty group; 4 others died from penetrating wounds received on maneuvers or accidentally.

Sixteen eyes were lost, including intraorbital injuries and enucleations. Twenty-five patients showed a cerebrospinal fluid leak or rhinorrhea. One hundred and sixty-one had severe residual neurological defects.

E.D.C. Comments: "Silk sutures," my notes say, "are doing better and cotton sutures appear satisfactory." Forward surgeons need the guidance that better x-ray films would afford. When retained bone fragments are demonstrated, Martin does not consider secondary debridement an emergency procedure. Many patients benefit by some delay for better delimitation of the area. Ten to 14 days is probably the optimal time.

(continued)

> "Martin has seen only a single example of what might be called the 'civilian' type of brain abscess. This had a thick wall, contained 2 ounces of pus with bone chips. Believes intrathecal use of penicillin questionable but thinks when used with diazene and given parenterally that penicillin has helped healing."

Henry G. Schwartz, neurosurgeon of the 21st General Hospital in the North African-Mediterranean Theater, made a consultant's tour to Southeast Asia January 14 to February 18, 1967. In his report to the Surgeon General he stated:

> "The work of the teams at the 3rd and 8th Field Hospitals is most impressive. They have taken to heart the historical experiences of past conflicts, have been assiduous in performing thorough débridement of head wounds (with particular emphasis on in-driven bone fragments) and have achieved an enviable record of survival and low infection rate."

Loyal Davis, in 1945, wrote:

> "It is agreed by neurological surgeons and neurologists that the principles which underlie the surgical treatment of peripheral nerve injuries are not well understood by the civilian surgeons who are in positions to give these patients the most advantageous early and primary care."

On the subject of peripheral nerve injuries, Schwartz reported from Vietnam that appropriate management was being carried out "with débridement of the wounds, followed by delayed primary closure. The nerve itself is left to be sutured three or four weeks later at a hospital in the communications zone or in the U. S. This lesson has been learned and reemphasized."

In the Mediterranean Theater, in 1944, Harvey Allen told me on October 29 that he had seen

> "no case suitable for suture at the time of reparative suture (three to six days). There is edema and reaction that would mean placement of the suture in the center of scar. In simple wounds secondarily closed, the conditions are suitable for suture in three weeks. When a wound is complicated by a fracture or a large tissue defect they are unsuitable for nerve suture . . . . Harvey Allen has done some 14 nerve sutures in arm and forearm after three weeks. All were minor types of lacerations without tissue defects or fracture."

Susanna D. Howard, Zarina S. Ali, and Daniel A. Hammer

This appendix describes an extraordinary number of penetrating cranial and ballistic peripheral nerve injuries that were managed by a single neurosurgeon, John Martin. Over a two-year period, Martin treated 200 penetrating brain injuries that had a mortality rate of 3%. Yet, this remarkably low mortality rate must be interpreted knowing that soldiers evacuated to the 12th General Hospital, who typically had already survived 3 to 10 days after the initial injury.

Not surprisingly, infection was the most common complication seen following cranial wounds in World War II. Contributing factors included the inability of achieving primary wound closure due to the large size of the soft tissue defect and the prolonged interval between injury and initial debridement. Infection rates decreased significantly with the routine use of penicillin, which started in the spring of 1944.

During World War II, neurosurgeons advocated for the increased use of radiographs at forward hospitals. The advent of computerized tomography (CT) since that time has revolutionized the management of penetrating brain injuries. In contrast to plain radiographs, CT scans clearly identify projectile trajectories. These trajectories and the pupil examination predict the patient's outcome and aid neurosurgeons in assessing the utility of decompressive craniectomy.

Technologic advances in vascular imaging, such as digital subtraction angiography, have also increased detection of traumatic aneurysms and cerebral vasospasm following blast injuries. In an analysis of patients with severe head trauma during Operation Iraqi Freedom and Operation Enduring Freedom, more than a third of them were found to have associated vascular injuries. The most common vascular injury observed was traumatic intracranial aneurysm, and in over half these patients, vasospasm was also seen. In addition to traditional open surgical clipping, modern endovascular techniques can now be used to manage traumatic aneurysms and vasospasm.

This appendix also addresses two aspects of peripheral nerve injury management: time to repair and repair technique. Surgeons often delayed repair for at least 3 to 4 weeks after the injury based on the assumption that peripheral nerve injuries were caused by ballistic weapons with associated soft tissue defects. After this delay, primary neurorrhaphy was performed in cases without tissue defects or fractures. However, we now know that this technique can lead to neuroma formation and less successful neurosensory and motor restoration. Today, nerve autografts, nerve allografts, and nerve conduits are commonly used to aid in repair and to enhance patient outcomes, although primary neurorrhaphy remains a mainstay for repair after a sharp laceration. With blunt or blast injury mechanisms, the zone of injury may not be immediately apparent. Therefore, delayed repair with full neuroma resection is preferred to facilitate reconstruction spanning the entire zone of injury.

The management of cranial and peripheral nerve injuries have made remarkable progress during periods of war. In World War II, neurotrauma care improved greatly with efforts to expedite medical evacuation along with the implementation of mobile neurosurgical units. In the recent conflicts in Iraq and Afghanistan, traumatic brain injury accounted for a larger proportion of casualties leading to significant neurologic morbidity. Subsequent effects on mood and cognition have also been increasingly recognized. Carrying forward lessons learned on and off the battlefield has optimized the likelihood that a brain-injured solider will return as a functional member of society.

SUGGESTED READINGS

Aarabi B, Howard E. Surgical management and prognosis of penetrating brain injury. In: Winn HR, ed. *Youmans and Winn Neurological Surgery*. Elsevier; 2022:3092-3104.

Bell RS, Ecker RD, Severson MA 3rd, Wanebo JE, Crandall B, Armonda RA. The evolution of the treatment of traumatic cerebrovascular injury during wartime. *Neurosurg Focus*. 2010 May;28(5):E5.

Gressot LV, Chamoun RB, Patel AJ, et al. Predictors of outcome in civilians with gunshot wounds to the head upon presentation. *J Neurosurg*. 2014;121(3):645-652.

Martin J, Campbell EH Jr. Early complications following penetrating wounds of the skull. *J Neurosurg*. 1946;3:58–73.

Rainone GJ, Zelmanovich R, Laurent D, Lucke-Wold B. How war has shaped neurosurgery. *World Neurosurg*. 2023 Jul 26;178:136-144.

Wounds of the Thorax

And they that lie in a pleurisy think that every time they cough, they feel a sharp sword snap them to the breast.

—Thomas More, 1530

THE ANNUAL meeting of the American Association for Thoracic Surgery was held in Toronto, in 1941, under the presidency of Fraser B. Gurd, and I succeeded him in this office. In accord with the desires of the government to reduce travel to an essential minimum, the 1942 and 1943 meetings were canceled. On my departure for active service with the Army, my abortive term as president came to an end and Frank S. Dolley, of Los Angeles, became president. The next meeting was held in Chicago in May, 1944.

I wrote the major part of the following account of the management of thoracic wounds in Italy and sent it to the secretary of the A.A.T.S., who read it at the 25th Annual Meeting in Chicago, May 5 and 6, 1944. It was published in the *Journal of Thoracic and Cardiovascular Surgery 13:*(#4) 307-311, August, 1944.[1] It reads as follows:

> TRENDS AND PRACTICES IN THORACIC SURGERY IN THE
> MEDITERRANEAN THEATER
> Colonel Edward D. Churchill
> Medical Corps, A.U.S.
>
> The change of the focus of attention from pleural space to lung stands as one of the important achievements of the military surgeon of World War II. The point of view that holds a chest injury to be progressing satisfactorily as long as pleural infection has not supervened is no longer tenable.

(continued)

---

[1]Reprinted from Churchill ED. Trends and practices in Thoracic Surgery in the Mediterranean Theater. *J Thorac Surg* 1944; 13: 307-315, with permission from Elsevier. Copyright © 1944 American Association for Thoracic surgery. Published by Mosby, Inc. All rights reserved.

The prime concern in the management of thoracic wounds in the combat zone has been the timing of operative intervention and the proper placement of various procedures in the line of hospitals from the front to the rear. In abdominal wounds, the early and fulminating complication of peritonitis leaves no question regarding the degree of urgency that demands immediate operation. In craniocerebral wounds, the complications of infection are slow to appear and a delay up to seventy-two hours for the initial operation can be accepted as a safe price to pay for the advantages of transportation to a hospital equipped and staffed for neurosurgery. In the management of thoracic wounds two distinct phases may be encountered —physiologic disturbance and infection. Profound physiologic disturbances must be corrected immediately, by operation if need be, in the most forward surgical installation. Not infrequently the hazards of infection can be eliminated simultaneously, but the two issues must not be confused. If a casualty is not subjected to early and complete operation on the indications of physiologic urgency, subsequent interference may be necessary three days to six weeks after wounding in order to prevent infection or minimize disability.

At the divisional clearing station casualties are diverted to the adjacent field hospital if urgent surgical indications are present. These are, for chest wounds, continuing hemorrhage, severe shock, sucking wounds, injuries associated with respiratory distress, or wounds in which the missile may have penetrated the abdomen. Continuing hemorrhage has been from the chest wall in the vast majority of instances and into the pleural cavity rather than external. Persistent shock, rapid pulse, and low blood pressure are not in themselves indicative of continuing hemorrhage. The diagnosis is made only by repeated aspiration and reaccumulation of blood. Aspirated blood is used for autotransfusion.

Sucking wounds are numerous, due to the predominance of high-explosive shell fragments as a cause of wounds. The wounds are usually small and the open pneumothorax is not in itself a common cause of embarrassment. Of course, larger defects are encountered from time to time. Closure of sucking wounds by suture before adequate débridement of the thoracic wall is performed was never sanctioned in this theater. Tight closure is likely to be followed by a pressure pneumothorax and surgical emphysema. A compress of petrolatum gauze held in place by adhesive plaster provides sufficient occlusion, and an escape for air is afforded if a bronchial leak exists. The surprising infrequency of pressure pneumothorax and subcutaneous emphysema can be attributed, at least in part, to this optimum size of wounds, too small to produce the phenomena of an open pneumothorax and too large to seal off the escape of air under pressure. Possibly pre-existing pleural adhesions, so important in the mechanism of pressure pneumothorax and emphysema, are less common today in our combat troops than they were when these sequelae of chest wounds terrified the military surgeons of the past.

The use of bronchoscopic or catheter tracheobronchial aspiration to clear the respiratory passages of blood and secretions has found increasing use. Unless this is done, oxygen administration and transfusion are of little avail. A great deal of enthusiasm has developed for novocain block of the intercostal spaces involved by the wound. Many surgeons consider this procedure specific for what is termed the wet lung that follows trauma. There is discussion as to whether novocain block interrupts a somatovisceral reflex and releases bronchospasm or whether relief from pain simply enables the man to cough more effectively. Until further evidence is presented the latter explanation would appear to account for the observations on record.

The urgent physiologic disturbances that attend wounds of the chest can be controlled by needle aspiration of air and blood, aspiration of blood and mucus from the tracheobronchial tree, novocain injection of intercostal spaces, insertion of a catheter with a flutter valve for pressure pneumothorax, oxygen therapy and transfusion, and débridement of sucking wounds with hemostasis of intercostal vessels and approximation of deep structures of the chest wall to close the pleural opening.

Immediate thoracotomy at a site of election is rarely indicated and is reserved for continuing intrathoracic hemorrhage uncontrolled by chest wall wound débridement (rare), large bronchopleural fistula not responding to conservative management (exceedingly rare), wounds of esophagus (if diagnosed), and thoracoabdominal wounds (common).

In intermediate position between the conservative methods of management and a radical thoracotomy at the site of election comes thoracotomy through the site of the wound. With large defects of the chest wall very little added exposure is needed; with small defects the aperture is increased by rib resection or intercostal extension of the incision. Carrying out intrathoracic procedures through the chest wall defect or an extension thereof is an operation of variable extent and indications. Both the indications and the procedure will vary with the experience of the surgeon, the condition of the patient, the prevailing tactical situation regarding hospitalization and evacuation, the location and size of the wound, and the presence or absence of retained foreign bodies. With so many variables it is not surprising that differences in opinion exist regarding its merits. The chief accomplishments lie in the recovery of foreign bodies from the pleural space, removal of rib fragments and readily accessible missiles from the lung, appraisal of perforations of the diaphragm with suture in some instances, control of bleeding from the chest wall at a point remote from the wound of

(continued)

entrance, and suture of wounds of the lung that are judged to be a source of continuing hemorrhage. In addition, an opportunity is provided to remove blood clots from the pleural cavity.

The dangers of this type of interference are those of any operation without a precise and predetermined goal, particularly if undertaken through an incision determined by the missile rather than chosen by the surgeon. Properly employed, it may save life as well as prevent infection and in many instances obviate the necessity for a delayed operation. Improperly employed, it may endanger life and delay the time when the patient is transportable to the rear. An important consideration is the likelihood that an extension of intrapleural operative procedures in the presence of a traumatized and partially collapsed lung will delay its re-expansion and by so doing invite pleural complications or render those that do occur more serious.

During the five- to ten-day period after wounding, surgery may be indicated for the prevention of infection. Foreign bodies in the pleura or lung over a size arbitrarily set at 1.5 cm. in greatest dimension are removed. At the same time residual clotted blood is removed from the pleural space. Wounds of the chest wall left open following débridement are sutured either previous to or at the time of operation.

Hemothorax is managed initially by repeated aspiration. Many cases, particularly those with minimal chest wall damage, clear up with this regimen. A considerable number of cases with collections of blood in the pleural space become static about the fourth week. Massive accumulations of fibrin with isolated pockets of serum resist further removal by aspiration. The chest wall becomes fixed and the interspaces narrowed. Doubtlessly some of these cases will eventually resolve spontaneously, others terminate in an organized or calcified hematoma, and still others are complicated by empyema. Microorganisms, particularly the staphylococcus, are demonstrable in the fibrin clot in many instances.

This chronic hematoma of the pleural space is rarely encountered in civilian injuries. It may be the result of the greater trauma that high-explosive missiles inflict on both the chest wall and the lung, with a prolonged period of plasma exudation. In civilian injuries with small caliber missiles, knife blades, and ice picks, the hemothorax appears to arise from the *initial* hemorrhage and is either absorbed spontaneously or yields to aspiration. In wounds from high-explosive fragments there appears to be a *continuing* exudation of plasma and red cells that builds up the fibrin clot to large dimensions. How great a role nonsuppurative infection plays in this continuing exudation is impossible to ascertain.

Between the third and sixth weeks careful appraisal is made of residual "clotted" hemothorax. If aspiration yields only a few cubic centimeters of bloody serum and serial x-ray pictures show no improvement, thoracotomy is advised. The pleural cavity is cleaned out and the dense layer of fibrin removed from the underlying lung to permit normal expansion. The lower lobe is often found distorted and folded upon itself, completely fixed by the fibrin envelope.

This early decortication of the lung in nonsuppurative or sterile clotted hemothorax will, it is believed, not only prevent many instances of chronic empyema at a later date but, conserve respiratory function in cases that do not go on to frank suppuration.

Posttraumatic empyema is treated in accordance with the same principle—the prevention of the serious and life-endangering chronic phase of pleural suppuration. Preliminary drainage is established when indicated, and when the patient's condition permits, decortication is carried out. The operation of decortication should be done before the tenth week following establishment of the infection, as after that time progressive organization of the inflammatory exudate on the visceral pleura obliterates a surgical line of cleavage.

Air replacement of blood aspirated from the pleural space is not done in this theater. It was recommended by the National Research Council Committee for continuing hemorrhage from a lacerated lung, not as a routine measure. This condition is rarely encountered, and should be approached by open thoracotomy.

Large hematomas of the lung are not uncommon but do not call for interference. Posttraumatic pneumatoceles may develop in the course of the missile tract. These may communicate with a hemothorax, or perforate into the pleura producing pressure pneumothorax as a late manifestation.

Asymptomatic foreign bodies in the lung, chest wall or mediastinal structures are not considered as disqualification for return to active duty within the theater. Return to active duty following chest wounds is measured by the functional capacity for exercise without embarrassing shortness of breath. Early decision regarding the removal of a foreign body should be made in each case so that the convalescence from the thoracotomy will fall within the time period of the convalescence from the wound.

Surgeons employing the low transthoracic approach for thoraco-abdominal wounds are enthusiastic about the exposure it affords and have extended its use to selected cases of left upper quadrant abdominal wounds. Wounds of the spleen, kidney, stomach, and splenic flexure of the colon are readily accessible by this approach. On the right side the transthoracic approach to the abdominal viscera is less free but many cases can be handled in this manner by extension of the incision far enough forward. Some surgeons still prefer a separate laparotomy incision.

Note: A collective review entitled "The Management of Chest Wounds" by Michael Debakey, was published in Surgery, Gynecology and Obstetrics 74:203-237, March, 1942. This was based on a bibliography of 474 references and provides an historic base line for the subject of chest wounds in World War II.

LECTURE AT UNIVERSITY OF LIVERPOOL

In the Mitchell Banks Lecture at the University of Liverpool on November 3, 1948, I presented some of the historic steps in the management of gunshot wounds of the thorax. The subject was developed further and, with the title "Wound Surgery Encounters a Dilemma," was delivered before the New York Society for Thoracic Surgery at the 40th Anniversary Dinner, November 8, 1957. It is reproduced here with some deletions and slight modifications.

If Michelangelo had fallen from the scaffolding while decorating the ceiling of the Sistine Chapel it is likely that he would have been treated by John of Vigo. John of Vigo was the first surgeon to record his views on gunshot wounds of the chest, and in fact his book *Practica Copiosa* printed in Rome in 1514 was one of the very early surgical texts to mention wounds by firearms. John of Vigo enjoyed a rich experience in wound surgery while attached to that fighting Pope, Julius the Second, and a nice legend perpetuated by Sir Clifford Allbutt places a French translation of the *Practica* in the hands of the young barber's apprentice, Ambroise Paré. At any rate, Paré, in 1575, quoted John of Vigo on the management of wounds of the chest.

"At first thought it might seem that the treatment of an open pneumothorax would have been a straightforward matter to the ancient wound surgeons. Such a wound presents what might appear to be a simple choice between two procedures: the wound can be closed or it can be left open. As a matter of fact, the several factors which are determinants to this decision puzzled surgeons for centuries and still crop up in one form or another in our own century. In my title I have referred to this choice as a dilemma and propose to identify some of the circumstances which made the choice between leaving the wound open and closing it a difficult one."

"Paré identified two major considerations. 'John of Vigo,' he wrote, 'said that there is a disagreement between the surgeons because some have a mind to close the penetrating wound as soon as possible . . . for fear that the cold air would penetrate into the heart and that vital spirits would depart and vanish; the others, contrary minded, recommend keeping the wound open . . . in order to evacuate the blood left in the thorax, fearing that this would decompose and putrefy; that would provoke fever, fistula and other complications. In truth, those who are of the mind to close the wound immediately . . . are entirely right, on condition that there is no blood or only a small amount inside the chest. . . . In the same manner are those quite right who have the mind to keep the wound open. . . .'"

"It is significant that Paré set out to define certain conditions or principles which were to distinguish between the two courses of action and point to the selection of the one better adapted to the particular circumstances. His text was written for the benefit of barber surgeons who, as workers in a practical art, desired to be guided by definite rules and precepts, preferably phrased in the imperative. They expected to be told either 'leave the wound open' or 'close the wound.' Such workers are particularly unhappy when the exercise of choice between alternative methods of procedure rests on conditions that they themselves may be unable to recognize. The condition which determined that the wound should be left open was indeed definite even though difficult to assess—blood in the chest. The concept of what would happen if blood were closed in the chest was straightforward and empirical. The blood would 'decompose and putrefy' and would 'provoke fever, fistula and other complications.'"

"Paré was on less certain ground when he attempted to define the conditions under which the wound should be closed immediately. He may have known that he was on unfamiliar ground, for he repeated the caution that there must be no blood or at least only a small amount of blood inside the chest if this course were to be elected. Then departing from his own surgical experience, Paré invoked a prevailing doctrine of ancient authority. 'Close the wound,' he wrote, 'for fear that the cold air will penetrate into the heart and the vital spirits depart and vanish.'"

"So the dilemma presented by an open chest wound as seen by the great surgeon of the Renaissance was: surgeons who close the wound to keep the vital spirits from departing may be right but experience shows that if blood remains in the chest, mischief will follow. Judging from the case reports of his own practice, it was Paré's custom to keep the wound open two or three days and allow the blood to trickle out by gravity; when the flow of blood ceased, the wound was closed. This compromise undoubtedly reflects Pare's estimate of the relative validity of the indications for the choice between closing the wound and leaving it open under the circumstances which actually prevailed. It is likely that the wounded of that period who survived to come under treatment by a surgeon had wounds of small cross-sectional area resulting from sword thrusts or low-velocity missiles."

"Let us now briefly trace the development of the more precise understanding of the two courses of action that confronted Paré as the two horns of a dilemma, first taking up the matter of blood in the pleural cavity. The untoward effects of the accumulation of blood in any wound are related in the legends of ancient wars, and many romantic stories can be found of friends who, having put their mouths to the flesh, sucked blood from the wounds of warriors. In the wars of the seventeenth and eighteenth centuries the sucking of wounds was so much in demand that it became a trade. Certain individuals in a regiment, frequently the drummer, became famous for their skill as wound suckers. There is adequate testimony in the old writings to establish the efficacy of this form of treatment, which of course is in principle a sound method in the light of present-day knowledge. Sucking was found particularly useful when quarrels were decided by duels with swords which terminated with the first flesh wound. The wounded swordsman after this form of treatment commonly was able to walk home and entirely conceal the affair. Today it is recognized that contaminated blood remaining in a wound track offers an inviting pabulum for the growth of pathogenic bacteria, and it is the usual practice with flesh wounds to leave them open with textile drainage and to close them on the fourth day by reparative suture."

"The activities of wound suckers finally fell into disrepute and the procedure itself became known as the *secret dressing*. To inflate their prestige and possibly in order to keep their trade to themselves the suckers pretended to make it a magical ceremony. They muttered cabalistic words, made strange motions, and drew the sign of the cross. It was understandable that the priests who also followed armies became outraged by such profanities and refused extreme unction or other sacrament to those who participated in these diabolical ceremonies. The suckers on the other hand refused to ply their art on those who had commerce with the priests under the pretense that Christian rites interfered with their incantations. La Motte, a surgeon of this period, was an eyewitness to many wonderful cures. He saw, for example, a soldier who had been run through the breast with a single lunge which passed, as he described it, 'in at the pap, and out at the shoulder.' By examining the wounds and noticing the length of the antagonist's sword La Motte was well satisfied that the weapon had pierced the lungs and gone quite across the chest. The drummer of the regiment first sucked one wound, then turned his patient and sucked the opposite wound. He applied a piece of chewed paper upon each and next day the soldier was seen walking in the streets."

"Wound sucking was thought to be particularly effective for wounds of the chest although some writers expressed doubt that retained blood actually could be removed from the pleural cavity. The question can be asked whether the phrase 'sucking wound' as it applied today to open chest wounds is a curious linguistic survival from this period because actually such a wound blows air out as much as it sucks air in."

"In 1707, And published in Amsterdam a small book on the art of sucking wounds without using the human mouth. A silver tube was the answer. One end could be attached to a piston syringe and the other applied to a wound. By this gadgetry the surgeon himself was able to take over the procedure of wound sucking, which then became known by the more refined term—aspiration. Improvements in the apparatus inevitably followed and one of these proposed by Birkholz, in 1771, introduced a reservoir into the suction line, producing in essence a Potain aspirator. Anel doubted that suction applied to the margins of the wound could actually evacuate the pleural cavity and so designed a cannula patterned after a female catheter which could be introduced into the pleural space through the wound. From this it was a short step to trocar and catheter."

"In 1772, Valentin published his small volume in which he declared that all wounds of the chest were to be closed as a measure to suppress hemorrhage and that when necessary a counter opening should be made to evacuate the effused blood at an early date. Guthrie, the great English military surgeon of the Napoleonic Wars and the Peninsular Campaign, closed wounds of the chest but followed them carefully with what he called 'unremitting attention in the use of the stethoscope,' and removed blood by trocar and cannula. 'The first object,' Guthrie wrote, 'is to save life. After that, if time be given, the next will be to relieve the loaded cavity.' Baron Larrey, Napoleon's surgeon, supposed that nine days should elapse before it was safe to evacuate blood without encountering the danger of renewed bleeding. If Guthrie, surgeon of the Duke of Wellington, could find an excuse to differ from Larrey he always did so; his recommended procedure was to wait until the patient reacted, when he concluded that bleeding had ceased. In following the situation he looked for the increase of serous effusion which usually came from the third to the fifth day. Then Guthrie either reopened the wound to evacuate blood or carried this out through another opening with a trocar and cannula. He placed great importance on relieving the lung from pressure at an early date so that it might expand and not be bound down by what he termed false membranes."

"Having traced these significant steps in the management of the retained blood, let us examine briefly the other horn of the dilemma, namely the disturbance in pulmonary ventilation which attends an open pneumothorax. In the view of Pare, disaster resulted from the cold air penetrating into the heart and the vital spirits departing the body through the wound and vanishing. Here, as with the complication of blood accumulating in the wound, the record of experience is lost in antiquity...."

"Little was understood about the lethal effects of an open pneumothorax until the early physiologists started a systematic analysis of the action of the organs of respiration. The phenomenon of pendulum air in open pneumothorax, a phenomenon which is customarily attributed in eponym to Brauer, was explained by Hoadley as early as 1737."

In expiration, the air in the unwounded side was condensed, and part of it, instead of going out at the windpipe, forced its way into the lung of the wounded side, and dilated it, till the air within it came into an equilibrium with the external air which surrounded it; and in inspiration, when the air in the lung of the unwounded side became rarer than the external air, the lung in the wounded side was compressed, and part of the air within it was, by the pressure of the external air, forced back into the lung of the unwounded side, till the equilibrium was again restored.

"On the basis of clinical observations, the brilliant young associate of the Hunters, William Hewson, observed in 1767 that with an open external wound the patient may hardly be able to breathe but he breathes easily when it is covered. Hew-son said the difficulty arose 'owing to the air getting into the cavity of the thorax in inspiration instead of entering the lungs by the trachea.' While such a wound is uncovered the patient is deprived of the use of the lobes of that side either partially or entirely 'according as the wound of the thorax bears a less or greater proportion to the branch of the trachea to that side.'"

"These concepts based both on physiologic experiments and on clinical observations in the eighteenth century stand today except for certain amplifications and minor corrections."

"It is difficult to be certain when wound surgeons closed a defect in the chest wall primarily to reestablish effective pulmonary ventilation rather than to control hemorrhage from the lung. The following story related in the memoirs of Baron Larrey, the surgeon of Napoleon, emphasizes the immediate and striking improvement in the condition of the patient that follows the closure of an open chest wound."

A soldier was brought to the hospital of the fortress of Ibrahym Bay, immediately after a wound . . . that penetrated the thorax, between the fifth and sixth true ribs, . . . it was about eight centimetres in extent: a large quantity of frothy and vermillion blood escaped from it with a hissing noise, at each inspiration. His extremities were cold, pulse scarcely perceptible, countenance discoloured, and respiration short and laborious; in short, he was every moment threatened with a fatal suffocation.

After having examined the wound, and the divided edges of the parts, I immediately approximated the two lips of the wound, and retained them by means of adhesive plasters, and a suitable bandage round the body.

In adopting this plan, I intended only to hide from the sight of the patient and his comrades, the distressing spectacle of a hoemorrhage, which would soon prove fatal: and I therefore thought, that the effusion of blood into the cavity of the thorax, could not increase the danger.

But the wound was scarcely closed, when he breathed more freely, and felt easier. The heat of the body soon returned, and the pulse rose; in a few hours he became quite calm, and to my great surprize, grew better. He was cured in a very few days, and without difficulty.

"Larrey then referred to two similar cases at the hospital of the Imperial Guard."

Since Ambroise Paré, all practitioners and authors, who have written on wounds of the thorax, advise not to close the wounds which penetrate this cavity, especially, when they are followed by hoemorrhage . . . . But the ancients closed such wounds, and even used sutures to make them more exact. . . .

The surprising success that attended these three apparently mortal wounds . . . led me to believe that this practice is preferable to that which is now adopted.

"Guthrie, whom I have already identified as the surgeon of the Duke of Wellington, remarked that Baron Larrey had received credit for advocating closure of chest wounds merely because he had so effectively supported the views of Valentin, and that although the precepts of Valentin may have been forgotten in France they were in existence and Larrey merely deserved the merit of having revived and confirmed them. Furthermore, Guthrie claimed that he himself had closed chest wounds long before he had seen any of Larrey's works and was not aware that he was acting out of the ordinary course of things except that he used a continuous suture instead of trusting to a compress and bandage. While Guthrie pointed to this as a trivial difference, far more weight would be put on this detail today, because until a surgeon can be certain that a wounded lung is not leaking air into the pleural space, the external wound should not be closed tightly with a suture. A lethal pressure pneumothorax may develop within a few minutes. Strapping the wound edges together as Larrey did permits the escape of air should pressure build up from a bronchopleural fistula."

"It was well known to Guthrie that closure of chest wounds relieved difficult breathing and he was familiar with the observations of Hewson to which he referred. Nevertheless his writings give the impression that his advocacy of closure of the wound was based primarily on the belief that in accord with the recommendation of Valentin this was the most efficacious means of arresting hemorrhage from the lung. Thus the two horns of Pare's dilemma became a point of issue between the surgeons of Napoleon and Wellington at Waterloo."

"There has been constant modification and duplication of detail in devices designed to suppress the in-and-out flow of air in an open chest wound. Hermetical seals were designed in World War I and, on the Italian front, Morelli used his occlusive rubber cuffs on tubes permitting suction drainage as well as closure of the defect."

". . . it may be of interest to review some of the circumstances that attended World War I and surrounded the task of the Empyema Commission of 1918."

"A beginning may be made in 1914, three years before the United States entered the War. At that time a fairly complete concept of the aerodynamics of pulmonary ventilation had been established; methods to maintain adequate ventilation during open chest operations had been devised, and techniques for applying these methods had been perfected. It was well into 1916 before the treatment of gunshot wounds of the chest by open operation in the combat zone had been undertaken except in the German army. Both French and British surgeons were submerged by an overwhelming load of casualties and preoccupied with the task of learning by bitter experience the surgical principles that must guide the management of flesh wounds from high-velocity missiles and high-explosive shell fragments."

"Then the Parisian surgeon, Pierre Duval, spearheaded what appeared to be a breakthrough on the surgical front":

> Surgery of the lung has undergone complete revolution in the war. The lung is no longer an organ inaccessible to the surgeon. One can open the chest widely, expose the lung, lobe by lobe, manipulate it, resect it, suture it, and treat it as one would a coil of intestine in a laparotomy. Surgery of the lung does not require any of those pressure chambers which the genius of the Germans invented and their persuasion made us think necessary.

"It is only fair to point out that Pierre Duval's claims were not widely accepted in France, where Grégoire and Courcoux maintained a far more conservative position. British surgeons were also skeptical although Moynihan and Gask were swept along on the tide of enthusiasm. H. Morriston Davies with his scholarly interest in thoracic physiology held to sound concepts, as did William Hutchinson of the Canadian army."

"The rash claims of Duval and his disciples and their scorn of differential pressure had more repercussions in the United States than in the theater of war. In the general exuberance over all things French and the condemnation of all things German, the fact was forgotten that scientific concepts recognize no national boundaries. Lord Moynihan, then Sir Berkeley, Colonel in the R.A.M.C., informed audiences in the United States that a surgeon might attack the lungs boldly, without heed to the danger of an open pneumothorax. Following the pattern of the triumphal tours of the victorious generals, Duval appeared before professional groups in the United States in the autumn of 1918...."

"And so patriotic fervor once again was to solve both horns of the old dilemma of John of Vigo and Paré."

"In reflecting upon the narrative of the experience of wound surgeons in the 1914-1918 War as compared with that of surgeons in previous and subsequent wars, I have become increasingly convinced that the outstanding feature of this period was the prevalence of hemolytic streptococcus infection both in Europe and in the United States. This epidemic assumed pandemic proportions when the hemolytic streptococcus rode the coattails of the influenza virus which swept around the world. For over a decade after the end of the war the hemolytic streptococcus haunted the surgical wards of our civilian hospitals and made return visits, particularly during the winter months. Those of us studying surgery during this period were weaned on the surgery of acute tenosynovitis, mastoiditis, primary streptococcal peritonitis, erysipelas, and the catastrophic infections of supposedly aseptic operative fields with this organism. The streptococcal pneumonia and empyema which accompanied the influenza epidemic of 1918 was a new disease to a generation of doctors. They had no precedents which defined it. In the past three decades, as far as my own experience is concerned, the disease is, for all practical purposes, extinct. During the 1914-1918 War, however, it gave rise to the Empyema Commission, which in the minds of thoracic surgeons is identified with Dr. Evarts Graham."

"Following the entrance of the United States into World War I, Dr. Graham was on duty as a captain in the Medical Corps assigned to take a course in neurosurgery in Chicago when he was visited by Dr. Allen Kanavel who was on duty as a consultant in the Office of the Surgeon General of the Army. Kanavel told Graham that there was growing apprehension about difficulties ahead with empyema as the country was then in the first year of an influenza epidemic which would undoubtedly increase in severity—would he be interested in working on the problem? Graham knew little or nothing about chest surgery at that time but was interested in nitrogen loss from massive exudation and had been selected because of this interest and his chemical training. Shortly after Kanavel's visit, Graham received orders to Camp Lee, there to team up with Dunham, who was working on the bacteriology of the disease. Graham and Dunham were joined by Captain Bell, a chemist of the Sanitary Corps who died a few years after the war. These three formed the hard nucleus of what became known as the Empyema Commission. With the help of Kanavel, a questionnaire was issued to camp hospitals and it was found that the average mortality rates attributed to streptococcal empyema were running approximately 30 per cent. The surgical staffs of the camp hospitals were stubbornly antagonistic to members of the Commission, whom they regarded as 'snoopers' from the Office of the Surgeon General. Opportunities for observation, however, could not be denied and disclosed that cyanotic patients, with pulmonary reserves crippled by massive and oftentimes bilateral bronchopneumonia, were being hurried to an operating room as soon as thoracentesis yielded fluid containing chains of streptococci. The operation was rib resection with open tube drainage. Death occurred quite regularly about a half an hour after the operation."

"It will be recalled that Sir Berkeley Moynihan had in the autumn of 1917 delivered the address in which he repeated the claims of Duval that the chest cavity could be opened as readily as the abdomen. When Graham, during his visits to Army camp hospitals, expressed apprehension about the open pneumothorax which attended rib resection for empyema he was asked who he thought he was to contradict the great Moynihan. When Graham cited an actual case in which a cyanotic and dyspneic soldier had died on the operating table that very morning and asked if the open pneumothorax might not have been a contributing factor, the reply was: 'No, he died because we didn't operate soon enough.'"

"Early evacuation of streptococcal pus was taught as a dogma of the surgery of the period; tendon sheaths were opened on the least suspicion of infection and oftentimes a spreading streptococcal cellulitis was slashed with multiple incisions long before fixation abscesses appeared. Graham was certain that the open pneumothorax was a factor in the deaths from empyema but at that time was not familiar with the literature on open pneumothorax, nor did he have sufficient observation or experiments to prove his point."

"In 1890, Bülau had advocated drainage of empyema by the 'closed' catheter technique, and the relative merits of closed drainage and open drainage by rib resection had been widely discussed in German-speaking countries. Emphasis, however, had been placed on the prevention of retraction of the lung and the quick healing which might be obtained, not on the immediate hazards of open pneumothorax nor on the reduction of functional lung volume to a point below tidal air requirements merely by the admission of air to the pleural space.

"In December, 1918, Evarts Graham wrote":

> During the past year the idea has become prevalent in this country that operations upon the thorax which permit of the free entrance and exit of air into the pleural cavity during the operation can be performed with about the same impunity as abdominal operations. In fact, the belief has arisen that surgeons at the front have found that alterations of the intrathoracic pressure by the admission of air through extensive incisions or large gaping wounds are in themselves not dangerous, and a feeling of optimism exists that now bold surgical intervention on the thorax may be carried out. It has been said consequently that the danger from creating an open pneumothorax in early operations for empyema with permanent drainage is negligible.

"Despite the developments and inventions and increased understanding of three and a half centuries, the Army surgeons of 1918 were caught off balance when confronted by the old dilemma of Pare. The same problem presented itself in a slightly different form: whether to accept an open pneumothorax with the danger that the vital spirits would depart and vanish or to strive for a closed chest cavity with its hazards of infection and increasing encroachment on pulmonary ventilation by fluid and air in the pleural space. The problem was solved in the same ways that were devised by those who followed Paré—the insertion of a catheter and evacuation of the pleural cavity by 'closed drainage' (Bülau); or repeated aspiration with needle and syringe until pleural adhesions localized an abscess that could be drained by rib resection without retraction of the lung. In the words of Guthrie, the first object became that of saving life; after that, if time were given, the next was to relieve the loaded cavity."

"This display of ignorance of the principles that form the foundation of thoracic surgery annoyed and dismayed the few surgeons in this country who were familiar with the progress which had been made in Germany prior to the 1914-1918 War. In his Presidential Address of 1922, Samuel Robinson spoke scornfully of those who would apply their war experience to that bugaboo of civilian surgery—bronchiectasis."

> It has always been my belief that the greatest triumph in thoracic surgery will be the surgical eradication of this deplorable disease. The enthusiast returns from the war who has often dragged a lung lobe into a spread thoracic wound, opened it, scraped it, washed it—yea, even removed it—and concluded, therefrom, that intrathoracic surgery is freed of its supposed dangers, and that the possibilities therein are comparable to those in the abdomen. Let him attempt the same performance in his home hospital in a case of lower lobe bronchiectasis. Then will he learn what real thoracic pathology means.

"There follows a vivid word picture of the surgical undertaking of lobectomy which ends abruptly with the ominous and cryptic statement: 'Suddenly, it is obviously time to return the patient to his bed. Not much has been accomplished.'"

"Samuel Robinson, an advocate of *überdruck*, had introduced the positive pressure cabinet for thoracic operations . . . in 1909. Dr. Willy Meyer worked with a chamber at the German Hospital in New York City in the same year. This universal chamber combined the principles of *überdruck* and *unterdruck* and allowed for a wide range of pressure conditions. Both Robinson and Meyer were scholars of the surgical literature and both were in close touch with the progress in Germany."

Carl A. Beyer, Jeffrey D. McNeil, and R. Stephen Smith

In Appendix B, Churchill includes two separate manuscripts addressing chest injury, a topic of particular interest to him since thoracic surgery was his primary civilian academic pursuit. The first article is a report on the management of chest wounds during the Italian campaign of World War II (WWII), which he wrote as the immediate past president of the American Association for Thoracic Surgery for presentation at the 1944 annual meeting. The second half of the appendix contains the edited transcript of a lecture Churchill delivered on multiple occasions, discussing the historical progression of treatment for penetrating thoracic trauma. Both manuscripts highlight the importance of decision-making and the timing of interventions to maximize success in patients with chest injuries.

The modern reader will recognize many parallels between the descriptions in the report from the Mediterranean Theater and the current management of thoracic trauma. Like the recent civilian multicenter studies and the military experience during the Global War on Terror, Churchill describes managing most chest injuries without surgery and reserves operation for patients with ongoing hemorrhage, severe shock, sucking chest wounds, and thoracoabdominal injury. Additionally, he emphasizes immediate bronchoscopy for airway clearance and endorses enthusiasm for intercostal nerve block to improve pulmonary toilet. Although he does not use the phrase "multimodal analgesia" from our contemporary jargon, the concept of adequate pain control and clearance of pulmonary secretions to prevent infectious complications is recognized as important. However, most of the manuscript discusses patient selection and timing for more ambiguous scenarios, including surgery via the tract of the traumatic wound and decortication for residual hemothorax. While modern surgeons are unlikely to explore an injury via the missile tract, and current retained hemothorax guidelines recommend much earlier thoracoscopic intervention than the "early" decortication at three to six weeks that Churchill describes, patient selection remains an ongoing topic of intense scrutiny for procedures related to chest trauma, such as resuscitative thoracotomy and surgical stabilization of rib fractures.

The second half of the appendix presents excerpts from Churchill's lecture on the treatment of chest wounds, delivered in final form in

New York on November 8, 1957. He traces a dilemma between open and closed management of wounds back to the first recorded care for thoracic firearm injuries by John of Vigo. The wound dilemma was initially understood as the choice between allowing cold air to penetrate to the heart, to the detriment of the "vital spirits," when left open, and the inability to evacuate blood with subsequent putrefaction when closed. Churchill then weaves this tale of patient selection for appropriate intervention on chest wounds from Paré to streptococcal empyema in the camp hospitals of WWI. While we now have a much better understanding of the pathophysiology of open pneumothorax and when "open" chest drainage, such as an Eloesser thoracostomy, can be utilized successfully, the dilemma of patient selection for retained hemothorax evacuation continues in our modern times, between thoracoscopic evacuation and thrombolytic therapy for those unable to tolerate an operation.

While this appendix focuses on the treatment of chest injuries from 1514 through WWII, the lessons from Churchill remain prescient today. Avoiding blind adherence to dogma, collecting observations of actual practice with outcomes, and analyzing the data to understand which patients will derive benefit from a particular procedure after injury are crucial. As technology advances, each new technique or piece of equipment must be evaluated within this framework. Much work remains for military and civilian surgeons to clarify the optimal implementation of resuscitative thoracotomy, pleural lavage, and other adjuncts to tube thoracostomy, the surgical stabilization of rib fractures, and early thoracoscopic surgery in the management of thoracic trauma. As Churchill describes in this appendix, a procedure "properly employed, may save life as well as prevent infection … improperly employed, it may endanger life and delay the time when the patient is transportable to the rear."

SUGGESTED READINGS

Beyer CA, Byrne JP, Moore SA, et al, EAST Multicenter Hemothorax Study Group. Predictors of initial management failure in traumatic hemothorax: a prospective multicenter cohort analysis. *Surgery.* 2023; 174(4):1063-1070.

Ivey KM, White CE, Wallum TE. Thoracic injuries in US combat casualties: a 10-year review of operation enduring freedom and Iraqi freedom. *J Trauma Acute Care Surg.* 2012 Dec;73 (6 Suppl 5):S514-9.

Joint Trauma System. *Wartime Thoracic Injury Clinical Practice Guideline* (CPG ID: 74). 2018. https://jts.health.mil/index.cfm/PI_CPGs/cpgs

Smith RS. Thoracic trauma and injuries to the diaphragm. *Fischer's Mastery of Surgery,* 8th Edition, Upchurch GR, Ellison EC, Eds. Walters Kluwer, Philadelphia, 2023.

Patel NJ, Dultz L, Ladhani HA, Cullinane DC, Klein E, McNickle AG, Bugaev N, Fraser DR, Kartiko S, Dodgion C, Pappas PA, Kim D, Cantrell S, Como JJ, Kasotakis G. Management of simple and retained hemothorax: a practice management guideline from the Eastern Association for the Surgery of Trauma. *Am J Surg.* 2021; 221(5):873-884.

APPENDIX C

Surgery of the Bowel

THE NORTH AFRICAN-Mediterranean Theater boasted of having two affiliated general hospitals from New Orleans—the 6th General Hospital from Louisiana State and the 24th General Hospital from Tulane. Dr. Munro Gage had organized the Tulane group. Dr. Frank Lahey called Munro Gage on the telephone and Bentley Colcock was added to the roster. At this time there was a conflict in ideas with respect to surgical procedures on the large bowel between Dr. Lahey and General Rankin. Ben Colcock contributed materially to the surgery of the large bowel by bringing the basic principles of Dr. Lahey to the theater.

The 24th General Hospital, set up for the first time in Bizerte, had Colonel Royles as its Commanding Officer and Frank Cox as its Chief of Surgery.

NOTES ON SURGERY OF THE BOWEL
By Bentley Colcock

North Africa

It was night, and the tiny electric bulb barely lighted the small plastered room which was part of the Commanding Officer's quarters. The several tired medical officers sat down on whatever chairs and boxes that were available. Their mind was on their visitor—the Surgical Consultant for the North African-Mediterranean Theater. Elsewhere a surgical consultant, on his infrequent visits, had told them all the things that were wrong with the hospital and their work. He told them so in a loud voice and he had no time to listen to explanations. They knew that many things they did were not according to War Department policy, but War Department policy, frequently, just didn't work under actual field conditions. They were new to this business (and so was he) and they knew it. After all, it was a new war. This was North Africa in 1943.

Nothing in the books that were available had much bearing on what they were faced with from day to day.

In a quiet voice, the visiting colonel turned to the head of the Orthopedic Section on his left, and said: "What are your problems?" So it went, from one man to the next, till each had a chance to voice his frustrations and to report his few successes. The major in charge of abdominal surgery was enthusiastic about the policy of exteriorizing all wounds of the colon, but all too often the colostomies that had been done, retracted. This had led to wound sepsis, dehiscence and abdominal abscesses. With each man in turn, the consultant would listen until he was finished, ask for his suggestions, and then discuss the problem until there was agreement. When the meeting broke up late that evening, each officer went back to his work with more peace of mind than he had known for many weeks.

Many surgeons still feel that exteriorization of the injured bowel is an excellent way to treat a lacerated wound of the colon even in peacetime. There was no doubt of it in North Africa, in 1943. For a soldier who had sustained such a wound, and had lain on a hillside for four to six hours, it was the only procedure which gave him a reasonable chance to survive. The principle was simple, but except for a few surgeons who had had experience with the Mikulicz procedure in treating cancer of the colon, the execution was not always simple. If the bowel was exteriorized under tension, it inevitably retracted and led to further complications. The opposite could occur if there was a redundant mesentery as in the transverse colon—the colostomy often prolapsed. If a Mikulicz's spur was constructed, the partition between the two could be divided with the clamp and the colostomy closed by an extraperitoneal procedure. All too often, however, the two limbs were not approximated and sometimes were widely divergent. To clamp such a spur was to risk injury to an interposed loop of small bowel.

The need for fighting troops was great in the theater early in 1943, and the surgeons began to close colostomies either by careful obliteration of the spur or by an end-to-end anastomosis. Until they were ready to go back to the line, these troops helped guard the many thousands of German prisoners taken on Cape Bon. Later, some of the men were casualties for the second time in Italy. The surgeons learned the hard way. They learned by experience. They learned how to treat shock before operating. They also learned that if shock did not respond to treatment, the intra-abdominal bleeding would have to be controlled without further delay. If there were eight or ten perforations in a localized

(*continued*)

segment of bowel, they learned not to laboriously close one after the other but to resect that segment and do an end-to-end anastomosis. They learned to look for small penetrating wounds in the back or flank, whenever there were signs of peritonitis, but no visible wound on the abdomen. They learned to look carefully along the lateral border of the second portion of the duodenum for a small brown stain or ecchymosis. If a wound of the flank or back had penetrated the retroperitoneal surface of the duodenum, it would lead to retroperitoneal sepsis and probably death, if it were not found and closed. One might roughly plot the course of a bullet or shell fragment by the wound of entrance and exit. But nothing short of a painstaking check of all of the abdominal viscera would prevent a tragic mistake. It was that one small hole in the small bowel or colon which had been overlooked that led to the death of the patient. A transverse incision might be fine for a laparotomy in peacetime. It was no good in this situation. They learned to exteriorize segments of colon which were ecchymotic but not penetrated. Three days later it was obvious that this area in the bowel wall was nonviable. How close they had come to leaving that segment inside the abdomen!

Complications not serious in themselves were often important because they could greatly delay a soldier's return to duty. Early in the war, excision of the coccyx was part of the recommended treatment for a perforating wound of the rectum. A persistent draining sinus from osteomyelitis of the tip of the sacrum occurred frequently. It was found that good drainage of the peri-rectal space could usually be obtained by incision the deep fascia. If it was necessary to remove the coccyx, it was better carefully to disarticulate it. They learned by experience—but they learned well. With no antibiotics and faced with fecal contamination in every patient with a perforating wound of the bowel—they fell back on fundamental surgical principles.

It is of interest to note that today—many years later—in spite of all our antibiotics, colon surgeons are warning that there is no substitute for adequate drainage — when indicated.

Slowly, but steadily, the mortality rate and the morbidity rate for battle casualties in the North African Theater improved.

Italy

It was late afternoon and the surgeon looked tired. He had operated upon a good many casualties during the last few weeks and this one had been a long, tedious job. He barely grunted when the nurse introduced the visitor to him. The shell fragments had produced multiple long lacerating wounds of the cecum and ascending colon. There had been no possibility of saving this segment of bowel and he had resected it. There had been a large amount of fecal contamination in the abdomen and the ecchymoses and hematomas in the mesentery had made control of the mesenteric vessels difficult. He was almost through his anastomosis of the ileum to the transverse colon, but this too, had not been easy. After all, most of his training before the war had been in obstetrics and gynecology. The worst of it was, the soldier also had a compound fracture of the femur which still had to be taken care of. The anesthetist leaned over to the visitor and whispered, "This boy isn't so good." He speeded up the transfusion.

Extensive wounds of the colon—particularly the right colon—were still a problem in 1944. They did not lend themselves to exteriorization except by creation of a complete small bowel fistula. All too often, the patient failed to survive resection of the bowel plus the anastomosis. Even if he lived through the procedure, the severe peritonitis from diffuse contamination of the peritoneal cavity often resulted in a fatality. Leakage occurred in spite of extreme care in suturing the bowel. These Mediterranean surgeons knew from experience that few patients would survive if there was continued soiling of the peritoneal cavity. One might close a dozen perforations, but if just one closure leaked, the patient usually died. The anastomosis could be avoided by resecting colon and exteriorizing both the terminal ileum and the transverse colon. However, the problems associated with an ileostomy were formidable. The rapid loss of fluid and electrolytes could lead to an irreversible situation unless they were promptly and accurately replaced. This was difficult to do in a field hospital. It became almost impossible during periods of evacuation. These patients required a tremendous amount of nursing care. If there were many casualties, it was sometimes not available.

The Mikulicz procedure for the resection of cancer of the colon had been modified to fit carcinoma arising into the cecum and ascending colon. A double barrel spur was constructed of the terminal ileum and the proximal transverse colon following resection of the tumor. This resulted in an ileostomy, it is true, but the construction of the spur enabled the ileostomy to be well fixed in position by the colon. With clamping of the spur (within a week or ten days) the fluid and electrolyte losses were sharply cut down. Later, the ileocolostomy stoma was closed by an extra-peritoneal procedure. *This operation could be used for the battle casualty with a destruction wound of the cecum and ascending colon.*

(*continued*)

The operating time would be reduced, and the danger of an intraperitoneal suture line in a patient with generalized peritonitis was eliminated.

The Surgical Consultant knew this suggestion was contrary to War Department policy, and probably would be rejected. But he also knew his surgeons since the early days in North Africa—and he kept a light hand on the reins. He read the recommendation—listened to its author patiently, and sent it to the Surgeon General's Office with the comment: "The writer defends his position vigorously and I am passing it along for further consideration". His intuition was correct. General Rankin read the paper and tossed it back to his aide, with the words, "This won't work. Doesn't the man who wrote this know that you can't clamp the colon and the small bowel together?" He fully appreciated, however, that something must be done about the high mortality rate associated with resection and anastomosis in these patients. The War Department policy was changed; from now on when the right colon had to be resected, the terminal ileum would be exteriorized in the right lower quadrant, and the transverse colon exteriorized in the left upper quadrant.

As had been suspected, this was not a happy solution. The intraperitoneal suture line was eliminated, but several other serious problems took its place. The transportation of the patient and the correction of the fluid and electrolyte loss in these patients with an ileostomy, was indeed difficult. Fixation of the mobile terminal ileum to avoid prolapse or retraction was a major problem—particularly in the presence of peritonitis.

There was however, a silver lining to this cloud. The GI's who fought and were wounded in Italy, were cared for by surgeons who had "come of age" in North Africa. Above all, at the top, they had the same quiet, confident Army officer as Chief Surgical Consultant. By repeated visits to every hospital, large or small in this theater, he knew his men and he knew what they could do. Because of this, many a soldier went up the gangplank carrying his own luggage and headed for home six to eight weeks following a Mikulicz resection of a lacerated right colon. With a well-healed incision he would require no nursing care on his way home. He was eating well, his strength was coming back and if there had been the same urgent need for manpower as there had been in North Africa, he could have gone back to duty.

In spite of the fact, that most of them had been overseas for one to two years or more, the morale of the surgeons working in the Mediterranean Theater was excellent. After many long hours spent at the operating table, both in Africa and Italy, they had learned a great deal about the treatment of battle wounds, including those of the small and large bowel. They had learned something more, even more precious than surgical skill, something that only comes with experience. They had learned good surgical judgment. The small perforating wound of the anterior wall of the colon was not always exteriorized. It frequently was sutured securely and the abdomen closed. A proximal colostomy was not always done for a small perforating wound of the rectum, which could be closed securely and well drained. The patients did well. These cases were carefully selected and it was good surgery.

In Florence, a unique situation developed. During the unsuccessful assault on the Gothic line in the autumn of 1944, many times the expected number of casualties occurred. The great majority of the wounded came down Highway 65 into Florence. A 1,500-bed general hospital which was located along the Arno River just outside the city received a large number of patients—some right from the battlefield.

At one period they had over 3,000 patients. By grouping casualties with wounds of the extremity in one section of the hospital, chest wounds in another, one 65-bed ward soon became completely filled with one type of patient. Every man in it had a penetrating wound of the abdomen. As soon as a patient was well enough to be sent along to Leghorn, another patient with an abdominal injury took his place. The majority of these patients had perforating wounds of the bowel. Rank was ignored. One bed might have a private or a corporal, the next bed a lieutenant colonel. The officer's ward was in another building 100 yards away but it was impossible to give officers the type of care they needed except by grouping them with other ranks. Throughout the three to four months' period when this ward remained filled, no officer was heard to complain because he was next to an enlisted soldier. Although some of the patients were admitted from the battlefield, the majority had had a laparotomy carried out at a field or evacuation hospital stationed in the hills above Florence. It was a rare day that the officer in charge of this ward, did not have the pleasure of making ward rounds with one or more surgeons from these field units. Thus, the operation surgeon learned which of his patients had developed abscesses and where they occurred. He found which wounds had dehisced and which had held. The surgeon doing the secondary surgery in Florence, received a firsthand account of the operative findings at the time of initial surgery. The close coordination of the surgical treatment, the devoted care of superb experienced nurses, and the morale of the sick patients in that ward,

(*continued*)

will remain an unforgettable experience for everyone connected with it. Many an abscess was drained, a fecal fistula resected, and a colostomy closed with one assistant—a tall, slender, dark-eyed nurse from the bayous of Louisiana, who had never cut a suture until she reached North Africa. The coffee pot at the end of the large operating room was never empty. The coffee was strong and it needed to be. If you could not drink it that strong liquid steam could be added from the nearby sterilizer. But it wasn't coffee that kept these nurses and corpsmen going until the surgeon ordered them to quit. It was "esprit de corps." Is it any wonder that ever after—they all just felt a little bit "different"?

It is quite possible that the treatment of abdominal injuries in wartime, including perforating wounds of the bowel, reached a height in Italy that was not surpassed during World War II. Many an American GI owes his life to the concentrated effort of a well-trained experienced surgeon, nurse and anesthetist, working over him all day and all night. It is a tribute to the U.S. Army Medical Corps that such care was made possible. In the German army, at that time in Italy, a soldier with an injury severe enough to make it obvious that he would never return to duty, even if he survived—often received no treatment at all. It has been said that in surgery there is no substitute for experience. To a large extent, this is true. Much of the splendid record compiled by surgeons working in Italy was attributable to the experience gained in the early days in North Africa. Like other troops, the Medical Corps was well fed, and wherever possible was well housed. This, however, could not account for the dedication to their work which was characteristic of almost every surgeon in the Mediterranean theater. He knew our problems and he knew his men. He never allowed them to be hamstrung by rules and regulations. They were encouraged to think. If it would help the patient, and it was based on sound principles, they would not be criticized for trying. They took pride in their work. They knew their surgical colleagues were "the pick of the crop." Most important of all, they took pride in their chief—the senior Surgical Consultant of the North African-Mediterranean Theater, Colonel Edward D. Churchill. Without him, they would have been a group of highly-trained temperamental individualists—the ""prima donnas" of the U.S. Army Medical Corps. With him they became a close-knit band of dedicated surgeons, inspired by the conviction that they were providing the finest surgical care the American soldier had ever received.

B. C.

COLOSTOMY DISCUSSION

This is from my diary:

E.D.C. Comments: November 1, 1944, I drove from Rome to Florence on Highway 2, a spectacular drive. After checking in at Fifth Army Rear I went directly to the 24th General Hospital. They had a tough time clearing the grounds of mines and booby traps and there are still sections taped off so it is necessary to stick to the paths.

I made rounds with Ben Colcock and discussed colostomies. He has had 50 cases of which 8 had the colostomy below the skin level. Four of these were the spur type, 3 were loop and 1 an exteriorized cecum. Five of the 50 cases were complicated by bladder wounds but 3 have healed both the fistula and the cystostomy. About half of the rectal wounds have coccygectomy, whereas last winter nearly all cases had the coccyx removed.

Ben feels very strongly that all colostomies should be done with spur construction and that the coccyx should never be resected. I still believe that the forward surgeon should be left free to do loop colostomies when desired—that one should not mix in too many considerations of reconstruction with what is primarily a life-saving emergency operation.

Ben and I agree that adequate mobilization of the large bowel and the selection of the site for exteriorization are more important than the type of colostomy performed. So far as resection of the coccyx is concerned, of course the pararectal space can be drained without excision of the coccyx, but here again, in dealing with surgeons who have not done peroneal resections, inadequate incision of the fascia propria may mean fatal retroperitoneal cellulitis. I do not want to forbid resection of the coccyx if a surgeon thinks he needs to in order to gain exposure.

It is important to close colostomies in the overseas theater. Transport can then be more completely ambulatory with use of latrines and improvement of morale. Also, the occurrence of fecal impaction on a long trip is avoided.

The colostomy question has caused a great deal of discussion and I am convinced that young American surgeons have had inadequate training in the principles of large bowel surgery. It was difficult to get them to accept exteriorization of large bowel wounds and colostomy for rectal perforations. Now it is difficult to get them done properly. The basic fault is a failure to mobilize the bowel by adequate division of the lateral peritoneal attachments.

Many of Colcock's abdominal cases showed vitamin deficiencies— rarely seen in other wounds even when complicated by sepsis.

Gary Alan Bass, Jeffrey D. Kerby, and Christopher J. Burns

Opening this section, Dr Churchill describes a tense conference call, hinting at how ingrained institutional practice patterns (anchored in elective civilian practice) could give rise to controversy between new colleagues thrust together in theater. The topic of disagreement was the optimal approach to the surgical management of penetrating intestinal injuries—centering on the thorny questions of resection, repair, and subsequent management. Dr Churchill, who shadowed Dr Bentley Colcock in the North African Theater, reproduces Dr Colcock's contemporaneous thoughts on this topic, documenting his observations in parallel.

Surveying his team of surgeons, Dr Colcock recognized their frustration that *"Nothing in the books that were available had much bearing on what they were faced with from day to day."* Specifically, he noted that the then-common practice of exteriorizing the injured colon wound onto the abdominal wall (as a repair in continuity or a trephined colostomy) was associated with surgical site infection, fascial dehiscence, and intra-abdominal sepsis. Recognizing this, some surgeons managing right-sided colon injuries opted for separate ileal and colonic ostomies placed on opposite sides of the abdomen. Deviating from War Department policy, Dr Colcock advocated instead for the use of the Paul-Mikulitz ileocolostomy procedure; superior outcomes in his patients were observed by Dr Churchill during ward rounds.

Modern trauma surgeons still grapple with decision-making around the management of destructive penetrating colonic injuries. Following resection or repair, the decision to restore bowel continuity should incorporate patient factors, intraoperative factors, and surgeon preference. Care advances that have improved outcomes in the interval since the book's first edition include hemostatic resuscitation and damage-control laparotomy, coupled with intensive care unit management aimed to repair deranged physiology through resuscitation, optimization, stabilization, and de-resuscitation (ROSE) phases. Cognizant that the art of surgery has been passed down through an apprenticeship model since antiquity, we must recognize that we are a product of our trainers, our colleagues, and our training experiences. Thus, we all hold biases anchored in that training that shape our practice and how we digest the evidence-base presented in the surgical literature. Indeed, we are often beholden to the comfortable college of our peers, found in medical professional societies, to provide the context and rationale in which we exercise surgical decision-making.

A synthesis of retrospective data in adult civilian patients with penetrating colonic trauma, and without signs of shock, hemorrhage, severe contamination, or delay to surgical intervention, led the Eastern Association for the Surgery of Trauma (EAST) to recommend that colon repair or resection and anastomosis be performed rather than colostomy, citing a high incidence of colostomy complications and a low rate of subsequent reversal. For high-risk civilian patients, including those receiving damage-control laparotomy, EAST conditionally recommends colon repair or anastomosis, while mandating colostomy for the most severe injuries. Injury patterns seen in modern urban warfare have changed from Churchill's time to include penetrating multifocal injury from mines, improvised explosive devices, and suicide drones. The polytraumatized battle casualty is likely best served by surgical options that are both time-efficient and mitigate risk effectively.

Framing this section in the context of inter-surgeon discourse and clinical cases, Dr Churchill describes the heterogeneity of surgical approaches to penetrating injuries and pelvic sepsis. These conversations remain salient today in civilian and military trauma surgery, where numerous approaches still permeate practice. Now, as then, the surgeon faced with these injuries ought to adapt as expansive and thoughtful an approach as Dr Churchill.

SUGGESTED READINGS

Cullinane DC, Jawa RS, Como JJ, Moore AE, et al. Management of penetrating intraperitoneal colon injuries: a meta-analysis and practice management guideline from the Eastern Association for the Surgery of Trauma. *J Trauma Acute Care Surg.* 2019 Mar;86(3):505-515.

McGuire R, Hepper A, Harrison K. From Northern Ireland to Afghanistan: half a century of blast injuries. *J R Army Med Corps.* 2019 Feb;165(1):27-32.

Ruscelli Paolo P, Georgi T, Renata P, et al. Modified Paul-Mikulicz jejunostomy in frail geriatric patients undergoing emergency small bowel resection. *Minerva Chir.* 2018;74:121-125.

Steele SR, Wolcott KE, Mullenix PS, et al. Colon and rectal injuries during Operation Iraqi Freedom: are there any changing trends in management or outcome? *Dis Colon Rectum.* 2007 Jun;50(6):870-877.

APPENDIX D

Thoracoabdominal Wounds

A TRANSDIAPHRAGMATIC approach that gave access to both major body cavities was not new in World War II, but came into widespread use for the first time. A brief excerpt from the 1945 history of the Fifth Army Medical Service (page 128) follows:

Thoracoabdominal wounds were discussed in some detail in last year's history. The development of surgery for these wounds in army hospitals has been a definite advance and contribution. At the beginning of the campaign it was the general opinion that the transdiaphragmatic approach to the abdominal part of the thoracoabdominal wounds might be desirable in some few cases . . . At the end of the campaign it was the opinion of most of the surgeons in Fifth Army hospitals that thoracotomy with transdiaphragmatic repair of all accessible abdominal wounds was definitely the procedure of choice, and that in those few cases in which laparotomy was essential because of wounds which could not be repaired transdiaphragmatically, that the thoracotomy should be done, the wounds in the left upper abdominal quadrant and other easily accessible areas dealt with, the diaphragm properly repaired, necessary intrathoracic surgery accomplished, the lung fully inflated, and the chest wall tightly closed before proceeding with the laparotomy. These general principles apply to wounds of the right diaphragm as well as to the left. The extent of the surgery possible in the right upper abdominal quadrant is, of course, much less than on the left side.

Thoracoabdominal Wounds
COMMENTARY

Omar A. Rokayak, Joseph J. DuBose, and Ernest E. Moore

In this section, Churchill describes thoracotomy with transdiaphragmatic exploration as the "procedure of choice" for thoracoabdominal wounds and hails upper quadrant intra-abdominal injury management through a primary thoracotomy incision as a "definite advance and contribution." In patients with inadequate visualization of injured intra-abdominal structures, he recommends completing all intrathoracic interventions including chest closure before proceeding with laparotomy.

In the modern era, we advise a completely different approach for thoracoabdominal wounds. Portable imaging, including focused assessment with sonography in trauma (FAST) and extended FAST (e-FAST), is now available to even the smallest and furthest forward surgical teams for triaging and managing multicavity injuries. Thus, the adjuncts to determine the operative approach to penetrating thoracoabdominal wounds include (1) plain radiographs to ascertain missile or fragment trajectory, (2) e-FAST to identify pericardial or intra-abdominal blood, and (3) tube thoracostomy to quantify intrathoracic bleeding or ongoing air leak. In rare instances without radiographs, the physical exam may provide clues as to the trajectory, although isolated or an odd number of wounds are both problematic. Tube thoracostomy is performed on the side of wounds penetrating the thorax simultaneous with e-FAST. The decision to explore the chest or abdomen first is then based on the collective information from these adjuncts. In general, the priorities are *thoracotomy* for pericardial blood or major ongoing blood or air from the chest tube and *laparotomy* for blood in the abdomen. Although controversial, in some instances, proximal aortic control using resuscitative endovascular balloon occlusion of the aorta (REBOA) may obviate entry into the chest.

These modern advancements allow for tube thoracostomy and laparotomy as the initial approach in most cases. Laparotomy with transdiaphragmatic pericardial window is used in patients with suspected intra-abdominal injury and equivocal cardiac assessment where a positive pericardial window would drive a sternotomy to rapidly address any cardiac injuries. Finally, if a cardiac or major pulmonary/vascular injury is suspected within the chest based on perceived trajectory, demonstrated on e-FAST, or indicated by high chest tube output, thoracotomy followed by laparotomy (as indicated) is the favored approach.

Typically, a lateral thoracotomy is preferred over sternotomy because it provides better access to the pleural space and can be extended into a clamshell for posterior cardiac or subclavian injuries. In a situation with life-threatening injuries in both the chest and abdomen, a sternotomy extended into a long midline sterno-laparotomy incision provides optimal access to manage severe multicavity injuries.

Churchill's recommendation to complete intrathoracic interventions including repair of accessible intra-abdominal injuries transdiaphragmatically, repair of the diaphragm, and complete chest closure prior to proceeding with laparotomy is one of interesting, historical significance. This recommendation predates the formalized concepts of damage control surgery (DCS) and damage control resuscitation (DCR). Now, complete closure of the first cavity is rarely performed prior to exploring a second cavity in most patients with concomitant thoracic and intra-abdominal injuries. Instead, the primary cavity is typically temporarily closed or left open until definitive hemorrhage control is secured in all cavities. Temporary closure then facilitates reassessment of the previously explored cavities in a controlled manner at the next level of care in the evacuation chain.

These recommendations by Churchill should be understood in their proper historic context—with limited portable imaging for triage, no ultrasound capability, and no formal description of DCR or DCS. Current recommendations for the management of thoracoabdominal injuries represent a highly dynamic and tailorable approach depending on patient presentation, suspected injury patterns, and operational considerations.

SUGGESTED READINGS

Bailey JA, Mullenix PS, Antevil JL. Thoracic Approaches and Incisions. In: Martin MJ, Beekley AC, Eckert MJ. *Front Line Surgery: A Practical Approach.* Springer International Publishing AG; 2017.

Blackbourne LH, Cancio L, Cap A, et al. *First to Cut: Trauma Lessons Learned in the Combat Zone.* US Army Institute of Surgical Research; 2012.

Hirshberg A, Wall MJ Jr, Allen MK, Mattox KL. Double jeopardy: thoracoabdominal injuries requiring surgical intervention in both chest and abdomen. *J Trauma.* 1995 Aug;39(2):225-229; discussion 229-231.

Skubic JJ, Haider AH. Penetrating chest injury. In: Dimick JB, Upchurch GR, Sonnenday CJ, et al, eds. *Clinical Scenarios in Surgery: Decision Making and Operative Technique.* Wolters Kluwer; 2019.

Wall MJ, Ghanta RK, Mattox, KL. Heart and thoracic vessels. In: Feliciano DV, Mattox KL, Moore EE, eds. *Trauma.* 9th ed. McGraw Hill; 2021:599-628.

The Surgical Management of the Wounded in the Mediterranean Theater at the Time of the Fall of Rome*

I would remind you again how large and various was the experience of the battlefield, and how fertile the blood of warriors in rearing good surgeons.

T. CLIFFORD ALLBUTT

Foreword

BY

BRIG. GEN'L FRED W. RANKIN, M.C.
DIRECTOR, SURGERY DIVISION, U. S. ARMY

The present-day health standards of our troops and survival rate among our wounded have been unequalled in the history of warfare. Perhaps one of the most important factors contributing to this highly gratifying record has been the role played by the professional consultants whose functions may be broadly described as administrative, correlative, advisory, educational and analytical. Consultants in the major fields of endeavor have been attached to every Service Command in the Zone of Interior and to all active Theaters of Operations. Selected on the basis of their special training and extensive background and on their eminent qualifications, they have been able to perform an incalculably valuable function in promoting higher standards of medical practice in this war.

(continued)

---

*From Churchill ED. The surgical management of the wounded in the Mediterranean theater at the time of the fall of Rome—[Foreword by Brig. Gen'l Fred W. Rankin, M.C.]. *Ann Surg.* 1944;120(3):268-283.

453

As Surgical Consultant to the North African and Mediterranean Theater of Operations and representative of this group, Colonel Churchill has done more than improve the quality of surgery performed in this Theater. Uniquely equipped to perform his mission and imbued with the true scientific spirit, he early recognized the inadequacy of certain preformed concepts in the surgical management of the wounded. With this flexibility of mind and with an elastic organization, he has utilized an investigative approach and drawn upon battlefield experience to evolve more rational and effective methods in the surgical care of the wounded. In this article, he has epitomized these observations and principles which constitute not only a contribution to war surgery but also to the advancement of medical science.

WOUND MANAGEMENT may be divided into three phases—initial, reparative and reconstructive. The first two are concerns of an overseas theater. The latter is the mission of the Zone of the Interior.

Initial Surgery

The initial surgery of the forward area is primarily directed toward the preservation of life and limb. The immediate physiologic disturbances incident to blood loss and the wound itself are corrected by both resuscitative and surgical measures. Wound infection is prevented or controlled by surgery and chemotherapy.

Resuscitation from shock has two goals: first, to render the casualty transportable and preserve his life until a hospital can be reached; and second, to prepare the casualty to withstand lifesaving surgical procedures. Shock as observed in the forward area is caused by whole blood loss except in burns, crushing injuries or rapidly advancing infection. Plasma is used in the divisional area to prepare the wounded for transportation and keep them alive until they can reach a hospital. Whole blood would be preferable, but it is not practical to use transfusions within the divisional area.

Plasma alone is not adequate to prepare a seriously wounded casualty to withstand the surgical procedures that are essential, or to carry him through the critical postoperative period. After admission to hospital a limited amount is used to augment the effects of whole blood transfusion. Plasma is a substitute for whole blood only in the sense that it can be packaged and stored in adequate quantity in areas where blood cannot be obtained. Plasma is not a substitute for whole blood in the physiologic sense. For these reasons a Blood Transfusion Unit procures and processes whole blood in the base and distributes it to the Army installations.

Shipments of blood were made by LST to the Anzio beachhead in February. As the front advanced and forward landing strips were opened, blood has been shipped each day by plane. In approximately four months, over 16,000 pints of whole blood have been drawn and processed for delivery to the Fifth Army. The blood is drawn by vacuum into bottles that are used only once. Glucose is added to the citrate as a preservative. Each flask of blood is triply checked for type, examined by smear for malaria and Kahn-tested.

Although Type "O" blood is commonly referred to as "universal donor" blood, its use in large amounts in patients of other types is hazardous unless the agglutinin titer is low. Every bottle of blood is titered and only those with an agglutinin titer less than 1 to 64 are issued as "universal donor" blood. All banked blood carries an expiration date of seven days.

To augment the supply of blood forwarded from the base, evacuation hospitals maintain their own unit blood banks. Responsibility for the supply of type specific blood other than "O" rests upon the individual hospital.

The initial wound operation is directed toward the prevention of infection by a complete excision of tissue devitalized by the missile. Procedures such as closure of a sucking wound of the chest or suture of a perforation of a hollow viscus restore physiologic equilibrium as well as arrest the dangers of infection. Recognition of all devitalized tissue is oftentimes impossible, particularly in a massive wound or one complicated by skeletal injury. Disturbances of blood supply and subtle changes that indicate impending death of tissues may not be detectable. In a certain number of these cases mixed anaerobic infection of residual dead tissues is the inevitable sequela. Others will develop invasive infection spreading from the wound to involve normal tissues. To minimize the incidence and hazards of infection, primary closure by suture is strictly avoided. Exact maintenance of the reduction of fractures by precise methods is precluded by the necessity for evacuation to the rear, so temporary or transportation splinting, usually with plaster of paris, is employed.

Chemotherapy is initiated in the field by local and oral administration of sulfonamides. The value of this procedure is questioned by many surgeons of experience. Preoperative penicillin therapy is started on all but the lightly wounded casualties on admission to hospital in the forward area. At operation, topical application of penicillin is carried out only in wounds penetrating the meninges, serous cavities and joints. Parenteral administration is continued beyond the period of the likelihood of infection or until established infection has been controlled. No patient is held in the forward area solely for the purpose of continuing penicillin therapy.

Just as plasma is not a substitute for whole blood in resuscitation, neither are sulfonamides and penicillin substitutes for the surgical excision of devitalized tissue. Chemotherapeutic agents cannot sterilize dead, devitalized or avascular tissues nor do they prevent the septic decomposition of contaminated blood clot.

In this war there have been two quite different approaches to the application of chemotherapeutic agents to military surgery. The first would utilize these agents to permit delay in wound surgery, and minimize the completeness of the excision of dead tissue. The second employs chemotherapy to extend the scope of surgery and achieve a perfection in results previously considered impossible. The latter policy has guided the surgery of the Mediterranean Theater. To reiterate the axiom that penicillin is not a substitute for surgery is not enough. Every surgeon must learn that chemotherapy opens new and startling possibilities in wound management.

The magnitude of the surgical problems that confront the forward surgeons when supported by adequate resuscitation therapy is difficult to visualize by one not having a first-hand acquaintance with their work. Highest standards of precision must be maintained if the potentialities of surgery are to be realized to full advantage. This precision must be attained in the use of the adjuncts to surgery as well as in operative technics. Initial surgery cannot be carried on as a hasty, slap-dash and bloody spectacle, with rapid evacuation of the patient to the rear if satisfactory results are to be achieved. The average operating times for certain types of cases recorded at an evacuation hospital were: one hour 49 minutes for penetrating wounds of the head; two hours for wounds of the abdomen; two hours and a half for wounds of the thorax. Many casualties have multiple wounds that require several major procedures in sequence or simultaneously. Postoperative care is as important as the operation and may demand holding the patient for ten days or longer.

Triage at the divisional clearing station based on the urgency of the wound and the condition of the casualty establishes a "three-point forward system," as described by Jolly in the Spanish Civil War. This provides a small surgical hospital for first priority casualties—in this theater a single platoon of a field hospital reorganized and equipped for this specific mission. Other casualties of less urgent types are transferred back to the chain of Evacuation Hospitals. An important modification of the system has placed the Field Hospital Platoon in physical conjunction with the clearing station triage point. This provides for the immediate transfer of wounded from the clearing station to the first priority surgical hospital by hand litter. No pause is required for resuscitation or interference with splinting or dressings. Expert surgical management that embraces resuscitation, operation and prolonged postoperative care, becomes immediately available. Cases with a continuing source of shock that cannot be made transportable without an operation are thus salvaged and the desperately wounded receive expert care as far forward as it can be provided.

Surgeons assigned the responsibility of caring for the wounded in a first priority surgical hospital must be highly trained and experienced, as their tasks are the most exacting of military surgery. The Auxiliary Surgical Group has been found ideal as a source for this personnel. The experience of the individual surgeon is augmented in the base during periods of an inactive front. Unity and uniformity in the control of this portion of forward surgical personnel has produced a high level of competence as well as economy in the deployment of specialized surgical skill and talent. If the achievements of surgery in this theater are ever judged noteworthy, they are attributable to the fact that expert rather than inexperienced surgeons are doing the work. All other measures are ancillary items.

A well-run first priority surgical hospital exerts a remarkably favorable effect on the morale of combat troops and their officers. The divisional medical service receives a stimulus to maintain its arduous task by firsthand evidence that the lives of the most desperately wounded may be saved by skillful first-aid measures and rapid evacuation. Splinting is improved, the use of plasma in Aid Stations is increased and the temptation for clearing or collecting companies to indulge in heroic surgical procedures for which they were never designed or equipped is removed.

Evacuation hospitals handle the great bulk of the wounded in the forward area, as the small group of first priority cases diverted to the Field Hospital Platoon constitutes approximately one-thirteenth of the total number. These institutions, with trained and experienced professional staffs, have attained a high degree of proficiency in the procedures of initial wound management and remain the backbone of the Army medical service.

Reparative Surgery

A highly significant and far-reaching advance in military surgery has taken place in the base hospitals with the development of what may be called *reparative surgery*. Wounds left unsutured at the initial operation are routinely closed by suture, usually at the time of the first dressing. With the use of penicillin as a safeguard against infection, the management of wounds complicated by fracture or joint involvement has been revolutionized. Surgical procedures in special fields of surgery—thoracic, craniocerebral, abdominal—have also been radically altered by the application of similar principles. The significance of this development and its effect on returning an increased number of wounded soldiers to duty and in preventing deformity, disability and death in the seriously wounded can hardly be overestimated.

Reparative surgery is not to be confused with the reconstructive surgery of the Zone of the Interior. Reparative surgery is designed to prevent or cut short wound infection either before it is established or at the period of its inception. Once established, wound infection is destructive of tissue and at times of life. In many instances it permanently precludes the restoration of function by the most skillful reconstructive efforts.

If the initial wound operation has been a complete one, wounds of the soft parts may be closed by suture on or after the fourth day. The dressing applied in the evacuation hospital is removed under aseptic precautions in an operating room of a general hospital at the base. Following closure, the part is immobilized preferably by a light plaster encasement, or if this is impractical, by bed rest.

Decision to close a wound by suture is based solely on an appraisal of the gross appearance at the time of removal of the dressing. Preliminary qualitative or quantitative bacteriologic analysis of the flora of the wound by smear or culture does not provide information pertinent to this decision or allow the prediction of the result. "Clean" wounds that heal by first intention after delayed closure may show a profuse and varied flora, both anaerobic and aerobic. Identification of species and tests for pathogenicity would require weeks of arduous laboratory procedure.

It is estimated that during the Italian Campaign alone, at least 25,000 soft-part wounds have been closed on the basis of gross appearance only. Healing has resulted in approximately 95 per cent, and no loss of life or limb or serious complications have been reported. Residual dead tissue in a deep recess of the wound is the most common cause of the failure in the 5 per cent that may be classed as unsuccessful closures. If the suture is not successful because of infection, appropriate studies and corrective therapy is instituted before resuture is attempted.

The presence of residual dead tissue or established invasive infection at the time of the first dressing is evidenced by discharge of pus and redness and edema of the wound margins. When these are present but minimal, the wound is allowed to "clean up" with moist dressings. Surgical excision of devitalized fragments or removal of retained foreign bodies may speed this process. Secondary closure may then be performed after a few days. If established infection is severe, or if the patient is toxic or anemic, a course of penicillin therapy and blood transfusions is instituted and followed by radical wound revision with staged closure.

The topical use of sulfonamides appears to contribute nothing to the favorable results of reparative wound surgery. Parallel series of closures show as satisfactory or better results without the topical application of sulfonamides at the time of suture, as with it. Penicillin therapy is entirely unnecessary as an adjunct to the usual reparative surgery of soft-part wounds. It is used parenterally for cases of established infection and in the reparative surgery of complicated wounds.

The reparative surgery of complicated wounds, including those with extensive muscle damage as well as those with skeletal or joint injury and penetration of the viscera, is a more major undertaking. It is in this group that both the incidence and hazards of infection may be expected to be greater. It is this group of cases that is kept on penicillin therapy during the interval between initial and reparative surgery and so maintained until the likelihood of infection is past. Immediate correction of secondary anemia on arrival at the base is an essential part of the program as the days are few during which the anemia from the initial blood loss may be projected into the anemia of chronic infection and indolent wound healing. The procedures of reparative surgery are frequently of great magnitude and the patients must be adequately supported by whole blood transfusions before, during and subsequent to operation.

Compound fractures are removed from transportation splints, the wound is revisioned for further removal of devitalized tissue, reduction of the fracture is secured and maintained by skeletal traction, internal fixation or other means as indicated. The original débridement incisions directly compounding the fracture site are closed by suture. Dependent stab wound drainage to the fracture site is usually established for a limited period of time.

Open arthrotomy is carried out for impending or early joint infection. Devitalized cartilage and retained foreign bodies are removed and the joint space closed. In a few cases when serious trauma or early established infection has irreparably ruined the joint architecture, resection of the joint has been performed and satisfactory healing in a position of maximum usefulness achieved.

Radical management of massive organizing hemothorax by thoracotomy, evacuation of the clot and decortication of the lung has proved its effectiveness in returning soldiers to duty and appears to have diminished the incidence of empyema. The same procedure applied to established posttraumatic empyema with penicillin therapy as an adjunct, is followed by immediate healing with a fully expanded lung. It is no longer acceptable to hold that a patient with a penetrating chest wound is making satisfactory progress as long as empyema has not made itself manifest. The focus has been changed from the management of posttraumatic pleural infection to the preservation of lung function. In the history of military surgery this will stand as one of the significant advances of World War II.

Early closure of small intestinal fistulae is a life-saving measure. Repair of exteriorized segments of large bowel returns a certain number of soldiers to limited duty and simplifies the nursing problems of the evacuation of others to the Zone of the Interior. Loop-sigmoid colostomy as an adjunct to the management of wounds of the perineum and anal regions has permitted early secondary suture followed by closure of the colostomy and return to full duty.

Skin loss in wounds comes from the missile, the over enthusiastic surgeon or infection. Skin defects attributable to tangential hits or the tearing action of the missile at the wound of exit are repaired by skin grafts as early as the fourth day following injury. In facial injuries, splinting of the bony parts and primary suture of soft parts with provision for drainage at the time of initial surgery is followed by meticulous wound management on arrival at the base. It is believed that there is a material reduction in the incidence of disfiguring mutilations. Extensive loss of skin and soft parts attributable to the missile is not commonly observed, and it seems likely that many of the facial mutilations of warfare are attributable to loss of tissue by sepsis and contracture—both preventable.

Revision of craniocerebral wounds when there is evidence of residual devitalized tissue or impending infection is followed by closure when feasible even if established infection is disclosed. Observations are being made relative to the earlier repair of peripheral nerve injuries. This is a procedure that may better be considered as early reparative surgery rather than late reconstructive surgery. The projected method of management includes revision and appraisal of the nerve injury at the time of secondary wound closure and in suitable cases repair as soon as satisfactory healing is established (two and one-half to three weeks).

To realize fully the potentialities of reparative surgery requires the introduction of a new concept in the organization of military surgery. The time-lag between wounding and initial surgery referred to as "the golden period" has been greatly reduced by the organization, of medical service in the forward area to this end. The time-lag between initial surgery and reparative surgery has now assumed an equal degree of importance. Just as every hour added to the time-lag between injury and initial surgery increases the loss of life and limb, so does every day added to the time-lag between initial and reparative surgery. Four to ten days is the "golden period" to close wounds, reduce and fix fractures, remove retained missiles and carry out other procedures to prevent or abort infection. To fail to take cognizance of the potentialities of early reparative surgery at the base in the future plans and operations will be as unthinkable as a failure to plan for the removal of the wounded from the field of battle.

Air evacuation between Army and Base, early establishment of general hospitals in close support of an advancing Army, sorting of casualties on arrival at Base so they may have the benefit of expert and specialized surgical management, are matters of administrative import. Education of surgeons to undertake new and unfamiliar procedures; the correction of anemia by whole blood transfusion so that essential surgery may be undertaken at an early date and increased attention to rehabilitation procedures are some of the major problems faced by professional personnel.

Particularly important is the concept that the surgical management of a wounded soldier from the field of battle to his ultimate hospital disposition within the theater demands continuity of policy and effort. A wounded man is not like a box of ammunition or a crate of rations that can be deposited at the boundary of an echelon and responsibility dismissed. Only by coordination of policy and methods between echelons can military surgery attain its full stature.

It is a satisfaction to note the contrast between the present concept of wound management and the doctrines in vogue scarcely a year ago. The closed-plaster management of wounds and fractures was designed to conserve life but exacted a high price in skeletal and soft-part deformity. Its use is now limited to certain cases with established infection of bone or with massive defects of soft parts compounding a fracture site. Recommendations that minimized the necessity for a complete initial wound operation or sought to delay it (wound trimming, "salting down with sulfa drugs," *etc.*) accepted suppuration as inevitable in a considerable proportion of cases and relied on chemotherapy to hold sepsis within bounds. Resuscitation measures that relied on plasma alone to compensate for loss of whole blood prolonged life but tied the hands of the surgeon in the performance of life-saving surgery. These and other earlier concepts were but faltering steps toward what will emerge as the ultimate scope of surgery as developed in the present war.

E. D. C.

Congratulatory Letter

The following is an extract from a letter received from Surgeon General Kirk:

"I have just read your article that you sent on for publication in the *Annals of Surgery*. . . . Fred Rankin and I are delighted with it. It is wonderfully written, describing the advances, which due to your great efforts, have been made during your tour in Italy. This article puts in writing some of the things that really count. The surgery that I saw a year ago in North Africa (May, 1943) is in no way comparable to what is being done now in Italy under your direction. My sincere thanks and congratulations to you. I am in hopes that you will have someone there write out in detail the various procedures that you have accomplished as separate entities so that we can immediately get this into print to inform other theaters as to what can be done if they know how."

Brian J. Gavitt, Donald H. Jenkins, and Peter M. Rhee

This appendix, penned by Dr. Churchill, provides a comprehensive executive summary of timeless surgical principles practiced by teams providing combat casualty care (CCC) in the Mediterranean Theater during the height of World War II. While the terminology and individual practices may differ, the principles are enduring and require repetition to ensure future surgeons are not left to rediscover them at the expense of the injured. A unique aspect of this chapter, and indeed its greatest strength, is its scope: in it Dr. Churchill provides key surgical principles for successful bedside CCC, but also reminds the reader of the combat surgeon's responsibility to organize and manage the CCC delivery system. We briefly discuss a selection of observations from Dr. Churchill's writings to encourage future generations of military surgeons to align the best bedside practice with robust trauma system management in order to save lives and accomplish the mission.

In his summary of the practice of surgical CCC, Dr. Churchill discusses several principles all surgeons would be wise to remember. The first principle is that antibiotics are never a substitute for aggressive surgical debridement of war wounds. While our knowledge about microbiology has advanced significantly since the 1940s, there are still no antimicrobial agents, whether used individually or in combination, that can compensate for inadequate surgical debridement. Expert and timely sharp soft tissue debridement is one of the most essential, but frequently overlooked, aspects of high-quality combat surgical care. A second related principle (that is a recurrent topic in performance improvement forums) is that war wounds should not be closed primarily. Generations of surgeons have rolled the dice attempting primary closure of war wounds only to reaffirm that in the expeditionary environment, primary closure of soft tissue wounds is dangerous and harmful. Third, patients in hemorrhagic shock should be resuscitated with whole blood. The surgical literature is replete with fervent efforts to find the ideal commercial fluid to resuscitate patients in hemorrhagic shock. The answer to this problem was clear at least as far back as 1944: bleeding patients do best when resuscitated with whole blood. The expeditionary surgeon must be fluent on all aspects of obtaining, storing, and administering whole blood in order to advise commanders of the risk they assume by allowing inferior substitutes. Sadly, these principles are frequently forgotten or neglected, yet they remain absolutely essential for surgical teams to provide optimal bedside care to combat casualties.

Second, Dr. Churchill provides organizing principles for the CCC system. The reader should recall that the content of *Surgeon to Soldiers* was written over a quarter of a century before the advent of Advanced Trauma Life Support. A common theme in this appendix involves surgeons standardizing the care for combat casualties across roles of care within a larger expeditionary trauma system. The importance of (evidence-based) standardization cannot be understated and underpins the effectiveness of more recent interventions like the implementation of Tactical Combat Casualty Care, or the clinical practice guidelines published by the Joint Trauma System. A second major theme is whole-team readiness. Dr. Churchill stresses the importance of having not just expertly trained and highly experienced surgeons, but rather all medical personnel across the entire spectrum of care must be trained, experienced, and ready as well. Shortsighted readiness plans focus narrowly on ensuring surgeons are ready to deploy; this is necessary but not sufficient. The literature consistently demonstrates most deaths early in a conflict occur in the prehospital setting—prior to the casualty ever encountering a surgeon. The ability to rescue wounded casualties therefore depends on the ability to project critical trauma care to the point of injury, and then throughout all roles of care. Readiness, therefore, must be holistic and encompass the entire CCC team, from the field medic to the rehabilitation team. All of these concepts—from system standardization to readiness—are (or will be) the responsibility of the trauma team clinical leader, namely the surgeon. Surgeons must not abdicate their responsibility to learn to organize and manage risk in an expeditionary trauma system; this an expected part of the scope of practice for expeditionary surgeons, in 1944 in the Mediterranean, now, and in all future conflicts.

In this chapter Dr. Churchill offers enduring principles of CCC practice every expeditionary surgeon should know and apply. Implementing these principles to build a robust CCC system provides a key collateral benefit according to Dr. Churchill: it emboldens the warfighter to aggressively prosecute the mission. CCC teams would do well to remember that their demonstrated ability to rescue injured warriors stiffens the spines and strengthens the resolve of those defending freedom and liberty; in this arena there is no room for mediocrity.

SUGGESTED READINGS

Borgman MA, Spinella PC, Perkins JG, et al. The ratio of blood products transfused affects mortality in patients receiving massive transfusions at a combat support hospital. *J Trauma.* 2007;63(4):805-813.

Eastridge BJ, Jenkins D, Flaherty S, Schiller H, Holcomb JB. Trauma system development in a theater of war: experiences from Operation Iraqi Freedom and operation enduring freedom. *J Trauma.* 2006;61(6):1366-1373.

Spinella PC, Perkins JG, Grathwohl KW, et al. 31st Combat Support Hospital Research Working Group. Risks associated with fresh whole blood and red blood cell transfusions in a combat support hospital. *Critical Care Med.* 2007;35(11):2576-2581